Praise for *The Lost Landscape*:

'As profound, as thorough and, at times, as dark as anything Oates has ever done'
Buffalo News

'Offers a window into a highly original mind. While it is never a given that a writer's personal story can illuminate her work, in Oates's case, it very much does'
Minneapolis Star Tribune

'A window into one of our most powerful writers' coming-of-age and the forces affecting how she sees and writes the world'
Christian Science Monitor

'Oates perfectly captures the unique confusion of childhood, brought on by the unsatisfying explanations of adults'
Elle (US)

'An exquisitely rendered g   ural
upstate New York'   *age*

NONFICTION BY JOYCE CAROL OATES

The Edge of Impossibility: Tragic Forms in Literature (1972)

New Heaven, New Earth: The Visionary Experience in Literature (1974)

Contraries (1981)

The Profane Art: Essays and Reviews (1983)

On Boxing (1987)

(Woman) Writer: Occasions and Opportunities (1988)

George Bellows: American Artist (1995)

Where I've Been and Where I'm Going: Essays, Reviews, and Prose (1999)

The Faith of a Writer: Life, Craft, Art (2003)

Uncensored: Views and (Re)views (2005)

The Journal of Joyce Carol Oates 1973–1982 (2007)

In Rough Country: Essays and Reviews (2010)

A Widow's Story: A Memoir (2011)

Joyce at her first desk, five years old. At home in Millersport, New York. (Fred Oates)

THE
LOST LANDSCAPE

A WRITER'S COMING OF AGE

JOYCE CAROL OATES

4th ESTATE • *London*

4th Estate
An imprint of HarperCollins*Publishers*
1 London Bridge Street
London SE1 9GF

www.4thEstate.co.uk

First published in Great Britain in 2015 by 4th Estate
First published in the United States by Ecco in 2015
This 4th Estate paperback edition published in 2016

1

A catalogue record for this book is
available from the British Library

ISBN 978-0-00-814661-0

Designed by Suet Yee Chong

Printed and bound in Great Britain by
Clays Ltd, St Ives plc

MIX
Paper from
responsible sources
FSC C007454

FSC™ is a non-profit international organisation established to promote
the responsible management of the world's forests. Products carrying the
FSC label are independently certified to assure consumers that they come
from forests that are managed to meet the social, economic and
ecological needs of present and future generations,
and other controlled sources.

Find out more about HarperCollins and the environment at
www.harpercollins.co.uk/green

To my brother Fred Oates
And in memory of those who have gone away

CONTENTS

III

AUTHOR'S NOTE

The Lost Landscape is not meant to be a complete memoir of my life—not even my life as a writer. It is, for me at least, something more precious, as it is almost indefinable: an accounting of the ways in which my life (as a writer, but not solely as a writer) was shaped in early childhood, adolescence, and a little beyond. Its focus is upon the "landscape" of our earliest, and most essential lives, but it is also upon an actual rural landscape, in western New York State north of Buffalo, out of which not only much of the materials of my writing life have sprung but also the very wish to write.

Because it is essential to *The Lost Landscape*, "District School #7, Niagara County, New York" has been reprinted from *The Faith of a Writer* (2003), in a slightly different form. In a more substantially altered form, an updated "Visions of Detroit" ([*Woman*] *Writer*, 1988) has been reprinted under the title "Detroit: Lost City 1962–1968." Other chapters have been revised significantly from memoirist pieces published in a variety of magazines, journals, and books, often in response to an editor's invitation.

To the editors of these publications, heartfelt thanks are due:

"Mommy & Me" originally appeared, in a shorter form, in *Civilization*, February 1997.

"Happy Chicken" originally appeared in *Conjunctions 61: A Menagerie*, 2013.

"Discovering *Alice*" originally appeared in *AARP Magazine*, 2014.

"Piper Cub" originally appeared, in a substantially different form, in *Rhapsody*, November 2013.

"After Black Rock" originally appeared in the *New Yorker*, June 2013.

"Sunday Drive" originally appeared, in a substantially different form, in *Traditional Home*, March 1995.

"They All Just Went Away" originally appeared in a substantially different form in the *New Yorker*, October 1995. Reprinted in *The Best American Essays 1996* and in *The Best American Essays of the 20th Century*. This essay incorporates "Transgressions," originally published in the *New York Times Magazine*, October 1995.

"Where Has God Gone" originally appeared, in a substantially different form, in *Southwest Review*, Summer 1995, and was reprinted in *Communion* edited by David Rosenberg, 1995 under the title "And God Saw That It Was Good."

"An Unsolved Mystery: The Lost Friend" originally appeared, in a substantially different form, in *Between Friends* edited by Mickey Pearlman, 1994.

"Start Your Own Business!" originally appeared in substantially different forms in the *New Yorker* under the title "Bound," April 2003; and in *Conjunctions* 63 (2014) under the title "The Childhood of the Reader," which will be reprinted in *Pushcart Prize: The Best of the Small Presses 2016*.

"The Lost Sister: An Elegy" originally appeared in *Narrative*.

"Nighthawk: Recollections of a Lost Time" appeared originally in *Yale Review*, 2001, and in *Conjunctions*, 2014; reprinted, in a substantially different form, in *Narrative*, 2015.

"Story into Film: 'Where Are You Going, Where Have You Been?' and *Smooth Talk*" appeared originally in the *New York Times*, March 23, 1986.

Detroit: Lost City 1962–1968" appeared originally, in a shorter form, in *(Woman) Writer*, 1988.

"Photo Shoot: West Eleventh Street, New York City, March 6, 1970" originally appeared, in a shorter form, under the title "Nostalgia" in *Vogue*, April 2006; reprinted in *Port*, 2014.

"Food Mysteries" originally appeared, in a substantially different form, in *Antaeus* 1991; reprinted in *Not By Bread Alone* edited by Daniel Halpern, 1992.

"Facts, Visions, Mysteries: My Father Frederic Oates, November 1988" originally appeared, in a substantially different form, in the *New York Times Magazine*, March 1989; reprinted in *I've Always Meant to Tell You*, edited by Constance Warloe, 1996.

"A Letter to My Mother Carolina Oates on Her Seventy-eighth Birthday, November 8, 1994" originally appeared, in a slightly different version, in the *New York Times Magazine*, 1995; reprinted in this version in *I've Always Meant to Tell You* edited by Constance Warloe and in *The Norton Anthology of Autobiography* edited by Jay Parini, 1999.

"My Mother's Quilts" originally appeared, in a slightly shorter form, in *What My Mother Gave Me: Thirty-One Women on the Gifts That Mattered Most*, edited by Elizabeth Benedict, 2013.

WE BEGIN . . .

WE BEGIN AS CHILDREN imagining and fearing ghosts. By degrees, through our long lives, we come to be the very ghosts inhabiting the lost landscapes of our childhood.

MOMMY & ME

Carolina Oates and Joyce, backyard of Millersport house, May 1941. (Fred Oates)

MAY 14, 1941. IT was a time of nerves. Worried-sick what was coming my father would say of this time in our family history but who could guess it, examining this very old and precious snapshot of Mommy and me in our backyard playing with kittens?

LOOKED LIKE I WOULD *be drafted. Nobody knew what was coming. At Harrison's, we were working double shifts. In the papers were cartoons of Hitler but none of it was funny.* The nightmare of Pearl Harbor is seven months away but the United States has been in a continuous state of nerves since Hitler executed his *blitzkrieg* against an unprepared

Poland in September 1939; by May 1941, with England under attack, the United States is engaged in an undeclared war in the Atlantic Ocean with Germany . . . But I am two years, eleven months old and oblivious to the concerns of adults that are not immediate concerns about *me*.

MY TWENTY-SEVEN-YEAR-OLD FATHER FREDERIC Oates, whom everyone calls "Fred" or "Freddy," is taking pictures of Mommy and me behind our farmhouse in Millersport, New York; it is a day when Daddy is not working on the assembly line at Harrison Radiator, a division of General Motors seven miles away in Lockport, New York, involved in what is believed to be "defense work." It is a tense, rapidly-shifting, unpredictable era before TV when news comes in terse radio announcements and in the somber pages of the *Buffalo Evening News* delivered in the late afternoon six days a week. But such global turbulence is remote from our farm in western New York where everything is green and humid in prematurely hot May and the grass in the backyard grows thick and raggedy. Here my twenty-four-year-old mother Carolina, whom everyone calls "Lena," is cuddling with me in the grass playing with our newborn black kittens, smiling as Daddy takes pictures.

TAKING PICTURES WITH THE blue box camera. Of dozens, hundreds of pictures taken in those years only a few seem to have survived and how strange, how astonishing it would have been for us to have thought, in May 1941—*These pictures will outlive us!*

How happy we are, and how good and simple life must have seemed to that long-lost child Joyce Carol—(who did not know that she was to be the "firstborn" of three children)—with little in her life more vexing than the ordeal of having her curly hair brushed and combed free of snarls and fixed in place with ribbons, and being "dressed up" for some adult special occasion.

You can see in the snapshot behind Mommy and me a young, black-barked cherry tree and behind the tree the somewhat dour two-storey wood frame farmhouse owned by my mother's step-parents John and Lena Bush. Built in 1888 on Transit Road, at the time a narrow two-lane country road linking the small town of Lockport with the sprawling city of Buffalo twenty miles away, and surprisingly large by Millersport standards (where some of our neighbors' houses were single-storey, lacking cellars, hardly more than cabins or shanties), this steep-roofed farmhouse was razed decades ago yet resides powerfully—indomitably!—in my memory, the site of recurring dreams. (In a dream of the old farmhouse in Millersport I recognize, not a visual scene, but a sensation: a tone, a slant of light. Often, details are blurred. If there are human figures, their faces are blurred. I seem to know where I am, and who is with me, though I might not be able to name anyone. Just that sensation, both comforting and laced with a kind of visceral dread—*Back home*.) Note the exterior cellar door, a common sight in this now-vanished rural America, like the rain barrel at the corner of the house where rainwater was collected—and used for all purposes except drinking.

Behind Daddy as he takes our picture (and not visible to the viewer) is the farmyard: weatherworn barn with pewter lightning rod atop the highest pitch of the roof; chicken coop surrounded by a barbed-wire fence to keep out raccoons, foxes, and the wandering dogs of neighbors; storage sheds; fields, fruit orchards. To the right of the sliding barn doors is a smaller door leading into the corner of the barn that houses my grandfather Bush's smithy with its anvil and hammer, blacksmith tools, small coal furnace and bellows that turns with a crank. Red-feathered chickens with no idea that they are "free range" are wandering about pecking in the dirt, oblivious of all else. *All these—lost.*

TAKING PICTURES HAS BEEN our salvation. Without *taking pictures* our memories would melt, evaporate. The invention of photography in the nineteenth century—and the "snapshot" in the twentieth century—revolutionized human consciousness; for when we claim to remember our pasts we are almost certainly remembering our favorite snapshots, in which the long-faded past is given a visual immortality.

TAKING PICTURES WAS AN adult privilege in 1941. My way of *taking pictures* was to scribble earnestly with Crayolas in coloring books and in tablets. Grass would be horizontal motions of the green crayon. Black kitten, black crayon. Chickens were upright scribbles, vaguely humanoid in expression. My parents, I would not attempt. No human figures would appear in any of my childhood drawings, only very deep-green grass and trees, kittens and cats with fur of many hues, Rhode Island Red chickens.

NO ROMANCE IS SO profound and so enduring as the romance of early childhood. The yearning we feel through our lives for our young, attractive and mysterious parents—who were so physically close to us and yet, apart from us, inaccessible and unknowable. Is this the very origin of "romance," coloring and determining all that is to follow in our lifetimes? I am drawn to stare at these old family snapshots lovingly kept in albums and in envelopes. And so I am drawn too to snapshots of strangers' families, sifting through boxes of old postcards and snapshots in secondhand shops—though these individuals are not "my" family, yet frequently they are not so very different from my family. Children in snapshots of long-ago, given a spurious sort of immortality by an adult's love, and all of them probably now departed. The almost overwhelming wish comes to me—*I want to write their stories! That is the only way I can know these strangers—by writing their stories. . .*

HAPPY CHICKEN 1942–1944

I WAS HER PET chicken. I was Happy Chicken.

Of all the chickens on the little farm on Transit Road in the northern edge of Erie County in western New York State in that long-ago time in the early 1940s, just one was Happy Chicken who was the curly-haired little girl's *pet chicken*.

The little girl was urged to think that she'd been the first to call me Happy Chicken. In fact, this had to have been one of the adults and probably the Mother.

Probably too it was the Mother, and not the little girl, who'd been the first to discover that of all the chickens, I was the only one who came eagerly clucking to the little girl *as if to say hello*.

Oh look!—it's Happy Chicken coming to *say hello*.

The little girl and the little girl's mother laughed in delight that, without being called, I would peck in the dirt around the little girl's feet and I would *seem to bow* when my back was lightly stroked as a dog or a cat might *seem to bow* when petted.

The little girl loved it, my feathers were *soft*. Not *scratchy* and *smelly* like the feathers of the other, older chickens.

The little girl loved hearing my soft, querying clucks.

Early in the morning the little girl ran outside.

Happy! Happy Chicken!—the little girl cried through small cupped hands.

And there I came running! Out of the shadowy barn, or out of the bushes, or from somewhere in the barnyard amidst other, ordinary dark-red-feathered chickens. A flutter of feathers, *cluck-cluck-cluck* lifting in a bright staccato *Here I am! I am Happy Chicken!*

The Grandfather shook his head in disbelief. Never saw anything like this—*Damn little chicken thinks he's a dog.*

It was a sign of how special Happy Chicken was, the family referred to me as *he*. As if I were, not a mere hen among many, a brainless egg-layer like the others, but a lively little *boy-chicken*.

For the others were just ordinary *hens* and scarcely discernible from one another unless you looked closely at them which no one would do (except the Grandmother who examined hens suspected of being "sickly").

Truly I was Happy Chicken! Truly, there was no other chicken like *me*.

My red-gleaming feathers bristled and shone more brightly than the feathers of the hens because I didn't roll in the dust as frequently as they did, in their (mostly futile) effort to rid themselves of mites. It wasn't just that Happy Chicken was young (for there were other chickens as young as I was, hatched from eggs within the year) but I was also far more intelligent, and more handsome; your eye was drawn to me, and only to me, out of the flock; for you could see from the special gleam in my eyes and the way in which I came running before the little girl called me, that I was *a very special little chicken*.

The yard between the barn and the farmhouse was cratered with shallow indentations in which chickens rolled and fluttered their wings like large demented birds who'd lost the ability to fly. Sometimes as many as a dozen chickens would be rolling in the dirt at the same time as in a bizarre coordinated modern dance; but the chickens were not coordinated and indeed took little heed of one another except, from time to time, to lash out with a petulant peck and an irritated cluck. When not rolling in the dirt (and in their own black, liquidy droppings) these chickens spent their time jabbing beaks into the dirt in search of grubs, bugs. Stray seeds left over from feeding time, bits of rotted fruit. Their happiness was not the happiness of Happy Chicken but a very dim kind of happiness for a chicken's brain is hardly the size of a pea, what else can you expect? This was why Happy Chicken—that is, I—was such a surprise to the family, and such a delight.

My comb was rosy with health, erect with blood. My eyes were unusually alert and clear. But each eye on each side of the beak, how'd you expect us to see *coherently*? We see double, and one side of our brain dims down so that the other side can see precisely. That's how we know which direction in which to run, to escape predators.

Most of the time, however, most chickens don't. Don't escape predators.

Sometime, they're so dumb they *run toward predators*. They do this when the predator is smart enough to freeze. They can't detect immobility, and they can't detect something staring at *them*.

I was not really one of *them*. To be identified as special, and recognized as Happy Chicken, meant that, though I was a chicken I was not *one of them*. And particularly, I was not a *silly stupid hen*.

SOMETIMES—AT SPECIAL TIMES—UNDER CLOSE adult scrutiny, and always held snug in the little girl's arms—Happy Chicken was allowed *inside the farmhouse*.

No other chicken, not even Mr. Rooster, was ever allowed *inside the farmhouse*.

Never upstairs but downstairs in the "wash-room" at the rear of the house—a room with a linoleum floor that contained a washing machine with a hand ringer, and where coats and boots were kept— this is where the little girl Joyce could bring me. But always held gently-but-firmly in her arms, or set onto the floor and held in place, in the wash-room or—a few special times—in the kitchen which opened off the wash-room, where the Grandmother spent most of her time. Here, the little girl was given scraps of bread to feed me, on the linoleum floor.

And here, I was sometimes allowed up in the little girl's lap, to be fussed over and petted.

The other chickens would've been jealous of me—except they were too stupid. They didn't *know*. Even Mr. Rooster didn't under- stand how Happy Chicken was privileged. Sometimes Mr. Rooster stationed himself at the back door of the farmhouse, clucking and preening, complaining, fretting, fluttering his wings, insisting upon the attention of everyone who went inside the house, or came outside, shamelessly looking for a treat, and when he didn't get a treat, squawking indignantly and threatening to peck with his sharp beak.

The little girl was frightened of Mr. Rooster, and hurried past him. The Mother and the Grandmother shooed Mr. Rooster away, for they were frightened of him, too. The Grandfather and the Father laughed at Mr. Rooster and gave him a kick. They thought it was very funny, a goddamn bird trying to intimidate *them*.

Sometimes Happy Chicken was allowed in the wash-room over- night, in a little box filled with straw, like a nest. And little Joyce pet- ted me, and fussed over me, and fed me special treats.

Happy Chicken! You are so pretty.

. . . you are so *nice*. I love you

Happy Chicken. *I love you*.

The little girl whispered to me, that no one else could hear. The little girl had many things to tell me, all kinds of secrets to tell me, whispered against the side of my head where (the little girl supposed) I had "ears"—and when I made a clucking noise, the little girl spoke to me excitedly, for it seemed to the little girl that I was *talking to her, and telling her secrets*.

What are you and Happy Chicken always talking about, the Mother asked the little girl, but the little girl shook her head defiantly, and would not tell.

(Sometimes, there was an egg or two discovered in Happy Chicken's little nest. The little girl took these eggs away to give to the Grandmother for they were *special Happy Chicken eggs* not to be mixed with the eggs of the hens out in the coop.)

(Yet still, though Happy Chicken produced eggs, it seemed to be taken for granted that Happy Chicken was a *boy-chicken*. For always, Happy Chicken was *he, him*.)

The little girl was given a gift of Crayolas! At once the little girl began drawing pictures of me on sheets of tablet paper. *Russet-brown* was the little girl's favorite Crayola crayon, for this was the color of my beautiful red-brown feathers. The little girl drew and colored many, many pictures of me, that were admired by everyone who saw them. With the help of the Mother, the little girl carefully printed, beneath the drawings

HAPPYCHICKEN

Sometimes, visiting relatives would peer at the little girl and me from the kitchen doorway, as the little girl sat on the floor beside my box drawing me, and I was tilting my head blinking and clucking at *her*.

The little girl would overhear people saying *Is that just a—chicken? Or some special kind of guinea hen, that's smarter?*

For it had not ever been known, that a "chicken" could be a pet, in such a way. At least, not in this part of Erie County, New York.

Between a chicken and a little girl there is not a shared language as "language" is known. Yet, Happy Chicken always knew his name and a few other (secret) words uttered by the little girl and the little girl always knew what Happy Chicken's special clucks meant, that no one else could understand and so when the Mother, or the Father, or any adult, asked the little girl what on earth she and the little red chicken were talking about, the little girl would repeat that it was a secret, she could not tell.

Sometimes, at unpredictable moments, I felt an urge to "kiss" the little girl—a quick, light jab of my beak against the girl's hands, arms, or face.

And the little girl had a special little kiss on the top of the head just for *me*.

I WAS A YOUNG chicken less than a year old at this time in the little girl's life when she hadn't yet learned to run on plump little-girl legs without tripping and falling and gasping for breath and *crying*.

If the Mother was near, the Mother hurried to pick up the little girl, and comfort her. If the Grandmother was near, the Grandmother was likely to cluck at the little girl like an indignant hen and tell her to get up, she wasn't *hurt bad*.

If the Father was near, the Father would pick up the girl at once, for the Father's heart was lacerated when he heard his little daughter cry, no matter that she hadn't been *hurt bad*. (But the Father was not often nearby for he worked in a factory seven miles away in Lockport, called Harrison Radiator.)

But always if an adult wiped the little girl's eyes and nose the little girl soon forgot why she'd been crying even if she'd bruised or scratched her leg—the little girl cried easily but also forgot easily.

When you are a little girl you *cry easily and forget easily*.

Nor is it difficult to appear *happy* when you are a *young chicken* and without memory as the smooth blank inside of an egg.

The Mother had chosen the little girl's name *Joy-ce Carol* because this seemed to her a happy name, there was *joy* in the name, when people spoke the name they smiled.

The Mother was a happy person, too. The Mother was not much older than a schoolgirl when the little girl was born but the little girl had no notion of what "born" was and so the little girl had not the slightest notion of how old, or how young, her pretty curly-haired Mother was, no more than Happy Chicken had a notion of anyone's *age*.

This was the time when the little girl was an only child and so it was a happy time for the little girl who had her own room (separated by just a walk-in closet from her parents' room) upstairs in the clapboard farmhouse. One day soon it would be revealed that the little girl was just the firstborn in the family. There would come another, a *baby brother with the special name Robin*, competing for attention and for love the way the squawking chickens competed for seed scattered in the barnyard at their feeding time.

The little girl had no notion of this amazing surprise to come. The little girl had no notion of anything that *was to come* except a promise of a drive to Pendleton for ice cream, or a visit with the Other Grandmother (the Father's mother) who lived in Lockport, or a holiday like Christmas or Easter, or the little girl's birthday which was the most special day of all June 16 when dark-red peonies bloomed in profusion along the side of the house as the little girl was told, *just for her*.

On her fourth birthday, the little girl was allowed to feed cakecrumbs to me, while the adults looked on laughing. Happy Chicken was allowed to sit on the little girl's lap, if the little girl held me snug, and my wings tucked in, inside her arms.

Pictures were taken with the Father's Brownie Hawkeye camera.

Pictures of *little Joyce Carol* and *Happy Chicken*, 1942.

With a frown of distaste the Grandmother would say, in her broken English, A chicken is *dirty*. A chicken should *stay on the floor*.

The Grandmother did not like me though sometimes the Grandmother pretended to like me. In the Grandmother's eyes, a chicken was never anything more than a *chicken*. And a *chicken* was only of use, otherwise worthless.

Outdoors, when the little girl was nowhere near, and the Grandmother approached, I knew to flee, and to hide. Always to flee and to hide away from the other chickens, so brainlessly scratching and pecking in the dirt, in the darkest corner of the barn or far away in the orchard.

A chicken is not *dirt-y*, the little girl protested. Happy Chicken is *nice and clean*.

And so when a small dollop of hot wet mess came out of my anus, which I could not help, and onto the little girl's shorts, the adults pointed and laughed, and the Mother quickly cleaned it away with wadded tissues as the Grandmother made her clucking-tsking noise.

The little girl was embarrassed, and ashamed. But the little girl always forgave me. And soon forgot whatever it was I'd done, because she was such a little girl, and forgot so easily, and was soon again stroking and petting me, and kissing the bone-hard top of my head.

Happy Chicken—*I love you*.

BECAUSE SHE WAS SUCH a little girl the little girl was always hoping that all the chickens would like her, and not just Happy Chicken

who was her pet. Naively the little girl hoped that the rooster—
(who was even more handsome than Happy Chicken, and much
larger)—would like her. And so the little girl was continually being
surprised—and hurt—when the rooster ignored her or worse yet
bristled his feathers indignantly and rushed to peck at her hands or
bare knees sharp enough to draw blood.

Many times this happened, that the little girl cried *Oh!*—and
ran away frightened, and sometimes Mr. Rooster would chase her,
and if the Grandfather was watching he would double over in laughter as if he'd never seen anything so funny. The Grandfather had a
loud sharp laugh like bottles popping corks. His barrel chest would
shake, his small shrewd eyes would shrink in the fleshy ridges of
his face, his laughter turned into snorts, wheezing, coughing. Such
loud, protracted coughing. And still, the Grandfather was laughing.
For nothing amused the Grandfather more than someone chased by
that goddamn bird unless it was the sight of the Grandmother's white
sheets billowing on the clothesline so hard, in such wind, clothespins
slipped and a sheet sank to the ground and the Grandmother came
running out of the house, furious, agitated, muttering in a strange
guttural speech the little girl did not understand and that frightened
her, like the loud shrieks and squawks of the chickens when something threw them into a panic, so the little girl stood very still and
cringing and shutting her eyes pressing her hands over her ears like
one who is waiting for something distressing to *go away, stop*.

If the little girl was inside the farmhouse, and heard a sudden
squabble outside, a sign that someone or something was agitating the
chickens, the little girl would run outside immediately to search for
me. Oh oh oh—where is Happy Chicken?

The little girl knew about foxes and raccoons and stray dogs that
might drag away chickens and devour them—(though it would be
very unusual for any creature to make such a foray in daytime)—and

so the little girl had to find me amidst the commotion, scoop me up in her arms and kiss the top of my head and smooth down my neatly folded wings and carry me quickly away promising that *nothing bad* would ever happen to Happy Chicken.

WE WERE RHODE ISLAND Reds. Three dozen hens and a single rooster.

Other male chickens in the flock had been squashed as soon as it was evident that they were *male*. Our rooster had not a clue that he'd come close to oblivion. Or, our rooster had not a care that he'd come close to oblivion. Through the day Mr. Rooster strutted in the yard and roosted in the lowermost limbs of trees showing off his spectacular tail feathers, and the ruff around his neck; bristling red-brown, dark-red, yellow-red feathers that shone in the sun. Yellow-scaly legs, and nasty-sharp spurs just above the talon-claws. Though Mr. Rooster was as stupid as any hen pecking brainlessly in the dirt, or rolling in the dirt in the (mostly futile) effort of getting rid of mites, yet Mr. Rooster was fascinating to watch for you never knew what Mr. Rooster would do next. (You never knew what any hen would do next, but anything a hen can do is of so little significance there is no point in observing her.) Mr. Rooster could leap into the air fluttering his wings, for instance, and devour a dragonfly three feet above the ground, and Mr. Rooster could rush in a blind rage at an unsuspecting hen, or two unsuspecting hens, or, as if he'd only just thought of it, and now that he was doing it, it was a significant thing to do, throwing himself down and rolling over vigorously in the dirt until his gaudy feathers were dull with dust like those of an ordinary chicken.

Mr. Rooster gave no sign of knowing who I was—who Happy Chicken was! Ridiculous how this stupid bird seemed not to notice even as the little girl singled me out for special attention and treats in his very presence. (I'd have liked to think that Mr. Rooster was jealous of me, but the fact was, Mr. Rooster was too vain and too stupid for jealousy.)

That is, Mr. Rooster was indifferent to me unless I stepped brashly in his way, or failed to get out of his way quickly enough when he charged forward into the midst of the chickens at feeding time.

Sometimes for a reason known only to Mr. Rooster's pea-sized brain he crowed loudly and irritably and flapped his wings in a show of indignation and flew clumsily to alight on a rail fence, like a person clumsily hauling himself up by a rope.

At dawn, Mr. Rooster woke everyone with his crowing. He was the first rooster to wake in all of Millersport—soon after Mr. Rooster crowed, you would hear roosters crowing at neighboring farms. No other rooster at any neighboring farm woke earlier than Mr. Rooster, and no other rooster crowed as noisily.

The hens took for granted that Mr. Rooster's crowing tore a rent in the silence of the countryside-before-dawn that allowed the sun to appear. The little girl may have thought this also, but only when she was very little.

The Grandfather who took little interest in the chickens—(these were the Grandmother's responsibility)—was yet proud of his *goddamn bird*. The Grandfather liked it that Mr. Rooster chased away other chickens and barn-cats who ventured too near and had to be disciplined.

How many dawns, the little girl was wakened by Mr. Rooster's cries. Through her life to come, long after she'd grown up, and gone away from the farmhouse on Transit Road to live, she would wake to the faint, fading cry of a rooster just outside in the dark-before-dawn.

Is a rooster a harbinger of the Underworld? Does a rooster wake you so that you have no choice but to follow him into the Underworld?

After she'd become an adult older than the Mother and the Father of her early childhood, and the little scabs and scars caused by the rooster's beak had long faded from her knees, frequently she would find herself touching her knees like Braille, when she was alone.

Very often, in bed. In the bright pitiless light of a bathroom she would examine her knees frowning and baffled, her childhood scars had so vanished as if they had never been . . . It is hard to disabuse yourself of the superstition that your skin is indelibly marked since childhood in a way known only to *you*.

Upsetting to remember how Mr. Rooster would single out a hen for no reason—(had she disrespected him? taunted him? dared to eat something meant for him?)—peck and jab at the terrified bird until she began to bleed, and chase her until she seemed to fall, or to kneel, before him. And then, Mr. Rooster might have mercy on her, and strut away. But a scab would form shiny and bright as a third eye on the hen's head, that would attract the attention of another hen, and so soon—for some reason—(the little girl could not understand this, it frightened her very much)—this hen would peck at the afflicted hen, and soon another hen would hurry over to peck at the afflicted hen, and another, and another; and sometimes Mr. Rooster, attracted by the squawking, might return for the *coup de grâce*—a series of rapid beak-stabs until the poor afflicted hen was bleeding, fallen over and unable to right herself beneath the frenzy of stabbing beaks . . . And hearing the barnyard commotion the Grandmother would hurry out of the house scolding and shooing with the intention of rescuing not the struggling live hen but the limp hen-corpse for the Grandmother's own purposes.

In her harsh guttural speech the Grandmother would curse the chickens and the rooster. Much of the Grandmother's speech had a sound of chiding and cursing. And the Grandmother would take up the limp blood-dripping hen-corpse into the kitchen and boil a pan of water on the stove and drop the hen-corpse into it, so that the feathers could be plucked more easily.

At these times the little girl had run away and hid her eyes.

The Mother would say to her, Don't pay any attention, help me in the kitchen, sweetie!

Mostly the little girl would not remember such things. The little girl's memory of the farm on Transit Road was very selective like the colander into which the Grandmother dumped boiling water containing her thin-cut noodles, made out of the Grandmother's noodle-dough, that trapped just the noodles but strained away the liquid.

In later years recalling with a fond smile very little of the farm, the barnyard, the flock of Rhode Island Reds—just, *me*.

THE LITTLE GIRL WAS so excited! She was *five years old*.

This was the summer the little girl was allowed to help the Grandmother collect eggs from the hens' nests in the chicken coop (where the chicken droppings were so smelly, you had to hold your breath especially after a rain) and soon then, the little girl was allowed to feed the chickens by herself, twice a day, their special chicken-feed. Like tiny pebbles the chicken feed seemed to the little girl, seized in handfuls to toss to the chickens; to get the seed you lowered a tin pie pan deep into the feed-sack, itself contained inside a larger, canvas sack to keep out rats and mice.

So exciting! Almost, the little girl wetted her panties, with anticipation.

And when she began to call to the chickens in her high, quavering voice as the Grandmother had taught her—*CHICK!-chick-chick-chick-chick-CHI-ICK!*—chickens came rushing in her direction at once, and made the little girl feel very special—very *powerful*. It was not ever the case that the little girl felt *powerful*—nor could the little girl have defined the sensation, at the time; but calling *CHICK!-chick-chick-chick-chick-CHI-ICK* provoked such a feeling in her, set her heart to pumping and a warm, rich sensation coursing through her veins, the little girl felt very special, and very proud.

Oh, she could see—(for she was a quick-witted, smart little girl)—that the chickens were oblivious of her, in their greed to devour seed they took not the slightest interest in her, or in their surroundings; yet still it seemed to the little girl that the chickens *must like* her, and *knew who she was*, for they came so quickly to her, colliding with one another, scolding and fretting, pecking one another in a frenzy to get to the seed the little girl tossed in a wide, wavering circle.

The Grandmother had instructed the little girl to distribute the seed as evenly as she could. You did not want all the chickens rushing together in a tight little spot, and injuring themselves. The little girl understood that she had to be fair to all the chickens, not just a few.

But the largest and most aggressive chickens rushed and pecked and beat away the others no matter how hard the girl *tried*.

Of course, Joyce Carol always fed *me*, specially. In a safe little area, by the side of the house. This was Happy Chicken's special meal, which was served ahead of the general feeding. If other chickens noticed, and ran clucking to this meal, the little girl stamped her feet and shooed them away.

Though he might have been prowling out in the orchard, soon there came Mr. Rooster running on his long scaly legs. Mr. Rooster could hear the *Chick-chick-chick!* call from a considerable distance. He pushed through the throng of clucking chickens knocking the silly hens aside and gobbled up as much seed as he could from the ground. Sometimes then pausing, looking up with a squint in his yellow eyes, and made a decision—(who knows why?)—to rush at the little girl and jab her bare knee with his beak.

So quickly this assault came, when it came, the little girl never had time to draw back and escape.

Ohhh! Why was Mr. Rooster so *mean!*

The little girl was always astonished, the rooster was so *mean*.

The rooster's beak was so *swift, so sharp and so mean.*

Worse yet, the rooster sometimes chased the little girl, trying to peck her legs. If the Grandmother saw, she shooed the rooster away by flapping her apron at him and cursing him in Hungarian. If the Grandfather saw, he gave the rooster a kick hard enough to lift the indignant bird into the air, squawking and kicking.

It was one of the mysteries of the little girl's life, why when the other chickens seemed to like her so much, and her pet chicken adored her, Mr. Rooster continued to be so mean. It did not make sense to the little girl that Mr. Rooster devoured the seed she gave him, then turned on her as if he hated her. Shouldn't Mr. Rooster be grateful?

The Mother kissed and cuddled her and said, Oh!—that's just the way roosters are, sweetie!

Plaintively the little girl asked the Grandmother why did the rooster peck her and make her bleed and the Grandmother did not cuddle her but said, with an air of impatience, in her broken, guttural English, Because he is a rooster. You should not always be surprised, how roosters are.

THE LITTLE GIRL WANDERED the farm. The little girl was forbidden to *step off the property*.

There was the big barn, and there was the silo, and there was the chicken coop, and there were the storage sheds, and there was the barnyard, and there was the backyard, and there were the fields planted in potatoes and corn, and there was the orchard and beyond the orchard a quarter-mile lane back to the Weidenbachs' farm where there were big nasty dogs that barked and bit and the little girl did not dare to go. In these places chickens wandered, and also Mr. Rooster, in their ceaseless scratching-and-pecking for food, though it was rare to see a chicken in one of the farther fields or in the lane. Happy Chicken only accompanied the little girl if she called him to these places, or carried him snug and firm in her arms.

The little girl placed me on the lowermost limb of the lilac tree by the back door of the house, so that I could "roost." The little girl urged me to try to "fly—like a bird." But if the little girl nudged me, and I lost my balance on the tree limb, my wings flapped uselessly, and I fell to the ground and did not always land on my feet.

At such a time I picked myself up and tottered away clucking loudly, complaining like any disgruntled hen, and the little girl hurried after me saying how sorry she was, and promised not to do it again.

Happy Chicken! *Don't be mad at me, I love you.*

(IT WAS TAKEN FOR granted, it was never contested or wondered-at, that our wings were useless. We could "flap" our wings and "fly" for a few feet—even Mr. Rooster could not fly farther than a few yards; though there were wild turkeys, fatter and heavier than Rhode Island Reds, who could manage to "fly" into the higher limbs of a tree, and there "roost.")

NOT JUST THE CHICKEN coop and much of the barnyard but the grassy lawn behind the house—("lawn" was a name given to the patch of rough, short-cropped crabgrass that extended from the barnyard and the driveway to the pear orchard)—was mottled with chicken droppings. Runny black-and-white glistening smudges that gradually hardened into little stones and lost their sharp smell.

You would not want to run barefoot in the backyard, in the scrubby grass.

And there was the ugly tree stump along the side of the barn, stained with something dark.

And surrounding the stained block, chicken feathers. Sticky-stained feathers in dark clotted clumps.

No chickens scratched and pecked in the dirt here. Even Mr. Rooster kept his distance. And the little girl.

GRANDMA WAS THE ONE, you know. The one who killed the chickens.

No! I did not know.

Of course you must have known, Joyce. You must have seen— many times. . . .

No. I didn't know. I never saw.

But . . .

I never saw.

In later years she would recall little of her Hungarian grandparents. Her mother's stepparents. For few snapshots remained of those years. She did know that the Grandfather and the Grandmother were something that was called *Hungarian*. They'd come on a "big boat" from a faraway place called Hungary years before the little girl was born and so this was not of much interest to the little girl since it had happened long ago. The grandparents seemed to the little girl to be *very old*. The big-breasted big-hipped Grandmother had never cut her hair that was silvery-gray-streaked and fell past her waist if she let it down from the tight-braided bun. The Grandmother had been eighteen when she'd come to the United States on a "boat" and at age eighteen it had seemed to her too late for her to learn English, as the Grandfather had learned English well enough to speak haltingly and to run his finger beneath printed words in a newspaper or magazine.

The Grandfather was a tall big-bellied man with scratchy whiskers who liked to laugh as if much were a joke to him. He had rough calloused fingers that caught in the little girl's curly hair when he was *just teasing*.

Worse yet was *tickling*. When the Grandfather's breath smelled harsh and fiery like gasoline from the cider he drank out of a jug. But the Mother insisted Grandpa loves you, if you cry you will make Grandpa feel bad.

The farm was the Grandfather's property. Of farms on Transit Road it was one of the smallest. Much of the acreage was a pear orchard. Pears were the primary crop of the farm, and eggs were second. The little girl and her parents lived on the Grandfather's property upstairs in the farmhouse. The little girl understood that the Father was not so happy living there, for the Father had been born in Lockport and preferred the city to the country, absolutely. The Father had tried his hand at farming and "hated" it. The little girl often overheard her parents speak of wanting to move away, to live in Lockport, where the Father's mother who was the little girl's Other Grandmother lived. Except years would pass, all the years of their lives would pass as in a dream, and somehow—they did not ever move away.

There was something strange about the Grandfather and the Grandmother but the little girl could not guess what it was. Later she would learn that the Grandfather and the Grandmother were not the Mother's actual parents but her stepparents and it was worrisome to the little girl, that in some way *steps* were involved. Like the long frightening *stepladder* that only Daddy could climb to pick pears, apples, and cherries from the highest limbs of the trees.

The little girl noticed that, when her parents were speaking together, or any adults were speaking together, if she came near they might cease speaking suddenly. They would smile at her, they would say her name, but they would not reveal what they had been saying.

The little girl ran away to hide, sometimes. When the adults were speaking sharply to one another. When the Grandfather cursed at the Grandmother in Hungarian, and the Grandmother wept angrily and hid her flushed face in her hands.

The little girl had several times seen the Grandmother's long coarse gray-black hair straggling down her back like something alive and livid. The little girl shut her eyes not wanting to see as she shrank from seeing the Grandmother's large soft melon-breasts loose inside a camisole, that was wrong to see for there were things, the little girl realized, that it was wrong to see and you would be sorry if you saw.

On a farm, there are many such things. Wild creatures that have crawled beneath a storage shed to die, or the bones of a chicken or a rabbit all but plucked clean by a rampaging owl in the night.

"Joyce Carol! Come *here*."

With a nervous little laugh like a cough the Mother would shield the little girl's eyes from something she should not see. Between the Mother's eyebrows, faint lines of vexation and alarm.

"Sweetie, I said *come here*. We're going inside now."

SOMETIMES THE LITTLE GIRL was breathless and frightened but why, the little girl would not afterward recall.

The little girl often took me with her to a special hiding place. Happy Chicken in the little girl's arms, held tight.

My quivering body. My quick-beating heart. Smooth warm beautiful chicken-feathers! The little girl held me and whispered to me where we were hiding in the old silo beside the barn, that wasn't used so much any longer now that the farm didn't have cows or pigs or horses. Smells were strong inside the silo, like something that has fermented, or rotted. The little girl's mother warned her never to play in the silo, it was dangerous inside the silo. The smells can choke you. If corncobs fall onto you, you might suffocate. But the little girl brought me with her to hide in the silo for the little girl did not believe that anything bad could happen to *her*.

Except the little girl began more frequently to observe that if a chicken weakened, or fell sick, or had lost feathers, other chickens turned on her. So quickly—who could understand why? Even Happy Chicken sometimes pecked at another, weaker chicken—the little girl scolded, and carried me away.

No no Happy Chicken—that is bad.

We did not know why we did this. Happy Chicken did not know.

It was like *laying eggs*. Like releasing a hot little dollop of excrement from the anus, something that *happened*.

Hearing a commotion in the barnyard, the little girl ran to see what was happening always anxious that the wounded hen might be *me*—but this did not happen.

Though sometimes my beak was glistening with blood, and when the little girl called me, I did not seem to hear. *Peck peck peck* is the action of the beak, like a great wave that sweeps over you, and cannot be resisted.

THE LITTLE GIRL GREW up, and grew away, but never forgot her Happy Chicken.

The little girl forgot much else, but not Happy Chicken.

The little girl became an adult woman, and at the sight of even just pictures of chickens she felt an overwhelming sense of nostalgia, sharp as pain. Especially red-feathered hens. And roosters! Her eyes mist over, her heart beats quick enough to hurt. *So happy then. So long ago...*

Still, she would claim she'd never seen a chicken slaughtered. Never seen a single one of the Rhode Island Reds seized by the legs, struggling fiercely, more fiercely than any human being might struggle, thrown down onto the chopping block to be decapitated with a single swift blow of the bloodstained ax, wielded by a muscled arm.

It was the Grandmother's arm, usually. For the Grandmother was the chicken-slaughterer.

Which the girl had not seen. The girl *had not seen*.

The girl did recall a time when Grandfather was not so big-bellied and confident as he'd been. When the Grandfather began to cough frequently. And to cough up blood. The Grandfather no longer teased the little girl, or caused her to run from him crying as she'd run from Mr. Rooster. The little girl stared in horror as the Grandfather coughed, coughed, coughed doubled over in pain, scarcely able to breathe. The Grandfather would scrape phlegm up from his throat, with great effort, and spit the quivering greenish liquid into a rag. And the little girl would want to hide her face, this was so terrible to see.

It was explained that the Grandfather was sick with something in his lungs. Steel-filings it was said, from the foundry in Tonawanda. The Grandfather had hated his factory-job in Tonawanda but the Grandfather had had to work there, to support the farm. For the farm would not support itself, and the people who lived on it.

The Grandfather had liked to say in his laughing-bitter way that he and the other workers should be running the foundry and not the goddamn owners. Until the terrible coughing spells overcame him the Grandfather would say how the workers of the world would one day rise against the goddamn owners but that was not to happen, it would be revealed, in the Grandfather's lifetime.

SELLING EGGS, SITTING OUT by the roadside. Sitting, dreaming, waiting for a vehicle to slow to a stop. Customers.

How much? One dozen?

Oh that's too much. I can get them cheaper just up the road.

Always there were eggs for sale. And, at the end of the summer pears in bushel baskets. Sweet corn, tomatoes, cucumbers, potatoes. Apples, cherries. Pumpkins.

With a faint sensation of anxiety the little girl would recall sitting at the roadside at the front of the house behind a narrow bench. When sometimes the Mother had to go inside for a short while and the little girl was left alone at the roadside.

Hoping that no one would stop. Hoping not to see a vehicle slow down and park on the shoulder of the highway.

Some of the anxiety was over chickens, that made their blind-seeming way down the driveway, to the highway. Chickens oblivious of vehicles speeding by on the road, only a few yards from where they scratched and pecked in the dirt.

Anxiously the little girl watched to see that no chickens drifted out onto the road. The little girl knew, though she wasn't altogether certain how she knew, for she'd never *seen*, that from time to time chickens had been killed on the road.

Sudden squawking and shrieking, and a flapping of wings. At first you rush to see what it is, and then you do not want to see what it is.

One of the constant fears of the little girl's life was that Happy Chicken might be hit on the highway for the little girl could not watch me all of the time.

Each morning running outside breathless and eager to call to me—Happy! Happy Chicken!

And I came running, out of the coop, or out of the barn, or out of a patch of grass beside the back door, hurrying on my scrawny chicken-legs to be stroked and petted.

"Happy Chicken! *I love you*."

THE LAUGHTER WAS KINDLY, and yet cruel.

Of course you ate chicken when you were a little girl, Joyce! You ate everything we ate.

No. She didn't think so.

You'd have had to eat whatever was served. Whatever everybody else was eating. You wouldn't have been allowed to *not-eat* anything on the table.

No! This was not true.

You hated fatty meat, and you hated things like gizzards, and we laughed at how you tried to hide these—beneath the rim of your plate!—as if, when the plate was removed from the table, the fatty little pieces of meat you'd left would not be discovered. But you certainly ate chicken white meat. Of course you did.

No. That was—that was not true . . .

Children ate what they were given in those days. Children ate, or went hungry. Your father would have spanked the daylights out of you if you'd tried to refuse chicken, or anything that your mother or grandmother prepared.

But *no*. She did not believe this.

It's true—she does remember her Hungarian grandmother preparing noodles in the kitchen. Wide swaths of soft-floury ghost-white dough on the circular kitchen table that was covered in oilcloth, and over the oilcloth strips of waxed paper. She recalls the Grandmother, a heavyset woman with gray hair plaited and fastened tight against her head, always in an apron, and the white apron always soiled, wielding a long sharp-glittering knife, rapidly cutting dough into thin strips of noodle. And the Grandmother's legs encased in thick flesh-colored cotton stockings even in hot weather. The surprise was, sometimes you could see a pleading girl's face inside the soft flaccid Grandmother-stern face. And the little girl remembers something white-skinned, headless in a large pan simmering on the stove, the surface of the liquid bubbling with dollops of yellowish fat.

You loved your grandmother's chicken noodle soup! You don't remember?

She hides her eyes. She hides her face. She is sickened, that terrible smell of wet feathers, plucked-white chicken-flesh.

Protesting, I had nothing to do with *that*.

Trying to recall in a sudden panic—what had happened to her pet chicken, she'd loved so?

Our memories are what remain on a wall that has been washed down. Old billboards advertising *Mail Pouch Tobacco*, in shreds. The faintest letters remaining that even as you stare at them, fade. The Hungarian Grandfather who'd been so gruff, so loud, so confident and had so loved his little granddaughter he'd been unable to keep his calloused fingers out of her curls had died at the age of fifty-three, his lungs riddled with steel filings from the foundry in Tonawanda. The Hungarian Grandmother lived for many years afterward and never learned to speak English, still less to read English. The Grandmother died in a nursing home in Lockport to which the granddaughter was never once taken, nor was the granddaughter told the name of the nursing home or its specific location.

Why was this? The Mother had wished to hide the little girl's eyes. Even when she was no longer a little girl, yet the Mother wished to shield her from upset and worry.

What happened to *me*? What happened to Happy Chicken?

Oh, the little girl did not know!

The little girl *did not know*. Just that one terrible day—Happy Chicken was not *there*.

She mouths the words aloud: "Happy Chicken."

There is something about the very word *happy* that is unnerving. Happy happy happy *happy*.

A terrible word. A terrifying word. *Hap-py*.

Waking in the night, tangled in bedsheets, shivering in such fright you'd think she was about to misstep and fall into an abyss.

Happy. Hap-py. We were so hap-py. . .

In the cold terror of the night she counts her dead. Like a rosary counting her dead. The Grandfather who died first and after whom the door was opened, that Death might come through to seize them all. The Grandmother who died somewhere far away, though close by. The Mother who died of a stroke when she was in her mid-eighties, overnight. The Father who died over several years, also in his mid-eighties, in the new, twenty-first century shrinking, baffled and yet alert, in yearning wonderment.

Wanted you kids to have the best you could have, but that didn't happen. We were just too poor. I worked like hell, but it wasn't enough. Things got better later, but those early years—! The only good thing was, we lived in Millersport. We lived on the old man's farm. You loved those animals. Remember your pet chicken—Happy Chicken? God, you loved that little red chicken.

Daddy brushing tears from his eyes. Daddy laughing, he wasn't the kind to be sentimental, Jesus!

She was thinking of how they'd found the rooster—not Mr. Rooster then, but just a limp, slain bird—beautiful feathers smudged and broken—out back of the barn where something, possibly a fox, or a neighbor's dog, had seized him, shaken him and broken his neck, threw him down and left him for dead. Poor Mr. Rooster!

Seeing the rooster in the dirt, horribly still, the little girl had cried and cried and cried.

And several hens, limp and bloody, eyes open and sightless. Flung down in the dirt like trash.

AND THERE CAME THE time, not long after this, or maybe it had been this time, when Happy Chicken disappeared.

The girl was stunned and disbelieving and did not cry, at first.

So frightened, the little girl could not cry.

For it seemed terrifying to her, that Happy Chicken might be—somehow—*gone*.

She'd run screaming to her mother who was upstairs in the farmhouse. The Mother who claimed to have no idea where the little chicken might be. Together they searched in the chicken coop, and in the barn, and out in the fields, and in the pear orchard. Calling *Happy Chicken! Happy Chicken!* Loudly calling *Chick-chick-chick-chick-CHICK!*

Other chickens came running, blinking and clucking. Yellow eyes staring.

And not one of these was *me*.

That morning the Mother had taken the little girl into Lockport to visit with the Other Grandmother, who was her father's mother, who lived upstairs in a gray clapboard house on Grand Street just across the railroad tracks. The highway that was Transit Road that ran past the little girl's house became Transit Street inside the Lockport city limits and was but a half-block away from the Other Grandmother's house.

The Other Grandmother was named Blanche: but she was also called "Grandma"—like the (Hungarian) grandmother. The little girl tried to understand why this would be so. *How could the two persons who were so different, be somehow the same—Grandma?*

The Other Grandmother, who lived in Lockport, was much nicer than the (Hungarian) Grandmother who lived in Millersport. This Grandmother did not smell of grease, or chicken gizzards, or wet chicken feathers, or any other nasty thing, but rather of something pale and creamy like lilies—did this Grandmother wear perfume? Were this Grandmother's hands soft from hand lotion? The little girl was always welcome to explore the Grandmother's rooms which included the Grandmother's bedroom that had such nice things in it—a shiny pink satin bedspread with white flowers, a "dressing table" with three mirrors and a mirror-top, many sweet-smelling jars and small bottles, a hairbrush with soft bristles that did not hurt the little girl's hair when the Grandmother brushed it.

Most importantly the Grandmother who was Blanche did not speak angry-sounding guttural words in Hungarian, and would never have raised her voice to scream at anyone; you could not imagine—(the little girl could not imagine!)—this nice Grandmother being cruel to any chicken.

This was the Grandmother whom Daddy loved—for this Grandmother was *Daddy's mother.* The little girl had been told this remarkable fact which she could not comprehend because Daddy was so much taller than the Grandmother it seemed to her *silly*—that her tall strong Daddy who was so forceful would have a *mother.*

This was the Grandmother who read books from the Lockport library, never fewer than three books each week. And these books smelling of the library in plastic covers. And these books smartly stamped in dark green ink LOCKPORT PUBLIC LIBRARY. This Grandmother took the little girl hand in hand into the children's entrance of the library, to secure a library card for the little girl. For here was the surprise, that would be one of the great, happy surprises of the little girl's life—"Joyce Carol" was old enough for a children's library card: six. And she was allowed to take out children's books, picture books, selected by the little girl herself, from shelves in the library—so many shelves! Such beautiful books! The little girl was so excited she could barely speak, to thank the Grandmother. Having her books stamped and discharged by the librarian made the little girl very shy but the Grandmother stood beside her so there was nothing to fear. And the little girl and the Grandmother-who-was-Blanche read these books together sitting on a swing on the front veranda of the gray clapboard house on Grand Street.

In all that day, the little girl did not once think of me.

Those hours, blinking and staring at the beautiful brightly colored illustrations in the books, turning the pages slowly, as the nice Grandmother Blanche read the words on each page, and encouraged the little girl to read too—the little girl did not once think of Happy Chicken.

But when the Mother took the little girl home again to Millersport, in the late afternoon of that day, and the little girl ran out into the barnyard to call for me, there was no Happy Chicken anywhere.

The little girl and the Mother would search the chicken coop, the barn, the orchard. . . . Oh where was Happy Chicken? The little girl was crying, sobbing.

The (Hungarian) Grandmother who was hanging sheets on the clothesline insisted she had not seen Happy Chicken.

The Grandmother had never really distinguished Happy Chicken from any other chicken—the little girl knew that. How ridiculous, the Grandmother thought, to pretend that one chicken was any different from any other chicken!

The Grandfather too insisted he hadn't seen Happy Chicken! Wouldn't have known what the damned chicken looked like, in fact. Anything that had to do with the chickens—these were the Grandmother's chores, and of no interest to the Grandfather who was worn-out from the foundry in Tonawanda and couldn't give a damn, so much fuss over a goddamn chicken.

When the father returned from his factory work in Lockport in the early evening he was in no mood either to hear of Happy Chicken. He was in no mood to hear his little daughter's crying, that grated on his nerves. But seeing his little girl's reddened eyes, and the terror in those eyes, the Father stooped to kiss her cheek.

Don't cry, he'll come back. What's his name—"Happy Chicken"? Sure. "Happy Chicken" will come back.

SHE IS CALLING HIM—HAPPY Chicken. *Her throat is raw with calling him*—Happy Chicken!

She has wakened in a sick cold sweat tangled in bedclothes. The little red chicken is somewhere in the room—is he? But which room is this, and when?

But here I am—suddenly—crouching at her feet. Eager quivering little red-feathered chicken at the little girl's feet. The little girl kneels to pet me, and kisses the top of my hard little head, and holds me in her arms, my wings pressed gently against my sides. And the little chicken-head lowered. And the eyelids quivering. Red-burnished feathers stroked gently by a little girl's fingers.

Where did I go, Joyce Carol? I flew away.

One day that summer, my wings were strong enough to lift me. And once my wings began to beat, I rose into the air, astonished and elated; and the air buoyed and buffeted me, and I flew high above the tallest peak of the old clapboard farmhouse on Transit Road.

So high, once the wind lifted me, I could see the raggedy flock of red-feathered chickens below scratching and pecking in the dirt as always, and I could see the roof of the old hay barn, and I could see the top of the silo; I could see the farthest potato field, and the farthest edge of the pear orchard, and the rutted dirt lane that bordered the orchard leading back to the Weidenbachs' farm where the big barking dogs lived.

For it was time, for Happy Chicken to fly away.

DISCOVERING *ALICE*: 1947

THE SINGULAR BOOK THAT changed my life—that made me yearn to be a writer, as well as inspired me to "write"—is Lewis Carroll's *Alice's Adventures in Wonderland* and *Through the Looking-Glass*. This beautiful, slightly oversized book published by Grosset & Dunlap in 1946 was a gift of my (Jewish) grandmother Blanche Morgenstern for my ninth birthday, in 1947. (My book-loving grandmother, my father's mother, gave me books for birthdays and Christmas and at other times as well, including Frances Hodgson Burnett's *The Secret Garden*. Grandma gave me my first typewriter—a toy typewriter—and she gave me a Remington typewriter at the age of fourteen as if foreseeing how I would need it.) To this day I treasure, and keep prominently on a bookshelf in my study, this gift book with its eerily beautiful quasi-"realistic" illustrations by John Tenniel.

The illustrations of Alice amid her bizarre wonderland world depict her as surprised and sometimes intimidated by that world but never overwhelmed by it. The great illustrator Tenniel gave to Alice a commonsensical gravity and a tender sobriety quite unlike most illustrations of children in American, contemporary children's books; Alice is recognizably a young girl, but she is not *childish*. There is something responsibly mature in Alice, an inclination to be skeptical, at times, of the adults who surround her; an unwillingness to be bossed around or frightened into submission. Alice is a girl who "speaks her mind"—as few children are encouraged to do, then or now. When I was nine, I was much too young to comprehend the underlying themes of Alice's astonishing adventures, which have to do with Darwinian evolutionary theory and the principle of "natural selection through survival of the fittest"—a controversial issue of the Victorian era that represented a challenge to conventional Christian theology, one not entirely resolved in the twenty-first century.

Like any child enraptured with a favorite book, I wanted to be the book's heroine—I wanted to be "Alice." It must have occurred to me that Alice was very unlike any girl of my acquaintance; she seemed to belong to a foreign, upper-class environment with customs (tea-time, crumpets, queens, kings, footmen) utterly alien to the farming society of Millersport, New York. I think that I learned from Alice to be just slightly bolder than I might have been, to question authority—(that is, adults)—and to look upon life as a possibility for adventures. If I'd taken Alice for a model, I was prepared to recognize fear, even terror, without succumbing to it. There are scenes of nightmare illogic in the *Alice* books—numerous dramatizations of the anxiety of being eaten, for instance—that suggest the essential gravity of the books, yet Alice never becomes panicked or loses her common sense and dignity.

It did occur to me that Alice is a character in a book—and that Alice was not telling her own story. The author of the book was named in gilt letters on the spine and on the title page: "Lewis Carroll." Being Lewis Carroll was an aspiration, like being Alice-in-Wonderland, and soon I was drawing stories in the mode of the Tenniel illustrations, not of adults or even children but of cats and red-feathered chickens. These were "novels" on lined tablet paper, that captivated me for long hours as a child. (Decades later I would see facsimiles of the Brontë children's miniature books, and feel a tug of kinship. The Brontë children may have been lonelier than I was in Reverend Brontë's remote windswept parsonage in Haworth on the moors of England, though probably they were not more fascinated by storybooks than I was.) Out of *Alice's Adventures in Wonderland* and *Through the Looking-Glass* have sprung not only much of my enthusiasm for writing but also my sense of the world as an indecipherable, essentially absurd but fascinating spectacle about which it is reasonable to exclaim, with Alice—"Curiouser and curiouser!"

DISTRICT SCHOOL #7, NIAGARA COUNTY, NEW YORK

I LOVED MY FIRST school!—so I have often said, and possibly this is true.

As a child I was filled with excitement, anticipation, apprehension, sometimes dread at the prospect of *school*. For the schoolhouse on the Tonawanda Creek Road in Niagara County, about a mile from my home, was a magical place to me, a place of profound significance, and yet it was not a place in which, as a young child, I could exert anything approaching what I would not yet have known to call "control."

I took for granted then what seems wonderful to me now: that, from first through fifth grades, during the years 1943 to 1948, I attended the same one-room schoolhouse that my mother, Carolina Bush, had attended twenty years before. Apart from the introduction of electricity in the 1940s, and a few minor improvements, not including indoor plumbing, the school had scarcely changed in the intervening years. It was a rough-hewn, weatherworn, uninsulated wood frame building on a crude stone foundation, built around the turn of the century at the approximate time my grandparents' farmhouse was built, twenty-five miles north of Buffalo and about six miles south of Lockport.

In late August, in anticipation of school beginning after Labor Day in September, I would walk to the schoolhouse carrying my new pencil box and lunch pail, gifts from my grandmother Blanche Morgenstern, to sit on the front, stone step of the school building. Just to sit there dreamy in anticipation of school starting: possibly to enjoy the solitude and quiet, which would not prevail once school started.

(Does anyone remember pencil boxes now? They were of about the size of a small lunch pail, with several drawers that, slid out, revealed freshly sharpened yellow "lead" pencils, Crayola crayons, erasers, compasses. The thrill of a compass with its sharp point! The smell of Crayolas! Lunch pails, which perhaps no one recalls either, were usually made of some lightweight metal, with handles; unlike pencil boxes which smelled wonderfully of crayons and erasers, lunch pails quickly came to smell awfully of milk in Thermos bottles, over-ripe bananas, peanut butter, jam, or baloney sandwiches, and much-used wax paper.)

The school, more deeply imprinted in my memory than my own child-face, was set approximately thirty feet back from the pebble-strewn unpaved Tonawanda Creek Road; it had three tall, narrow windows in each of its side walls, and very small windows in its front wall; a steeply slanting shingle board roof that often leaked in heavy rain; and a shadowy, smelly, shed-like structure at the front called the "entry"; nothing so romantic as a cupola with a bell to be rung, to summon students inside. (Our teacher Mrs. Dietz, standing Amazon-like in the entry doorway, rang a handbell. This was a sign of her adult authority; the jarring noise of the bell, the thrusting, hacking gesture of her muscled right hand as she vigorously shook it. In my memory, Mrs. Dietz's sturdy face was usually flushed.)

Behind the school, down a slope of briars and jungle-like veg-etation, was the "crick"—the wide, often muddy, fast-moving

Tonawanda Creek, where pupils were forbidden to play or explore; on both sides of the school were vacant, overgrown fields; "out back" were crudely built wooden outhouses, the boys' to the left and the girls' to the right, with drainage, raw sewage, virulently fetid in warm weather, seeping out into the creek. (Elsewhere, off the creek bank, children, mostly older boys, often swam. They dived from the sides of the bridge when the water was high enough. There was not much consciousness of "polluted" waters in those days and even less fastidiousness on the part of energetic farm boys.)

My memory of the outhouses is a shudder of dread. But lately, I am apt to feel an alarmed sort of sympathy for poor Mrs. Dietz, who had no choice but to use the girls' outhouse, too.

At the front of the school, and to the sides, was a rough playground of sorts, where we played such improvised games as "May I?"—which involved "baby-" and "giant-steps"—and "Pom-Pom-Pullaway" which was more raucous, and rougher, where one might be dragged across an expanse of cinders, even thrown into the cinders. And there was Hide-and-Seek, and Tag, which were my favorite games, at which I excelled, at least with children not too much older than I was.

Joyce runs like a deer! certain of the older boys, chasing me, as they chased other younger children, to bully and terrorize, would say, admiring.

Inside, the school smelled of varnish, chalk dust, and woodsmoke and ashes from the potbellied stove. On overcast days, not infrequent in western New York in this region south of Lake Ontario and east of Lake Erie, the windows emitted a vague, hazy light, not much reinforced by ceiling lights. We sat in rows of seats, smallest at the front, largest at the rear, attached at their bases by metal runners, like a toboggan; the wood of which these desks were made seemed beautiful to me, smooth and of the red-burnished hue of horse chestnuts. The floor was bare wooden planks. The blackboard stretched across the front of the room. An American flag hung limply at the far left of the blackboard and above the blackboard, running across the front of the room, so positioned to draw our admiring eyes to it, to be instructed, were cardboard squares of the alphabet showing the beautifully shaped script known as Palmer Method.

All of my life, though my handwriting has changed superficially, it is the original Palmer Method that prevails. In an era in which handwriting scarcely exists, and most signatures are unintelligible, those of us who came of age under the tutelage of the Palmer Method can be relied upon to write not just beautifully, but legibly.

Perhaps Palmer Method carried with it an (unwitting, unconscious) moral bias? If beauty and clarity and a wish to communicate are your intention in writing, are you not likely to be *good*?

Mrs. Dietz, of course, had mastered the art of such penmanship. She wrote our vocabulary and spelling lists on the blackboard, and we learned to imitate her. We learned to "diagram" sentences with the solemn precision of scientists articulating equations. We learned to read by reading out loud, and we learned to spell by spelling out loud. We memorized, and we recited. Our textbooks were rarely new, but belonged to the school district and were passed on, year after year until they wore out entirely. (How I would love to examine those textbooks, now! I have not the vaguest memory of what we were actually being made to read, and what our arithmetic books were like.) Our school "library" was a shelf or two of books including a *Webster's* dictionary, which fascinated me: a book comprised of *words*! A treasure of secrets this seemed to me, available to anyone who cared to look into it.

Some of my earliest reading experiences, in fact, were in this dictionary. We had no dictionary at home until, as the winner of a spelling bee sponsored by the *Buffalo Evening News*, when I was in fifth grade, I was given a dictionary like the one at school. This, like the prized *Alice* books, remained with me for decades.

My early "creative" experiences evolved not from printed books but from coloring books, predating my ability to read. I did not learn to read until I was in first grade and six years old, though by this time, comically precocious as I seem now in retrospect, I'd already produced a number of "books" of a kind in tablet form, by drawing, coloring, and scribbling in what I believed to be a convincing imitation of adults. My earliest fictional characters were not human beings but zestfully if crudely drawn upright chickens and cats engaged in what appeared to be dramatic confrontations; of course, Happy Chicken figured predominantly. The title of one of these tablet-novels was allegedly *The Cat House*, which was set in an actual house in which cats lived as human beings might live. (When I was an adult my father would joke with me about this title, whose *double entendre* humor had escaped me. For years my mother saved the tablet-novel among her things, but I think *The Cat House* must be lost to posterity by now.)

In addition to the *Alice* books which I'd soon memorized we had, at home, the daunting *The Gold Bug and Other Tales* by Edgar Allan Poe, which was my father's book: the title was in dull-gold letters on the book cover which was made of some odd, thick, dim material resembling mossy tree bark. What I could make of Poe's belabored gothic prose, I can't imagine. Though Poe's classic tales seem to move, in our memories, with the nightmare rapidity of horror films, the prose in which Poe cast most of these tales is highly formal, tortuous, turgid if not opaque; his masterpiece "The Tell-Tale Heart" is unique in its head-on fluency. Yet, somehow, perhaps because I had few other books close at hand, I persevered in reading Poe as a young child, and must have absorbed, along with the very different prose-consciousness of Lewis Carroll, something of that writer's unique sensibility. (No wonder my immediate kinship with Paul Bowles, whose first story collection, *The Delicate Prey*, is dedicated to his mother, who had read Bowles the tales of Poe as a young child.)

My child's logic, which was not corrected by any adult because it would not have occurred to me to mention it to any adult, was that the mysterious world of books was divided into two types: those for children, and those for adults. Reading for children, in our grade-school textbooks, was simpleminded in its vocabulary, grammar, and content; it was usually about unreal, improbable, or unconditionally fantastic situations, like fairy tales, comic books, Disney films. It might be amusing, it might be instructive, but it was not *real*. Reality was the province of adults, and though I was surrounded by adults, as an only child for five years, it was not a province I could enter, or even envision, from the outside. To enter that reality, to find a way *in*, I read books.

Avidly, ardently! As if my life depended upon it.

One of the earliest books I read, or tried to read, was an anthology from our school library, an aged *Treasury of American Literature* that had probably been published before World War II. Mixed with writers who are mostly forgotten today (James Whitcomb Riley, Eugene Field, Helen Hunt Jackson) were our New England classics—though I was too young to know that Hawthorne, Emerson, Poe, Melville, et al. were "classics" or even to know that they spoke out of an America that no longer existed, and would never have existed for families like my own. I believed that these writers, who were exclusively male, were in full possession of *reality*. That their *reality* was so very different from my own did not discredit it, or even qualify it, but confirmed it: adult writing was a form of wisdom and power, difficult to comprehend but unassailable. These were no children's easy-reading fantasies but the real thing, voices of adult authenticity. I forced myself to read for long minutes at a time, finely printed prose on yellowed, dog-eared pages, retaining very little but utterly captivated by the strangeness of another's voice sounding in my ear. I tackled such a book as I would tackle a tree (a pear tree, for instance) difficult to climb. I must have felt almost physically challenged by lengthy, near-impenetrable paragraphs so unlike the American-English language spoken in Millersport, and totally unlike the primer sentences of our schoolbooks. The writers were mere names, words. And these words were exotic: "Washington Irving"—"Benjamin Franklin"—"Nathaniel Hawthorne"—"Herman Melville"—"Ralph Waldo Emerson"—"Henry David Thoreau"—"Edgar Allan Poe"—"Samuel Clemens." There was no Emily Dickinson in this anthology, I would not read Emily Dickinson until high school. I did not think of these exalted individuals as actual men, human beings like my father and grandfather who might have lived and breathed; the writing attributed to them was them. If I could not always make sense of what I read, I knew at least that it was true.

It was the first-person voice, the (seemingly) unmediated voice, that struck me as *truth-telling*. For some reason, children's books are rarely narrated in the first-person; Lewis Carroll's Alice is always seen from a little distance, as "Alice." (Yet we see everything through Alice's amazed eyes, and we never know anything that Alice does not know.) But many of the adult writers whom I struggled to read wrote in the first person, and very persuasively. I could not have distinguished between the (nonfiction) voices of Emerson and Thoreau and the (wholly fictional) voices of Irving and Poe; even today, I have to think to recall if "The Imp of the Perverse" is a confessional essay, as it sets itself up to be, or one of the *Tales of the Grotesque*. I may have absorbed from Poe a predilection for moving fluidly through genres, and grounding the surreal in the seeming "reality" of an earnest, impassioned voice. Poe was a master of, among other things, the literary *trompe l'oeil*, in which speculative musings upon human psychology shift into fantastic narratives while retaining the earnest first-person voice.

One day I would wonder why the earliest, most "primitive" forms of art seem to have been fabulist, legendary, and surreal, populated not by ordinary, life-sized men and women but by gods, giants, and monsters? Why was reality so slow to evolve? It's as if, looking into a mirror, our ancestors shrank from seeing their own faces in the hope of seeing something other—exotic, terrifying, comforting, idealistic, or delusional—but distinctly *other*.

Of Mrs. Dietz, I think: how heroic she must have been! Underpaid, undervalued, overworked. (I am guessing that a female teacher in this rural outpost in the 1940s was "underpaid.") Not only was it the task of a one-room schoolteacher to lead eight disparate grades through their lessons, but also to maintain discipline in the classroom, where most of the older boys attended school grudgingly, waiting for their sixteenth birthdays when they were legally released from attending school and could work with their fathers on family farms; these boys were taught by older male relatives to hunt and kill animals, and they were without mercy in "teasing" (the more accurate term "harassing" had not yet been coined) younger children. Mrs. Dietz was also in charge of maintaining our wood-burning stove, the school's only source of heat, in that pitiless upstate New York climate in which below-zero temperatures weren't uncommon on gusty winter mornings, and we had to wear mittens, hats, and coats through the day, stamping our booted feet against the drafty plank floor to keep our toes from going numb . . . I can only imagine the emotional and psychological difficulties poor Mrs. Dietz endured, and feel now a belated kinship with her, who had seemed to me a very giantess of my childhood. No other teacher looms as archetypal in my memory, for no other teacher taught me the fundamental skills of reading, writing, and doing arithmetic, which seem to me as natural as breathing. I am grateful to Mrs. Dietz for not (visibly) breaking down, and for maintaining a certain degree of good cheer in the classroom. The schoolhouse for all its shortcomings and dangers became for me a kind of sanctuary: a precious counter-world to the chaotic and unbookish roughness that existed outside it.

Years later, revisiting the Lockport area, giving a talk sponsored by the Lockport Public Library, I was approached by a woman of my approximate age who looked familiar to me, to a degree; when the woman introduced herself, I remembered her at once, as a girl who'd lived on a farm a few miles away on one of the creek-side roads; she spoke of how, outside the school at recess, I would sometimes "teach" her and a few other children, who hadn't understood our teacher Mrs. Dietz . . . What a pleasure to meet again, after so many years, Nelia Pynn! I love the name, out of that lost past, and must write it again: *Nelia Pynn*.

FOR A LONG TIME vacant and boarded up, District #7 school was finally razed in the late 1970s. And for a long time afterward, when I returned to Millersport to visit my parents, I would make a sentimental journey to the site, where a collapsed stone foundation and a mound of rubble were all that remained. Soon such one-room schoolhouses will be recalled, if at all, only in photographs: links with a mythopoetic "American frontier past" that, when it was lived, seemed to us, who lived it, simply life.

PIPER CUB

"DON'T BE AFRAID. DADDY is right here."

Yet, Daddy was not visible to me, for Daddy was behind me. It did not seem natural to me that my father, who always drove our car from the position of authority behind the steering wheel, was seated behind me in the Piper Cub that was a beautiful bright yellow like a butterfly's wings.

It was a summer day in the late 1940s. I would have been nine or ten years old. My young, adventurous father Fred Oates had earned a pilot's license a few years before, and this was my first trip with him.

Daddy had not been drafted into the army as he'd feared. He had not served in World War II due to deferments he and his fellow workers at Harrison Radiator had been given, since they were involved in "defense manufacturing." And now, after the war, planes belonging to the government had passed into private ownership, and men like my father began to take flying lessons.

How and why my father took flying lessons at Lee's Airfield on Transit Road north of Buffalo, New York, I have no idea. There wasn't much money in any household in which he'd ever lived. To help with expenses my father not only worked at Harrison's but also painted signs for commercial businesses in the area. Yet somehow he'd been able to afford flying lessons as early as 1935 (when he was twenty-one) and had acquired a pilot's license by 1937, the year before I was born, which enabled him to fly not only small planes like Piper Cubs, Cessnas, and Stinsons but also eventually the sporty Waco double-winged biplane, and even ex–Air Force trainers—a Fairchild with 175 horsepower, a Vultee basic trainer, 450-horsepower, with a canopied open cockpit that could fly at twelve thousand feet.

My first time in the Piper Cub would be one of the great memories of my life.

Initially, immediately, there was the strangeness of my father "dressing" me—(which he never did; only my mother dressed me)—as I was outfitted with goggles and a helmet, which were much too large for me. (My father wore a parachute, but I did not, which might have seemed ominoua if I had thought about it. But of course—I could not have used a parachute.) Next, I was half-lifted by Daddy into the single front seat of the plane, and buckled in; the door which seemed to be made of some metal much lighter than a car door was shut and secured. Next, the Piper Cub propeller was turned manually by a boy who worked at the airfield until it began to spin with a loud roar, and the motor kicked in. Next, I was being driven along the bumpy airstrip, past rows of larger planes, at an ever-accelerating speed, totally terrified, dry-mouthed and astonished as I stared through the windshield at a world that was rushing at me much too quickly, and without any adult to shield me from it as if I, and not my father behind me, were the pilot.

Suddenly then, and sickeningly, the quaking little plane was in the air—rising above a row of trees, and above open fields.

Like any ten-year-old I trusted my father, absolutely. As I trusted my mother. (And now I wonder what my young mother must have been thinking, watching us from the runway. Did she, too, have complete trust in my father? Was she frightened when he took her up into the air, and did she really want to accompany him?—or was she, perhaps subtly, coerced? Should my father, with his newly acquired pilot's license, have taken up a ten-year-old child?) There was a daredevil recklessness to life in those days which seems in our more cautious era, in which children are likely to be over-protected by their parents, very remote indeed. Recall that this was a time when seat belts in vehicles were unknown and virtually everyone (including my parents) smoked.

Through his life my father would always say, "Flying is safer than driving a car." Statistically, this is (evidently) true, yet not quite a consolation for some of us.

My most vivid memories of that first trip are the fields opening beneath the plane, the blur of the spinning propeller close in front of me, the buffeting rush of the wind, and the quaking of the plane. In small aircraft you are very conscious of the wind. You are very conscious of the sky. Below, every detail seems heightened. You have suddenly an entirely new, unexpected perspective—you are looking down, bizarrely, from above. It is something of a miracle to see the roofs of houses and barns not so very far below as you pass over.

Pilots of small planes invariably head for home to fly over their houses and property. My father never failed to do this, a quick trip of only a few minutes, since our farmhouse was no more than three miles away. What is more pleasurable than to "buzz" the houses of friends and relatives?

Such playfulness suggests the youth of my father at this time, as it suggests the youth of the era. "Buzzing" low over houses and property was viewed as a sort of practical joke and not a dangerous annoyance as we would be inclined to see it today.

In the Piper Cub my father was likely to fly us to Lockport, where we could see the Erie Barge Canal stretching out below; he was likely to fly us in the direction of Niagara Falls, and the Niagara River; we would never fail to see the Tonawanda Creek, that stretched past our house on Transit Road and would enter my dreams for a lifetime. All these waterways were fascinating to me like the wind-buffeted airborne perspective itself. *Safety is a small price to pay for such a perspective!*—so my father might have said.

To be in the air—airborne! There was nothing like it for my father and his pilot-friends.

Returning to the airfield: that thrill in the pit of the stomach as the Piper Cub circles the runway and begins to dip down. (Sometimes, if the plane isn't in the ideal position, the pilot decides not to land. And so you sweep up again, rapidly up into the air again, the nose of the plane lifting into the sky so that for an unnerving moment there is nothing to see but sky.) Then, circling back, and trying again as the nose of the plane is lowered by a movement of the pilot's stick.

Landing is the most dangerous maneuver. A mistake at that time can be fatal. . .

A reassuring jolt as the plane's wheels strike the runway and within an instant the plane is on the ground, bouncing and bumping along the runway.

Returning to the hangar in a kind of triumph. And my mother hurrying forward to greet us with a tight embrace and a little sob of relief as if to say *Thank God! You are returned to me safely.*

IN SUBSEQUENT YEARS MY father would take me up in some of the larger and more intimidating airplanes at Lee's Airfield. There was at least one picture of Daddy and me in the Fairchild PT-19 with its cockpit open and both of us, in helmet and goggles, smiling and waving at the camera, presumably held by my mother—but this precious snapshot (for which I continue to search) seems to be permanently lost. It is embarrassing to recall that within a year or two of the first Piper Cub flight I had become so habituated to flying with my father, and so utterly trusting of him, that I dared to bring a tablet with me into which I scribbled "stories" while airborne . . .

(What was I always scribbling in those days? My mother would keep a selection of my school tablets that were filled with drawings of chickens and upright cats like human figures; I have seen these, but through a haze of embarrassment I lost a clear memory of them. There seemed to have been in my life as a writer a seamless transition from pre-literate activities of vigorous drawing in tablets with Crayolas to my first childish "stories" when I'd learned to write as adults write; from there, a seamless transition to my first typed stories when I was fourteen, and beyond.)

Though my father could never afford to own his own plane he remained an avid flier for decades; eventually he would log over two hundred hours of flying time. Indeed, "Fred Oates" was famous in Millersport and environs for his love of flying. Only reluctantly, when his eyesight began to weaken in his late sixties, did he give up flying.

(In the mid-1970s when a West German film crew preparing a documentary on my writing career for public television came to Millersport to interview my parents, the director arranged for my father to fly him and his cameraman over the terrain of my childhood, in a Cessna 182 horsepower single-prop plane. How courageous these Germans were! Or did they not quite comprehend how courageous they were being to entrust their lives to a stranger, Fred Oates, who could claim only a pilot's license from a rural upstate New York airfield? And how truly bizarre it was for me to see the film footage of my father in the cockpit of the plane flying again over that familiar landscape!)

Many times Daddy has said that for the pilot there is nothing in life on land to quite compare with life in the cockpit, at his instruments, aloft.

IN LATER LIFE, MY father and mother often visited my husband Raymond Smith and me in Princeton. On these trips they always flew, and sometimes they flew in a small plane to the small Princeton airfield about ten miles from our house.

Though *being flown* is nothing like *flying*—(as my father insisted)—these flights were exhilarating to him. Daddy never failed to comment on the pilot's performance and, if he had the opportunity, he congratulated the pilot on a "good landing."

Sometimes, when I am alone, and aloft, in my window seat staring out at a sea of clouds, or at land or glittering water far below, I feel a sudden pang of loss—for what, I don't know.

For Lee's Airfield, perhaps. For the shining little Piper Cubs and the boys who'd helped to start their propellers. For my beloved father, a young father, with tufted dark hair and a widow's peak, laughing as he adjusted helmet strap beneath my chin, for I must have looked very silly in my flying gear, as a child. And for my beloved mother, scarcely daring to breathe until the shining little yellow plane returned to the airstrip, and made a "successful" landing.

The long-ago romance of small planes. Daddy as pilot.

But I have only to shut my eyes to see the airfield bumping and jolting outside the windows of the Piper Cub and to feel again how we are being lifted into the air, wind-buffeted but bravely continuing to rise . . .

AFTER BLACK ROCK

DO ALL FAMILIES HARBOR secrets? Do all families conspire in secrets, if not cultivate secrets? The family is the social unit that seems to depend crucially upon a clear separation of those who are *in power* and those who are *subordinate*; those wielding power are required to know more than those who are subordinate to them, and there almost seems, at times, a kind of taboo in sharing such knowledge. *Before you were born* is both a neutral designation and a way of shutting a door in your face which you would wish to open at your own risk.

Of course, all that children are not told, children somehow *know*. Not the words to the song but its melody, and its tone. A writer might be one who, in childhood, learns to search for and decipher clues; one who listens closely at what is said, in an effort to hear what is not being said; one who becomes sensitive to nuance, innuendo, and fleeting facial expressions.

And there are the abrupt silences among adults, when a child comes too near.

IN HIS PREFACE TO *What Maisie Knew*, Henry James ponders the "close connection of bliss and bale"—the irony of "so strange an

alloy, one face of which is somebody's right and ease, the other somebody's pain and wrong." Nowhere is this paradox more true than in
the matter of a premature and violent death, for example the murder
of my mother's father which was also, in effect, the murder, as it was
the irrevocable dissolution, of a family.

All this happened long before I was born, in 1917. In a Hungarian community in Black Rock, now a part of Buffalo, New York. My
mother's father was in his forties at the time, a Hungarian immigrant
from the countryside near Budapest, who worked in a factory in Buffalo; one night, in a tavern in Black Rock, he was killed by another
Hungarian immigrant, allegedly "beaten to death with a poker."

Beyond these blunt bare facts, nothing more seemed to be
known. The killer must have been identified, maybe even arrested
and charged, and very likely the killing would have been described
as "self-defense"—possibly, this was true. All I would ever know
of my mother's father was that he was, like other Hungarian males
in the family, an individual of whom it might be said that he was
not slow to flare up in anger, if not rage, and that he was a "heavy
drinker." The word *peasant* is a disallowed word, a shameful usage
to contemporary ears, but *Hungarian peasants* is probably the most
objective description of my mother's relatives who'd immigrated to
western New York in the early 1900s. By contemporary standards
these immigrants were desperately poor people of the class of those
about whom Upton Sinclair wrote so compellingly in *The Jungle*
(1906), set in the Chicago slaughterhouses.

The sudden death of my mother's father left her family desti-
tute. Her parents had had eight children, the older of whom were
already working. (Recall that this is 1917, when immigrant children
rarely went to school but worked in factories, mills, and slaughterhouses, for wages much less than those of adult men.) My biological
grandmother, whom I would never meet, nor even see a photo of,

gave away at least one of her children at this time, the youngest, my mother, who was nine months old.

The infant was given to the couple whom I would know as Grandma and Grandpa Bush—Lena and John Bush. ("Bush" was the name the immigrant couple had been given at Ellis Island, as it is an approximation of their Hungarian name "Bus.") One day it would be told to me, or suggested, in the casual way in which such genealogical information was likely to be provided, that John Bush may have been a brother of my mother's deceased father—in which case, my mother had been sent to live with an uncle and his wife, which does not seem quite so desperate as being given away to strangers. There were no "adoptions" in those days—at least, no government agencies that were concerned with the fate of immigrant children of whom, in heavily Roman Catholic communities like Black Rock, there were many. My mother was taken in by a couple who not only wanted a child, but also needed another farm-helper in their household; as soon as she was old enough, she was given farm chores; for a few years she attended a one-room schoolhouse a mile away from the small farm in Millersport, across Tonawanda Creek in Niagara County—the very one-room schoolhouse I would attend years later.

Briefly too my mother attended a Roman Catholic school taught by nuns, in Swormville, from which she graduated after eight grades, at which time her education ceased. Eight grades were considered more than sufficient at this time in our history, in rural communities especially, where the designation "high school graduate" was a matter of pride.

When my mother Carolina Bush was eighteen or nineteen years old, and working part-time as a waitress in a restaurant on the Millersport Highway, she and my father Frederic Oates met. This would have been 1935 or 1936. Fred Oates was three years older than Carolina; he'd been born in Lockport, a small city seven miles north of Millersport, on the Erie Canal. Like my mother's early life, my father's early life had been shaped by the premature and violent death of a relative, in this case his maternal grandfather, a German Jewish immigrant who'd tried to kill both his wife and his fourteen-year-old daughter (my grandmother-to-be) with a shotgun, and ended up killing only himself. My father, too, had had to quit school young, and began work in a "machine-shop" (Harrison Radiator) in Lockport. He would work at Harrison's for an astounding forty years before retiring, though by degrees he was to be promoted from the assembly-line machine shop to tool and die design.

Since such family secrets were shrouded in mystery, as in mortification and shame, I never knew, nor had I any way of substantiating, whether these two (very attractive) young people confided in each other, or commiserated with each other; both sides of my family were notable for reticence, and a stubbornness in reticence; these were not individuals for whom openness came easily, still less anything approaching "full disclosure." The ardor of confession for which our era is known would have been astonishing to them, scarcely believable and in no way desirable. There seemed the fear among my adult relatives that something misspoken could not be reclaimed; if you spoke heedlessly, you would speak unwisely and you would regret it. In much of my fiction there is a simulacrum of the "confessional" but to interpret it in these terms is misleading. Not literal transcription but emotional transcription is the way of the writer.

While we were growing up, my brother Fred, Jr., and I had no idea of our parents' backgrounds. We had no idea that my mother had been given away by her mother, after her father's murder; we had no idea that my father's mother had nearly been murdered by her raging father. We had no idea that my father's mother Blanche Morgenstern was Jewish. (In western New York State of those days, we had no idea what "Jewish" was.) We would be adults before we learned even the skeletal outline of these old, shameful secrets that had both altered the trajectories of our parents' (impoverished) lives but also made our births, in 1938 and 1943 respectively, possible.

It was fascinating—I suppose. To live among adults who must have frequently spoken to one another in a kind of code. (My mother's stepparents with whom we lived would certainly have talked about my mother's biological mother and her siblings, who lived less than ten miles away; there were Bush uncles and aunts and cousins who appeared at a little distance, and gradually became known to me in my teens.) Much of adult life was forbidden of entry to children— not just family secrets of this sort but financial crises, health crises, problems with work. Outside the brightly-lit "home" there is the murky penumbra of adults who don't especially care about you, and are not obliged to wish you well. It may be that the writer/artist is stimulated by childhood mysteries or that it is the childhood mysteries that stimulate the writer/artist. Sometimes in my writing, when I am most absorbed and fascinated, to the point of anxiety, I find myself imagining that what I am inventing is in some way "real"; if I can solve the mystery of the fiction, I will have solved a mystery of my life. That the mystery is never solved would seem to be the reason for the writer's continuous effort to solve it—each story, each poem, each novel is a restatement of the quest to penetrate the mystery, tirelessly restated.

The writer is the decipherer of clues—if by "clues" is meant a broken and discontinuous subterranean narrative.

I WAS WELL INTO adulthood and living far from Millersport by the time the Bush family secret came to light, and even then it was a faint, glimmering light, about which no one wished to speak without averted eyes, an air of embarrassment and shame, and a wish to change the subject. Growing up in their household, on that farm in Millersport, my brother and I may have had a vague awareness that John and Lena Bush were not my mother's "real" parents—beyond that we couldn't know, and in the way of family reticence, which is a kind of dignity, we could not ask, any more than children of that era would have boldly asked their fathers what their incomes were and their mothers whether they'd really wanted children.

But here is the surprise: my mother's account of that traumatic time in her early life did not center upon the murder of her father (whom she had not known—after all she'd been an infant at the time) but on the mortifying fact of having been "given away." When for a special feature in *O, The Oprah Magazine* in the late 1990s several women writers were commissioned to interview their own mothers, I learned of some of this old, sad story, still upsetting to my mother so many decades later. All my mother seemed to know was: her father had been murdered, her mother had given her away. Several times she said, "My mother didn't want me. I used to cry and cry . . ." I was stricken to the heart—my mother was eighty years old! This trauma of 1917 was as recent and fresh to her as if no time had intervened.

Of all the relatives on both sides of our family my mother Carolina Oates had the reputation of being the most generous, the most kind, the warmest and "sunniest"—I did not want to think that, in her innermost heart, Mommy thought of herself as a child whose mother had not wanted her.

Crimes reverberate through many years, and through many lives. It is a rare homicide that destroys only one person. And it is a paradox to accept that, had a Hungarian immigrant not been murdered in 1917, I would not be alive today; how many of us, many more than would wish to speak of so sordid a fact, owe our births to the premature deaths of others whom we have never known but to whom we are linked by that mysterious shared fate called "blood."

Here is the ironic equipoise of which Henry James wrote: this catastrophe that was for my mother, through her life, a source of acute sorrow and shame was for me, her daughter, the very genesis of my life.

SUNDAY DRIVE

ONCE UPON A TIME, the Sunday drive.

In our succession of Daddy's wonderful cars!

(Were Daddy's cars wonderful, or did my brother and I just imagine this? They were all American cars of course and all built by General Motors for my father worked for Harrison Radiator in Lockport, New York, an automotive supplier for GM. Though technically these were not "new cars" but "used" they were always "new" and spectacular to us.)

Where are we going, I would ask.

And the answer was enigmatic, Wait until we get there. You'll see.

Our car was our principal means of adventure, exploration, and entertainment; our lengthy, looping, seemingly uncalculated Sunday drives with sometimes my father, sometimes my mother, at the wheel were our primary means of experiencing ourselves as a *family*.

Of course, we did not know this. We would scarcely have articulated such a notion, at the time.

Where weekday drives were always purposeful, Sunday drives were spontaneous and improvised. If Daddy was driving it was not unlikely that we might drive south on Transit Road in the direction of Lee's Airfield just to see who was there; if Mommy was driving it was not unlikely we might drive west or east on narrow curving country roads along the Tonawanda Creek, where Mommy knew who lived in every house. Our car was like a small boat, or maybe a small plane, blown like the perpetual cumulus clouds of the sky above the Great Lakes, in any of these directions, by chance and not choice; the drives were familial daydreams, dreams somehow made conscious and translated into landscape. Unknowing, we were enchanted by the mystery of the (familiar) landscape and our place in it.

The writer is one who understands how deeply mysterious the "familiar" really is. How strangely opaque, what we've seen a thousand times. And how inconsolable a loss, when the taken-for-granted is finally taken from us.

IT WAS A BEAUTIFUL landscape in some way haunted.

Millersport Rapids Swormville Getzville East Amherst Clarence Rapids Pendleton Wolcottsburg Lockport Middleport Wrights Corners Gasport Ransomville Royalton Medina Wilson Newfane Olcott—a strangely comforting poetry these place-names of our Sunday drives. Open, uncultivated countryside; stretches of dense deciduous woods; pastures bounded by barbed wire in which dairy cows, beef cattle, sheep and horses grazed; fields planted in corn, wheat, potatoes, soybeans; miles of fruit orchards—apple trees, pear trees, cherry trees, peach trees; farmhouses that resembled my grandparents' house, large hay barns, dairy barns, silos and corncribs. Single-span wrought-iron bridges over the Tonawanda Creek or the Erie Barge Canal whose planks rattled as we crossed high above the water; smaller bridges over narrow streams, only just wide enough for a single vehicle. (The particular terror of the larger bridge was the possibility that a wide vehicle—truck, tractor—might be crossing at the same time, in the other lane; the driver of our car might then be required to back up, slowly and laboriously, to let the other pass. The fear of the smaller bridge was that another vehicle might suddenly appear around a blind curve and collide head-on with us.) Two-lane blacktop roads sticky as licorice in hot summer; narrow rutted dirt roads winding like strips of fraying ribbon between plowed fields; those attractive and beguiling unpaved roads through dense countryside that dwindled into mere lanes bordering farmers' fields, bumpy and eventually impassable ending in what my parents called *dead ends* . . . We learn our awe of the world as children staring eagerly out the windows of a moving vehicle.

If we began our Sunday drive along the Erie County side of the Tonawanda Creek to Pendleton a few miles away we might cross the wrought-iron bridge at Pendleton and enter Niagara County; if the drive was to be a relatively short drive we might turn right, or west, onto the Tonawanda Creek Road, return to Transit Road a few miles away and cross the bridge into Millersport, and so to our house which was the first on the right, beside a small Esso gas station (operated by my mother's brothers Frank and Johnny Bush). Or, we might drive along the creek to Rapids, a few miles in the other direction, cross the bridge there and so return to Transit Road along a more circuitous route following the curves of the Tonawanda Creek, past the single-room schoolhouse which I attended for five grades, and which my mother had attended twenty years before, and so home. ("Tonawanda Creek Road" is a confusing term because, in effect, there were four roads with the same name, that might more accurately have been designated "Tonawanda Creek Road North-East"—"Tonawanda Creek Road North-West"—"Tonawanda Creek Road South-East"—"Tonawanda Creek Road South-West." These were country roads narrow and minimally paved, bisected by the wider Transit Road running north and south.)

When my father drove, my mother sat beside him in the passenger's seat. But whenever my mother drove, it meant that my father wasn't coming with us because my father would never have consented to be a passenger in any vehicle in which he was not the driver.

(In this Fred Oates was the quintessential American male of his time. It wasn't a question of "equality"—that my mother was a woman was not the issue; it was a question of who had authority in a vehicle, and this was likely to be the man of the family, in whose name the vehicle had been purchased.)

These least adventurous/most familiar Sunday drives nonetheless intrigued my brother Robin (Fred, Jr.; born on Christmas Day 1943) and me, for our mother knew the inhabitants of virtually all of the houses along the Tonawanda Creek, if not personally then by reputation, or rumor; my fascination with people, as with their houses and "settings," surely began with these Sunday drives and my mother's frequent, often quite startling and elliptical commentary. Six years in the one-room schoolhouse containing eight grades of often unruly "big boys" had enabled my mother's generation of young people to know one another intimately, if not always fondly; sometimes my mother's reticence was all that was forthcoming as we passed a house. ("Yes. I know who lives there.")

This was an era memorialized by Edward Hopper of shingle-board houses with front porches and people sitting on these porches keen to observe people driving past in vehicles observing them. Narrow, winding creek roads were best for such sightings, for vehicles were likely to be driven at unhurried speeds on these roads; sometimes my mother would be stuck behind a slow-moving tractor or even a horse-drawn hay wagon.

Once, on the creek road to Rapids, when my father wasn't with us, my mother behind the wheel suddenly said: "In that house, a terrible thing happened."

Mommy slowed the car. No one appeared to be visible in the house, observing us.

(Had this been an ordinary-seeming dwelling? Not a farmhouse but a smaller, shanty-like structure with a tar paper roof, set back from the road on a badly rutted driveway. In the front yard, straggly trees. Rusted hulks of cars in the scrubby grass. Decades later the name of the family who lived there is still vivid in my memory—not *Reichling* but a name that slant-rhymes with it.)

A man had been murdered, my mother said. The father of a girl with whom she'd gone to school.

At first it was believed that the man had "disappeared"—his wife claimed not to know where he was. But then his body was discovered in the creek behind the house; it had been forced inside a barrel, and the barrel had been nailed shut, and rolled down to the creek where it only partially sank in about five feet of water close to shore.

"The wife and her man-friend murdered him. Stabbed him. It was a terrible thing."

Why did they kill him, I wanted to know. Were they arrested, were they in prison, who had discovered the body in the barrel— many questions sprang to my lips which my mother was vague about answering, whether because Mommy thought I should not be so curious, or because she didn't know. Enough for our mother to have surprised us by saying—*It was a terrible thing*.

(I HAVE TO CONCEDE that I scarcely remember myself as a child. Only as an eye, an ear, a ceaselessly inquisitive center of consciousness. For instance, I can remember my mother's tantalizingly brief account of the murder on the Tonawanda Creek Road in the direction of Rapids only a few miles from our house but I can't fit this memory into a sequence of memories of that drive, that day, that week or even that year; our memories seem to lack the faculty for chronological continuity, in which case an episodic and impressionistic art most accurately replicates the meanderings of memory, and not chronological order. What is vivid in memory is the singular, striking, one-of-a-kind event or episode, encapsulated as if in amber, and rarely followed by the return home, that evening's dinner, exchanged remarks, the next morning; not routine but what violates routine.

Which is why the effort of writing a memoir is so fraught with peril, and even its small successes ringed by melancholy. The fact is—*We have forgotten most of our lives. All of our landscapes are soon lost in time.)*

WHEN MY FATHER TOOK us on Sunday drives, it was more likely that he would take us much farther, as he drove faster; on Transit Road, which Daddy traveled all too frequently, he was inclined to drive above the speed limit, and to pass slower cars with some measure of irritation. My sense of maleness, based solely and surely unfairly upon my father Fred Oates, is that the male more than the female is inclined to *impatience.*

Where Mommy drove us on country roads never very far from the Tonawanda Creek, that cut through her childhood, as through mine, and fixed us comfortingly in place, Daddy had little interest in the familiar countryside of Erie County, apart from his visits to Lee's Airfield. The landscape of Fred Oates's boyhood was Niagara County: he'd been born in Lockport, in the least affluent area of the small city known informally as "Lowertown," and had lived in Lockport all of his life until he'd married my mother and came to live with her in Millersport. (There had been an earlier domestic life in Lockport, about which I knew nothing, and which had always seemed to me romantic, as it had to have been short-lived. Only a scattering of snapshots allowed me to see my young parents, an infant bundled in their arms, photographed in a waste of snow behind a rented apartment in Lowertown near the canal. *Where we lived before Millersport*—was the terse description. *Before we came to live with your grandparents.*)

Daddy's drives may have reflected his restlessness. The same restlessness that motivated him to fly airplanes, even to experiment one summer with a glider at Lee's Airfield. (Gliders are far more dangerous than small aircraft and Daddy may have had some close calls with this glider, about which my brother and I would not have been told.) Though Daddy did not drive slowly past houses and name to us their inhabitants and hint to us of the mysteries of lives within, yet Daddy's drives into Niagara County were more interesting than Mommy's drives in Erie County, as they were farther-ranging, and fraught with the kind of urgency my father brought to most things.

Daddy liked to follow the Erie Barge Canal westward in the direction of the beautiful turbulent Niagara River or eastward into hilly Orleans County, in the direction of Brockport and Rochester; he liked to drop in on a small airfield in Newfane, where he had friends; he liked to drop in at the Big Tree Inn near Newfane, or the Inn at Olcott Beach on Lake Ontario; there was the excitement of the Niagara County Fair at the Fairgrounds, and the excitement of volunteer firemen's picnics scattered through the county where food and drinks—especially beer—were served. Daddy's drives were not without direction like Mommy's but intended to bring him to places where, when he approached, voices lifted happily—"Fred! Jesus, here's Fred Oates."

In such places there were jukeboxes. Clouded mirrors behind the bar where men who resembled my father turned to welcome him. Pervading smells of beer, cigarette smoke. Plastic ashtrays filled with ashes and butts. Small bowls in which greasy fragments of potato chips remained. If such places were on the vast, wind-lashed lake, there was a sandy beach littered with broken shells. There were picnic areas with tables, benches. Summertime smell of wet sand, wet bathing suits and towels. Burnt charcoal, grilling hamburgers, hot dogs and mustard and ketchup. Broken rinds of watermelon on the ground, corncobs buzzing with flies. Discarded Coke bottles, beer bottles. Music from car radios.

If summer, and if near Lake Ontario, there was always a chance of lightning and thunderstorms. You started off in Millersport on a sunny blue-skied summer day, you ended at Lake Ontario in pelting rain beneath a boiling-black sky in autumnal chill. Even when we had plenty of time to return home, Daddy tended to ignore our pleas and continue driving. Or, if we were already at Lake Ontario, and the sky began to darken ominously, Daddy was likely to delay leaving until the last possible moment.

There came flashes of heat lightning, soundless. Then actual lightning, thunder. Deafening thunder like cymbals crashing. We were chastened waiting for the storm to pass beneath the overhangs of strangers' roofs, beneath tall windswept trees.

At the Big Tree Inn on a promontory above the lake there was indeed an enormous tree—probably an elm tree. The novelty of the "big tree" was that it had been many times struck by lightning. My mother feared lightning, as her older sister Elsie (my "Aunt Elsie" who lived in Lockport) had in fact been injured when lightning struck a doorway in which she was standing: Elsie's face, throat, and arm were riddled with slivers from the shattered doorframe; but my mother could not prevail against my father who thought a thunderstorm was an occasion for rejoicing and not cowering indoors.

My mother was not an assertive person. Especially she was not assertive with my father. Mommy might suggest turning back to avoid a storm but she could not insist, and if she had, our father would have ignored her; if she'd insisted more adamantly, our father would have defied her.

Once, not at the Big Tree Inn but at a place called Koch's Paradise Grove, by chance on my way to a women's restroom adjacent to the bar, amid a barrage of loud music, a din of voices, laughter, I came across a sight that was shocking to me, and that I have never forgotten: my father speaking with another man, a man of about his age, a stranger whom I was sure I'd never seen before, and they were standing close together, faces flushed and voices raised in anger, and the frightening thought came to me—*They are going to fight, they are going to hurt each other*; but in the next instant my father turned, and saw me, and the expression on his face altered, and the moment passed.

A child is very frightened—viscerally, emotionally—by the raised voices of adults. Even when anger isn't involved but rather excitement, hilarity.

I might have registered—*They have been drinking. But Daddy is not drunk!*

It was not unknown, that men became *drunk*. But that was very different from being classified as a *drunk*.

So often it seemed to happen in my life as a child and a young girl, such arrested and abbreviated moments—the scene that is interrupted by the girl blundering into it. If there were words exchanged the intrusion of the girl silenced these words and so it is not words that remain but the sound of a voice or voices, uplifted in anger or in hilarity, essentially indecipherable. It is the child's experience to blunder into scenes between adults and to become a witness to something inexplicable to her though it is (probably) a quite ordinary episode in what are not extraordinary lives after all; it remains that the child or young adolescent will make of these broken-off and mysterious fragments some sort of coherent narrative. What is fleeting and transient in time, no doubt soon forgotten by the adults, or rendered inconsequential in their lives, may burrow deep into the child-witness's soul, whatever is meant by "soul" that is not fleeting and transitory but somehow permanent, and inextricable. And so, decades later I am still seeing my father and the unknown, unnamed man, a man who resembled my father, and both of them flush-faced and prepared to fight; I am remembering how my mother's father died, in a tavern fight in Black Rock in 1917, though long before I was born; I am remembering a casual remark of my father's—*A man never backs down from a fight. You just can't.*

And there were other occasions, like this. Like the Sunday drives, beyond estimation. A child sees her father at a little distance, a figure among other figures; a man among men; a child is baffled and thrilled by her father in precisely those ways in which the father eludes the child. It is as if my father had said to me—*You will not ever know me, but it is allowed that you can love me.*

The mother is the *known*, or so the child imagines. (This would turn out to be not exactly true, or not true in the fullest degree, but it was not the case that my mother was inaccessible to me emotionally, as often, in those years, my father was.) But the father is the *lesser-known*, the more obvious figure of romance.

How many times returning late from Sunday drives into the countryside beyond Lockport, in Niagara County; a nighttime drive back to Lockport and up the long steep glacier hill to the wide bridge over the Erie Canal at the junction of Main Street and Transit Street; and so onto Transit Road (NY Route 78) and another long, steep glacier hill and our house seven miles away in the countryside just across the Tonawanda Creek. Often, my brother and I would drift off to sleep in the backseat of the car. Often, it seemed to be raining. We would hear the slap of windshield wipers, and my parents' lowered voices in the front seat. Headlights of oncoming cars sweeping into the back of our car, across the ceiling and gone . . .

On a map of the region—(I would not examine a detailed map of Erie and Niagara counties until 2014 while composing this memoir)—the space of our Sunday drives is compressed like something in a children's storybook. Lake Ontario, that had seemed so romantically far from our home, is fewer than twenty miles away, to the north; Niagara Falls is only twenty-five miles away, to the west. The landscape of my childhood that had seemed so vast, so fraught with mysteries, could be contained within something like a thirty-mile radius.

Sunday drives! You'd think they would continue forever but nothing continues forever. Like gas selling for twenty-eight cents a gallon, that's gone forever.

FRED'S SIGNS

"DADDY! CAN I TRY?"

And your father will hand you one of his smaller brushes, its thick-feathery tip dipped in red paint, and a piece of scrap plywood, and on the plywood you will try conscientiously to "letter" as your father lettered—precisely and unhesitatingly, with deft twists of his wrist. But in your inexpert hand the paintbrush wavers, and the lettering is wobbly—childish. The bright red flourish of Daddy's letters, the subtle curls and tucks of his brushstrokes, will be impossible for you to imitate at any age.

This evening after supper in a season when the sky is still light. When you have left your room upstairs in the farmhouse and crossed to your father's sign shop in the old hay barn—not a "shop" but just a corner of the barn that has been converted to a two-vehicle garage with a sliding overhead metal door. The shop isn't heated of course. Your father seems virtually immune to cold (never wears a hat even in winter when icy winds lower the temperature to below zero, often doesn't wear an overcoat) though he has to briskly rub his hands sometimes when he's painting signs. When he isn't working at Harrison Radiator in Lockport, forty-hour weeks plus "time-and-a-half" on Saturdays, Fred Oates is a freelance sign painter whose distinc-

tive style is immediately recognizable in the Lockport/Getzville/
East Amherst area, particularly along the seven-mile stretch of rural
Transit Road from Lockport to Millersport.

It is fascinating to you, to observe your father preparing his signs.
Some are so large they have to be propped up on a bench against a
wall, smooth rectangular surfaces on which he has laid two coats
of shiny white paint. Then, bars straight-penciled with a yardstick,
between which he will inscribe his flawless letters:

GARLOCK'S FAMILY RESTAURANT
5 Miles

EIMER ICE
We Deliver

FULLENWEIDER DAIRY

KOHL'S FARM PRODUCE
2 Miles

CLOVERLEAF INN

He'd begun as a sign painter for the Palace Theater in Lockport,
when silent movies were shown there. In fact, he'd begun as an usher
at the Palace, and a Wurlitzer player. (Silent movies were not "silent"
of course but required live music initially.) How, at age fourteen, had
Fred Oates been hired for such responsibilities? Soon he was work-

ing at the Palace and painting signs for local businesses—"I don't remember how I got started. Just one thing led to another."

The lives of our parents, grandparents, ancestors—*Just one thing led to another.*

Vertiginous abyss between then and now.

After the Palace, Fred Oates went to work in the machine shop at Harrison's, a short block or two from the Palace Theater on Main Street, Lockport. There he would work for the next forty years until retiring at sixty-five, all the while painting signs in his spare time, to amplify his income.

Difficult not to feel unworthy of such parents, who'd come of age as young adults in the Great Depression. Their lives were work. Their lives were deprivation. Their lives have led to *you*.

As he paints, Daddy hums. He has never complained of the circumstances in his life for possibly it has not occurred to him that there might be legitimate grounds for complaint. Work has been much of his life, and in this, his life is hardly uncommon for its time and place. Painting signs is work of a kind but it is also pleasurable, like playing the organ at the country church or, when he'd been a boy, playing the piano at the Palace Theater. *Work to do* is not, as some might think, a negative but rather a strong positive for *work to do* means purpose, and the pleasure of having completed something. In this case, something for which Fred Oates will be paid.

You must be quiet when Daddy is wielding the paintbrush, and you must be still. A restless child isn't wanted here in Daddy's "sign shop." You are fascinated by your father's utter concentration as he paints. You can see that there is a distinct pleasure in precisely shaping the subtly curving letters and you will absorb this pleasure in precision, in "lettering," that might translate into a pleasure in "writing"—for a writer is after all someone who *writes words* in succession, and words are shaped out of *letters*.

In the sign shop there is a strong smell of paints, turpentine. And a smell of damp earth—(the barn's floor is hard-packed dirt). On Daddy's work bench are paintbrushes of varying sizes, and all kept in good condition. For Daddy can't afford to use brushes carelessly; each brush is valuable. There is no excitement quite like taking a camel's-hair brush from your father's fingers and dipping it into paint to "letter" on a piece of plywood—*Joyce Carol Oates*.

Is it a magical name, that Daddy and Mommy have given you? That has often seemed a gift to you, out of the magnanimity of their love.

"Can I try?"—not once but many times.

As long as you can remember as a girl, the landscape within an approximate fifteen-mile radius has always contained your father's signs. Mommy will point as we drive past—"See? That's Daddy's new sign." In a vehicle with others, someone might say—"See? That's one of Fred's signs." To a neutral eye these signs are of no special distinction. One would not even know that they are hand-painted and not rather manufactured in some way. They are mere signs, distractions that interrupt the mostly rural landscape of Transit Road. Yet, to you, the sign-painter's daughter, these signs are beautiful. There is something bold and dramatic about a hand-painted sign nailed to a tree. On the side of a barn. You can pick out Fred Oates's signs anywhere—the curve of the *S*'s and *O*'s that suggest almost human figures. The way Daddy crosses his *T*'s. Once you asked your father, "Why is there a dot over the *i*?" and your father gave this childish question some thought before saying, "Maybe because without the dot the *i* would look too small, like something was left out."

For many years after he'd ceased to paint them Fred Oates's signs remained on Transit Road. Then, one by one, they were removed, or replaced, or faded into the oblivion of harsh weather and time. And now, I have not driven along Transit Road in years in fear and dread of what I will not see.

"THEY ALL JUST WENT AWAY"

I MUST HAVE BEEN a lonely child. I know that I was a secretive child.

Yet I must have loved my aloneness. Until the age of twelve or thirteen my most intense, happiest hours were spent tramping desolate fields, woods, creek banks near my family's farmhouse in Millersport, New York.

No one knew where I went. No one could have guessed how far I wandered. Did my parents inquire, and if so, what did I say? *Just walking. Back the lane. Down by the creek.* Our answers are vague and self-protective. We learn young to obfuscate the truth even when the truth is not harmful to us.

My father would never have asked me where I'd been, because my father was away much of the time. If my mother inquired where I'd been, I would have answered in a way to deflect her curiosity. I was an articulate, verbal child for whom language was both a means of communication and a scrim behind which I might hide, unseen. Of course like all children of that era I had numerous chores—feeding chickens, gathering eggs, even mowing the lawn (with a hand-mower, no joke in tough sinewy crabgrass) as well as more common household chores like helping with meals and dishes.

Still, I seemed to have had ample time to be alone. I could not have explained to any adult what drew me to descend the steep hill to the Tonawanda Creek and to walk for miles along the rocky bank—if to the right, I would have to make my way beneath the bridge, on a crumbling concrete ledge just above the water, surely no more than twelve inches wide. Overhead were exposed rusted girders and the desiccated nests of birds (barn swallows?); when vehicles passed on the bridge the entire structure shook and echoed in a way that made the hairs at the nape of my neck rise. In the fast-moving, rippling creek, the bridge's reflected underside quavered like something that is forbidden to see, which is yet seen. There was a certain fearfulness involved in inching across the ledge beneath the bridge—a quickening of the heartbeat. Was there danger? The water beneath the bridge wasn't as deep as elsewhere—concrete and other debris had been left there by the construction crew. The water's surface was luridly broken by rusted shafts and rods which had become dulled by time. Once on the other side of the bridge I could follow a faint, worn path, a fisherman's path, that would continue for a few hundred yards until it disappeared into underbrush.

Often there were men fishing on the creek bank beside the bridge. There might be two men, or there might be a solitary man; they were not likely to be residents of the area. You would see their cars parked on the grassy shoulder of the road by the bridge. My memory of these strangers is utterly blank—I can't think that I approached them, yet I don't recall turning back to avoid them. It is possible that, from time to time, one of the solitary men spoke to me, asked my name and where I lived—that would not have been unusual, and it would not have been alarming. But beyond that, I have no memory.

Did my mother think to warn me—*Joyce, don't go near the fishermen! Stay on our side of the bridge*.

To recall the sight of an individual fishing on the creek bank is to feel a thrill of apprehension. The graceful arc of a fishing line cast out into the creek, the sound of the hooked bait and sinker dropping into the water—these are exciting to me, somehow fascinating, suffused with a kind of dread.

In the fisherman's plastic bucket near shore, live fish, rock bass, trapped and squirming in a few inches of bloody water.

Our side of the bridge was the safer side. The other side of the bridge was the "other" side.

On the safer side was a similar path along the creek bank but it was wider, more defined. This was an area in which as a young child I had played with other children amid a scattering of large boulders and rocks that extended well out into the creek. Close by was a makeshift dam of rocks built by a neighboring farmer across which, if we were very careful, we could make our way to the other side.

At any point where a path led up from the creek, usually up a very steep hill, I could ascend and explore fields, woods, stretches of land that seemed to belong to no one. Within a mile's radius from our house on Transit Road was this other, deeply rural, uncultivated and "wild" place containing abandoned houses, barns, silos, corncribs. There were badly rusted tractors, hulks of cars with broken windows and no tires, rotted hay wagons, piles of rotted lumber. A kind of dumping-ground, at the edge of an overgrown and no longer tended pear orchard. Why NO TREPASSING signs exerted such a powerful fascination, I don't know; even today such signs are complex signifiers that stir atavistic memories and cause my pulse to quicken. Yet more attractive because more forbidding was the sign WARNING— BRIDGE OUT. Or, DANGER—DO NOT TRESPASS. Everywhere were NO HUNTING NO FISHING NO TRESPASSING signs and many of these were riddled with buckshot, for adults too were contemptuous of such admonitions.

An early memory divorced of all context and explanation as a random snapshot discovered in a drawer is of trying to walk, then crawling on hands and knees across the skeletal rusted girders of an ancient bridge across the creek, tasting fear, fear like the swirling foam-flecked water below, trying not to glance below where jagged rocks and boulders emerged from the water. A possibly fatal place to fall, a place that might have left me maimed, crippled for life, yet a kind of logic demanded that the girders had to be crossed and, more fearfully, recrossed. I could not have said why such a mad feat of daring had to be performed, as if it were a sacred ritual, unwitnessed.

In the company of other children, I was compelled to be the most reckless. Once, I jumped from the roof of a small, boarded-up shanty-house to land on hard, grassless ground fifteen feet below. What an impact! I remember the sledgehammer blow that reverberated through my legs, spine, neck, head. My companions changed their minds about jumping and I was left with a dazed, headachy elation.

The stupidity of childhood, that reverberates through decades.

The realization——*How close you came to killing yourself, and how unknowing you were!* In adulthood we have no way of measuring the illogic of our young selves except to hope that we have outgrown it.

Close by our property, on the far side of a dirt lane, was a boarded-up old cider mill on a sloping bank of the creek. ("Millersport" is named for this mill, whose owner went bankrupt in the Depression.) Within my mother's memory the mill was operated but I never knew it to be otherwise than abandoned and haphazardly boarded up as if in haste or in disdain—planks crossed like giant *X*'s over empty windows, through which any child or teenager could crawl very easily. Of all places the cider mill was forbidden and was festooned with signs warning DANGER—NO TRESPASSING. Yet how many times alone or in the company of others I would push through a cellar window at the rear of the mill that was hidden by tall grass and debris, crawling into the wreck of a building with no heed that

I might cut myself on broken glass or exposed nails. What a wonderland this was! The very odor—chill, dank, sour-rotten on even
the freshest days—was exhilarating. No children's play-world could
be more fascinating than the cider mill where fantastical machines
(presses? conveyor belts?) in various stages of rust and decrepitude
dwarfed me as if I were no larger and of no more significance than a
prowling cat. Here was a stillness in which no adult had set his foot
in years.

Though steps were missing from the rotted staircase it seemed
necessary to climb to the second floor. And to walk—slowly,
cautiously—across this swaying floor, to stare out a high window
at the creek. Behind the mill was an immense compost pile of rotted apples like an avalanche. In this rich dark pungent-smelling soil
fishermen sought worms to use for bait on their hooks. From the
high window I might watch them, unseen and waiting until they had
safely departed.

Or maybe I had been hiding there. The memory is blurred like
newsprint in water.

BUT IT WAS ABANDONED houses that drew me most. A hike of
miles in hot, muggy air through fields of spiky grass and brambles,
across outcroppings of shale steeply angled as stairs, was a lark if the
reward was: an empty house.

Some of these empty houses had been recently inhabited as
"homes"—they had not yet reverted to the wild. Others, abandoned
during the 1930s, had long begun to collapse inward engulfed by
morning glory and trumpet vines.

To push open a door to such silence: the emptiness of a house
whose occupants had departed.

Fire-scorched walls, ceiling. A stink of wet smoke. Part of the house has been gutted by fire but strangely, several downstairs rooms are relatively untouched.

Broken glass underfoot. Drone of flies, hornets. Rapid glisten of a garter snake gliding silently across the floorboards. It is hurtful to see the left-behind remnants of a lost family. Broken child's toy on the floor, mucus-colored baby bottle. Rain-soaked sofa with eviscerated cushions as if gutted by a hunter's knife. Strips of wallpaper like shredded skin. Broken crockery, a heap of smelly tin cans in a corner, beer cans, whiskey bottles. Scattering of cigarette butts. A badly scraped enamel-topped kitchen table. Icebox with door yawning open. At the sink, a hand-pump. (No "running water" here!) On a counter a dirt-stiffened rag that, unfolded like precious cloth, is revealed to be a girl's cheaply glamorous "see-through" blouse.

When I was too young to think *The house is the mother's body. You can be expelled from it and forbidden to re-enter.*

It seemed that I would steel myself against being observed. A residue of early childhood when we believe that adults can see us at all times and can hear our thoughts. In an empty house, a face can appear at a high window, if but fleetingly. A woman's uplifted hand in greeting, or in warning. *Hello! Come in! Stay away! Run! Who are you?* Often in an empty house there would be a glimmer of movement in the corner of my eye: the figure of a person passing through a doorway. He had hurt her badly, we knew. And the children. For they were his to hurt.

We knew though we did not know, for no one had told us.

The sky in such places of abandonment was of the hue and brightness of tin. As if the melancholy rural poverty of tin roofs reflects upward.

No one had told me and yet I knew: it was a dangerous place to be a woman if you were not a woman protected by a man or men. If you were not a child protected by a father, a mother. If you were not of a family that owned a house—a "home."

A *HOUSE* IS A structural arrangement of space, geometrically laid out to provide what are called rooms, and these rooms divided from one another by walls, ceilings, floors. The *house* contains the *home* but is not identical with it. The *house* anticipates the *home* and will survive it, reverting again to *house* when *home* has departed.

In my life subsequent to Millersport I have not found the visual equivalent of these abandoned farmhouses of western New York in the north country of Erie County in the region of the Tonawanda Creek and the Erie Canal. You are led to think most immediately of Edward Hopper: those unsettling stylized visions of a lost America, houses never rendered as "homes," and human beings, if you look closely, never depicted as anything other than mannequins. There is Charles Burchfield who rendered the landscapes of western New York and his native Ohio as visionary and luminous and excluded the human figure entirely. The shimmering pastel New England barns, fields, trees and skies of Wolf Kahn are images evoked by memory on the edge of dissolution. But the "real"—that which assaults the eye before the brain begins its work of selection, rearrangement, censure—is never on the edge of dissolution, still less appropriation. The "real" is raw, unexpected, unpredictable; sometimes luminous but more often not. Above all, the "real" is gratuitous. For to be a "realist" (in life as in art) is to acknowledge that all things might be other than they are. No design, no intention, no aesthetic, moral, or teleological imprimatur. The equivalent of Darwin's vision of a blind, purposeless, and ceaseless evolutionary process that yields no ultimate "products"—only temporary strategies against extinction.

How memory is a matter of bright, fleeting surfaces imperfectly preserved in the perishable brain.

Where a house has been abandoned, too wrecked, rotted, or despairing to be sold, very likely seized by the county in default of taxes and the property held in escrow, there is a sad history. There have been devastated lives. Lives to be spoken of cautiously. How they went wrong. When did it begin. Why did she marry him, stay with *him*. Why, when he'd so hurt her. Why, when he'd warned her. Those people. Runs in the family. Shame.

For the abandoned house contains the future of any house. The tree pushing like a tumor through the rotted porch in sinewy coils, hornets' nests beneath sagging eaves, a stained and rain-soaked mattress on a floor of what was once a bedroom, a place of intimacy and trust; windows smashed, skeletal animal remains and human excrement dried in coils on what had once been a parlor floor. On a wall in what had once been the kitchen, a calendar of years ago with blocks of days exactingly crossed out in pencil, discolored by rain.

I SEEM TO HAVE suggested that the abandoned houses were all distant from our house and that we did not know the families who were unfortunate enough to have lived in them. In fact, the fire-gutted house, the Judds' house, was less than a mile from ours and so by the logic of rural communities, the Judds were—almost—"next-door neighbors" and Helen Judd was my "next-door friend."

The Judds lived on the Tonawanda Road between Millersport and Pendleton. If you took a shortcut to their house behind our barn and through our cornfield and a marshy stretch of trees, it was a walk of no more than ten minutes.

This is a walk I often take in dreams. A stealthy walk. For my parents did not like me to "play" with Helen Judd.

The Judds' dog Nellie, a mixed breed with a stumpy energetic tail and a sweet disposition, sand-colored, rheumy-eyed, hungry for affection as for the food scraps we sometimes fed her, trotted over frequently to play with my brother and me, for the Judds did not feed their dog but expected her to hunt and scavenge food like a wild animal. Robin and I were very fond of Nellie but my grandmother would shoo her away if she saw her. None of the Judds was welcome at my grandmother's house.

The *Judd house* it would be called for years. The *Judd property*. As if the very land (which the Judds had not owned in any case but had only rented) were somehow imprinted with the father's surname, a man's identity, infamy.

For tales were told in Millersport of the father who drank, beat and terrorized his family, "did things to the girls," at last set the house on fire either deliberately or in a drunken stupor and fled on foot and was arrested by Erie County sheriff's deputies and caused to disappear forever from the community. There was no romance in Mr. Judd though he "worked on the railroad"—at least, in the railroad yard in Lockport. My father knew him only slightly and despised him as a drinker, a wife- and child-beater. Mr. Judd seemed to work only sporadically though he always wore a railway man's cap and work clothes stiff with dirt or grease. His face was broad and sullen, vein-swollen and flushed with a look of alcoholic reproach. He chewed tobacco and craned his head forward to spit between his booted feet. He and his elder sons were hunters, owning among them a shotgun and one or two deer rifles. He was of moderate height, shorter than my father, heavyset, with straggly whiskers that sprouted from his jaws like wires. Often, he was to be seen walking at the roadside. His eyes swerved in their sockets seeking you out when you could not escape quickly enough. *H'lo there little girl! Little-Oates-girl, eh? Are you?*

The name *Oates* was hostile and jeering in his mouth.

Mrs. Judd was a woman at whom we never looked directly. There was something hurt and abject about Helen's mother, it would pain you to see. She had been a "pretty" woman once—(my mother said)—but seemed bloated now as with a perpetual pregnancy. She had had seven or eight babies—even Helen wasn't sure—of whom six had survived. Her bosom had sunk to her waist. Her legs were encased in flesh-colored support hose. *How can that poor woman live with him. That pig.* There was disdain, disgust in this frequent refrain. There was pity, indignation, disapproval. *Why doesn't she leave him. Did you see that black eye? Did you hear them, the other night? She should take the girls away, at least.* For Mrs. Judd was the only one of the family who worked regular shifts, as a cleaning woman in the Bewley Building in Lockport and later in a canning factory north of Lockport.

A shifting household of relatives and "boarders" lived in the Judd house. Of the six children remaining at home, four were sons and two daughters and all were under the age of twenty. Helen was a year older than I was, and Dorothy two years younger. There was an older brother of Mr. Judd's who walked with a cane, said to be an ex-convict from Attica. (What was Attica? A men's maximum security prison in upstate New York.) The oldest Judd son had been in the navy briefly, had been discharged and returned to Millersport where he worked from time to time in Lockport as a manual laborer; he owned a motorcycle, which he was always repairing in the driveway. There were frequent disputes at the Judds' house. Tales of Mr. Judd chasing his wife with a butcher knife, a claw hammer, the shotgun. Threatening to "blow the bitch's head off." Mrs. Judd and the younger children fled outside in terror, hid in the hayloft of a derelict old barn behind the house where Mr. Judd couldn't climb to find them.

Sheriff's deputies were summoned to the Judd house. No charges were pressed against Mr. Judd for Mrs. Judd refused to speak with any law enforcement officers, nor would any of the children speak with them. Until the fire that was so public that it could not be denied.

There was the summer day, I was eleven years old. When Mr. Judd shot Nellie.

At first we had no idea what was wrong, what creature was it wailing, moaning and whimpering intermittently for hours somewhere at the rear of our property. For sometimes in the orchard and woods behind our house there were wild creatures—raccoons, we thought—that sent up strange, caterwauling cries. There were shrieking cries of rabbits seized by owls. But finally we realized, the cries were Nellie's, and we remembered having heard several rifle shots earlier in the day.

When my father came home from work that evening he went to speak to Mr. Judd though my mother begged him not to. By this time poor Nellie had dragged herself under the Judds' cellarless house to die. Mr. Judd was furious at my father's intrusion, drunk, defensive—Nellie was his "goddam dog" he said, she'd been "pissing him off," whining and whimpering, she was "old." But my father convinced him to put the poor dog out of her misery.

Mr. Judd commanded one of his sons to drag Nellie out from beneath the house, which was set on concrete blocks. He then loaded his rifle, panting and wheezing as he straddled the bloodied dog and shot her a second, and a third time, at close range. My father who had never hunted, who'd never owned a gun and felt contempt for those who did, backed off, a hand over his face.

Afterward my father would say of that occasion that walking away from "that drunken son of a bitch with a rifle in his hands" was the hardest thing he'd ever done. Daddy expected the shot to hit between his shoulders.

THE FIRE WAS THE following year, just before Thanksgiving.

After the Judds were gone from Millersport and the part-collapsed house stood empty, I discovered Nellie's grave. I'm sure that it was Nellie's grave. Beyond the dog hutch in the weedy back-yard, a sunken patch of earth measuring about three feet by four with one of Mrs. Judd's whitewashed rocks at the head and on this rock, in what appeared to be red crayon, NELY.

It was Helen's writing, I was sure. Helen had always loved Nellie. In wild clusters vines grew on the posts of the sagging front porch. Mrs. Judd had had little time for gardening but she'd planted holly-hocks and sunflowers in the scrubby yard beside the house. Flowers that were beautiful and tough as weeds, that would survive for years.

We'd played Parcheesi, Chinese checkers, and gin rummy on that porch. Helen and me, and sometimes one or another of Helen's sisters. Helen was only a year older than I was but looked two or even three years older for she was a big-boned husky girl with a face that appeared to be sunburnt, her mother's face, with her mother's wide nose, thin-lipped mouth, chin. It had been said of Helen Judd and her sister Dorothy that they were "slow" but I did not think this was true of Helen who was a shrewd player of games, and who sometimes beat me fairly. (At other times, Helen cheated. I pretended not to see.) Helen was certainly not slow to fly into a rage when teased by boys at school or by her own older brothers. She waved her fists, rushed at the boys cursing and stammering—*Fuck! Cocksucker!*—words so shocking to me, yet thrilling, it was as if my friend was jabbing a knife at her tormentors.

For only boys and men could utter such words—such savage gleeful syllables.

At such times Helen's face darkened with blood and her thin lips quivered with a strange sort of pleasure like the quivering of a cat's jaws when it has sighted prey.

The house the Judds rented was like a number of other, small wood-frame houses in the neighborhood. It was not a farmhouse like my grandparents' house—it did not have an excavated cellar, nor did it have running water. (There was a small hand-pump at the kitchen sink.) At the rear of the property was an "outhouse" that smelled so fiercely, you would not want to come near.

The Judds' house had a small upstairs, just two bedrooms. No attic. No insulation. Steep, near-vertical stairs. The previous tenant had started to build a front porch of raw planks, never completed or painted. The roof of the house was made of sheets of tin scarred and scabbed like a diseased skin and the front of the house was covered in haphazard pieces of asphalt siding. Through all seasons windows were covered in translucent plastic and never opened. From a distance the house was the fading dun color of a deer's winter coat.

Unlike the Judds' house ours had both a cellar and an attic. We had a deep well with a solid stone foundation, its water was pure and cold even in summer. There was pride in the upkeep of our house: my father did all of the carpentry, even the roofing, the painting, the masonry; even the electrical wiring.

I would not know until I was much older that Fred Oates came from what is called a "broken home"—the image is a lurid one of a house literally broken, split in two, its secrets spilled out onto the ground like entrails.

Yet, I was superior to Helen Judd. For I had a father who loved me.

Think of the frail lifeline! It is all that separates us from heartbreak and chaos.

Unlike Mrs. Judd who had to drive to Lockport in a battered old car to work as a cleaning woman to support her family, my mother could remain at home. *At home* was a continuous responsibility.

Preparing meals, serving and cleaning up after meals. Cleaning house. Laundry. Hanging damp clothes on the clothesline in the backyard. Tilling the hard soil, planting rows of tomatoes, pepper plants, lettuce, strawberries, beds of flowers. Every day I helped my mother, especially in the kitchen.

Now, it is sometimes lonely. In a kitchen. In a garden.

Along the edge of our property were peony bushes which my mother had planted. Enormous crimson peonies my mother told me blossomed just in time for my birthday—June 16. For a long time I'd believed that this was so.

At Christmas, my father brought home a fresh-cut evergreen tree that smelled of the forest. Our nostrils pinched, this smell was so strong and so wonderful.

In a corner of our living room, upstairs in my step-grandparents' farmhouse where our family lived, we decorated the tree with ornaments kept wrapped in tissue in a large cardboard box. Each Christmas, the same glass ornaments that seemed to me beautiful, wonderful—but breakable. Strings of colored lights. "Bubble lights." And beneath the tree, wrapped presents. There are snapshots that bear record to these wonders.

My mother, and my father. Mommy, Daddy.

How hard my parents worked, and my Bush grandparents! A small farm, even a farm that is not very prosperous, is ceaseless work. Just to keep fences in repair, for a farmer, is ceaseless work. Just to maintain outbuildings, vehicles. To keep chickens from dying, from pecking one another to death. To maintain fruit orchards, devastated after a storm. There was happiness here of course and yet how fierce the need to declare *We are not the Judds*.

VIVIDLY I REMEMBER THE night of the fire. A festive occasion to which children were not invited.

Like all great events of long ago it was an adult occasion. Possessed, interpreted, judged by adults.

Out of the night came suddenly the sound of a siren on Transit Road. And then, turning onto the creek road near our house. A fire siren! How few times in my life I've been wakened in such alarm and excitement, in dread of a frenzied world beyond my control and comprehension. I was wakened by shouts, uplifted voices—the frightening sound of adults shouting to one another. At a window I stood staring in the direction of the Judds' house—an astonishing burst of flame. It was very late, past midnight. It was a summer night. The air was moist and reflected and magnified the fire like a nimbus. Hurriedly my father threw on clothes and ran to help the volunteer firemen of whom several were men from Swormville he knew. My mother told me to go back to bed, there was no danger to us. Yet my mother watched what she could see of the fire from an upstairs window of our house and did not send me away as I watched beside her.

The fire had begun at about midnight and I would not get back to bed until after 4:00 A.M., stunned and exhausted.

Do you think Helen could come live with us?—though I knew the answer, such a question must be asked.

ABRUPTLY, THE JUDDS HAD disappeared from Millersport and from our lives.

There was no question of neighbors *taking in* any of the Judds.

It was said, and would be reported in the Lockport newspaper, that Mr. Judd had fled the fire "as a fugitive" and was being sought by police. Soon after, Mr. Judd was arrested in Cheektowaga, a small city near Buffalo. He was charged with arson, several counts of attempted murder, aggressive assault, endangerment of minors. The

Judd family was broken up, scattered. The younger children were placed in county foster homes.

That quickly. The Judds were gone from us.

For a long time the smell of woodsmoke, scorch, a terrible stink of wet burnt wood, pervaded the air of Millersport. Neighbors complained that the *Judd house* should be razed, bulldozed over and the property sold. And good riddance! No one wished to say *There is a curse on that house*. And so the *Judd house* was one of the abandoned and condemned properties we were warned against. *No Trespassing— Danger.*

It was a lesson, I think I have never forgotten. How swiftly, in a single season, in fact within a few hours, a human habitation, a *home*, can turn wild.

The rutted dirt driveway over which the oldest Judd boy had ridden his motorcycle, only a few days before the fire. In time, overgrown with weeds.

What had happened to Roy Judd? (That was his name: I would murmur aloud, in secret—"Roy Judd.") It was said that he'd joined the navy—but no, he had already been in the navy and had been discharged "for health reasons." It was said that he'd gone to live with relatives in Olcott Beach but then he'd disappeared. He had given a sworn statement to the Erie County sheriff about the night of his father's "arson"—he was to have been a material witness—but he'd panicked, and disappeared.

We waited to hear of Mr. Judd. Such cases involve long waits.

Eventually, Mr. Judd was sentenced to prison. There was disappointment in this—the brevity of such a statement. For there had been no trial, no public accountability. *Pleaded guilty to charges, sentenced twenty years to life, Attica.*

NOW THEY WERE GONE, the Judds haunted Millersport.

No Trespassing—Danger.

Property Condemned by Erie County.

My brother and I were warned never to wander over onto the Judd property. There was known to be a well with a loose-fitting cover, among other dangers.

Even, in the back, a sinkhole—a smelly cesspool that had not been cleaned in decades.

Of course, neighbor children explored. Even my young brother explored. As if we would fall into a well! We smiled to think how little our parents knew us.

Have I said that my father never struck his children, as Mr. Judd struck his? And did worse things to them, to the girls—"When he was drunk. And afterward he'd claimed he didn't remember."

And Mrs. Judd who'd seemed so vague-minded, so apologetic and ineffectual—it was revealed that Mrs. Judd too had beaten the children, screaming and punching them when she'd been drinking— (for it was revealed that Mrs. Judd drank too)—and Helen bore the mark of her mother's rage, a fine white scar in her left eyebrow.

County social workers came around to question neighbors in Millersport. Few neighbors knew anything of the Judds apart from what other neighbors had told them yet much seemed to be revealed, and was assiduously recorded. *Once you tell them something, it will never be erased*—this was my father's warning.

My father did not speak much with the authorities. My father did not trust authorities. But others spoke, including my mother. And my grandparents who'd known Mr. Judd from when he'd been young— younger. *He got that way from something that happened to him, not all of it was his fault. That's why they drink.*

Like most children of that era I was disciplined sometimes—

"spanked." Like most children, I remember such episodes vaguely. As if they'd happened to another child, not me.

How would you know if you'd been a bad girl, if you were not spanked? Specific *badness* is lost in memory but *spanking* remains.

Once I happened to see Mr. Judd urinating at the roadside. Might've been drunk, or anyway he'd been drinking, returning on foot from a country tavern on Transit Road. Afterward I would confuse the blurred stream of his urine with the flying streams of kerosene he'd flung about his house before setting the fire with a single wooden match. The one I had seen, the other I had to imagine. *Joycie-Oates c'mere! That your name, eh?—Joycie?*

Had Mr. Judd really wanted to burn up his family in their beds? It was said that he'd sprinkled the kerosene haphazardly, sloppily— drunk and staggering on his feet.

Mrs. Judd insisted to police that they'd all been awake—they had all had time to run outside before the fire really started. Mrs. Judd insisted that they'd never been in any danger not even the youngest who was four years old.

Still, they were hospitalized. Trauma of the fire, smoke inhalation. For a while, Mrs. Judd was hospitalized in a psychiatric ward.

Yet for years afterward the *Judd house* remained standing. Something defiant about the ruin like an individual who has been killed but will not die.

The "see-through" blouse had not belonged to Helen but to an older relative. Some of Helen's clothes I'd recognized, in one of the back rooms. Socks, old shoes. Broken Christmas tree ornaments in a heap of broken things. Each time I dared to enter the house I discovered more things, for always there is more to be seen. One of the stained and water-soaked mattresses drew me to it with the fascination of horror. The most terrible punishment for a bad girl, I thought, would be to be forced to lie down on such a mattress.

It was in the ruin of their house that I thought of Helen, and of Dorothy. Mr. Judd had "done things" to them—what sort of things? Mrs. Judd with her swollen blackened eyes, bruised face. In Millersport hatred for Mrs. Judd was as fierce as hatred for Mr. Judd and possibly fiercer for there is the expectation that the mother will protect the children against the *goddamn no-good drunk son-of-a-bitch father.*

Shouts and sirens in the night. The shock of a fire in the night. And nothing ever the same again, after that night.

No charges were ever filed against Mrs. Judd, in any case. The county social worker who knew my mother told her how Mrs. Judd continued to insist that her husband had not meant for the fire to hurt anyone, he had not done anything wrong really, he should not be in prison. Screaming, cursing at the woman. The names she'd called the nurses! A woman would not want to repeat such names even to another woman, even in a whisper.

Mrs. Judd was the wife of Mr. Judd. They'd had babies together made from their bodies. What right has the law to interfere? The law has nothing to do with what passes between a man and a woman.

As a woman whose primary expression is through language, I have long wondered at the wellsprings of female masochism. Or what, in place of a more subtle and less reductive phrase, we can call the predilection for self-hurt, self-erasure, self-abnegation in women. The predilection is presumably learned—"acquired"—"culturally determined"—but surely they must spring from biological roots, neurophysiological states of being. Such predilections predate culture. Indeed, shape culture. It is tempting to say, in revulsion—*Yes but the Judds are isolated, pathetic individuals. These are marginal Americans, uneducated. They tell us nothing about ourselves.* Yet they tell us everything about ourselves and even the telling, the exposure, is a kind of radical cutting, an inscription in the flesh.

Yet: what could possibly be the evolutionary advantage of self-hurt in a woman? Abnegation in the face of another's brutality, cruelty? Acquiescence to another's (perverted, mad) will? This terrifying secret of which women do not care to speak, or in some (religious, fundamentalist) quarters even acknowledge.

Don't speak. Don't ask. They will rise against you, they will tear you to pieces. Run!

SEVERAL YEARS LATER IN junior high school, in Lockport— (where those of us from Millersport who'd gone to the one-room schoolhouse were now bused since the school no longer taught eight grades, as in my mother's time, but only five)—there Helen Judd appeared one day! It would turn out that Helen had gone to live with relatives in Newfane. And now, she'd moved, or had been moved, to Lockport. If I was fourteen now, Helen was fifteen. Like an adult woman she appeared, if you saw her at a little distance: big-hipped, big-breasted, with coarse hair inexpertly bleached.

Helen's homeroom was "special ed."—in a corner of the school beside the boys' vocational shop classroom—but she was assigned to some classes with the rest of us, presumably because she was considered one of the brighter of the special ed. students.

We had home economics in common but if Helen recognized me she was careful to give no sign. Rarely did she look at any of us—at our faces—girls from "normal" classes.

(Home economics! For girls like us, a class so ridiculous with its instructions in the proper making of a model bed, the proper ironing of men's "dress shirts," the preparation of simple meals involving a stove and an oven, the skills of vacuum-cleaning, even our teacher seemed embarrassed.)

"Helen?"—one day I dared to speak to her, my voice barely audible.

Barely audible too was Helen's reply as she turned quickly away with a cringing smile, a gesture of her hand that was both an acknowledgment and a rebuff, a tacit greeting and a plea to be invisible, let-alone, unnamed.

I would protect Helen, I thought. I would tell no one about her family. When we encountered each other at school, I gave no sign of knowing her. I saw that she was relieved, though she did not fully trust me. I thought—*She doesn't know what has happened to her, or she doesn't remember. She doesn't want me to remember.*

There seemed to be a tacit understanding that "something had happened" to Helen Judd. Her classmates and her teachers treated her guardedly. She was "special" as a handicapped person is special. She was withdrawn, quiet; if she was still susceptible to sudden outbursts of rage, she might have been on medication to control it. Her eyes, like her father's, seemed always about to swerve in their sockets. Her face was round, somewhat coarse, fleshy as a pudding, her wide nose oily-pored. In her expression, her mother's meekness, and the baffled fury of such meekness. She wore dark lipstick, she wore "glamorous" clothing—nylon sweaters with rhinestone glitter, gauzy see-through blouses, patent leather belts that cinched in her thick waist. In gym class her large soft breasts strained at her T-shirt and the shining rippled muscles and fatty flesh of her thighs were amazing to us who were so much thinner and less female, as of another species.

We did not think—*She is of childbearing age. And we are children.*

The actions of adolescents are inexplicable even to them, and even in retrospect. I remember baffling my friends by going out of my way to be cordial to Helen Judd whom they knew only as one of the special ed. students. The pretense was that I did not know Helen but was coming to know her, greeting her warmly—"Helen! Hi"—as if such behavior were altogether normal on my part, and not an elaborate imposture.

If Helen could be urged to smile, her face lost its slack, sallow look, and so it was a challenge to me, to induce Helen Judd to smile. She appeared to be lonely, and miserable at school, and flattered by my attention. For "normal" students rarely sought out special ed. students except to tease or torment them. At first she may have been suspicious of my motives but by degrees, over a period of weeks and months, she became trusting. I saw her sitting alone in the cafeteria, and sat with her, when I might have sat with other girls, and she understood this, and must have been surprised as others were surprised. I thought of Nellie: trust shows in the eyes. I asked her where she lived now and she told me she lived on Niagara Street, but that she might be moving soon. I asked her about the house on the Tonawanda Creek Road, hadn't she lived there with her family, and they'd moved out, and Helen blinked at me, and creased her forehead as an adult might do, and told me that she had not ever lived there but only stayed for a while, it had been her uncle's house in Millersport. I said, "There was a fire, wasn't there? How did it start?" and Helen said, slowly, each word like a pebble sucked in the mouth, "Lightning. Lightning hit it. One night in a storm."

I asked if she was living with her mother now and Helen shook her head vehemently, no. I asked her if she saw her mother and Helen shrugged and said she "wasn't sure" where her mother was. I considered asking about her father but did not for I knew that Helen would lie about him, and I did not want her to lie, and to see in my face that I knew she was lying, for I wanted to be her friend.

I asked about Dorothy. With a pained cringing smile Helen said that Dorothy was "somewhere else."

I told Helen that my mother had always liked her mother and missed her when they'd moved away. Helen continued to smile at me without seeming to hear me. She had a nervous habit of scratching at her arms, which she was doing now.

(It did not go unobserved that each special ed. student had some habit, some mannerism, some tic or compulsion that set him or her apart from "normal" individuals. Helen Judd was one of the least conspicuous of these.)

"We miss you. We wonder how you are. I wish—I wish you would visit me, Helen."

These words came spontaneously. I wanted to be Helen Judd's friend. And then a kind of slow horror came over me, for I seemed scarcely to know what I was saying.

Helen shrugged, and laughed. She gave me a sidelong glance, almost flirtatiously. Almost inaudibly she muttered what sounded like *OK*.

"You will? You'll come to visit? Sometime . . ."

But Helen was distracted now. Vigorously she was scratching at her forearm in a way nearly to draw blood. If I'd scratched myself in such a way in my mother's presence, Mommy would have leaned over to clasp and stop my hand. *Honey, no. Don't hurt yourself.*

Helen's nails were polished a shiny peach color, but were badly chipped and even bitten. And her hair, that had always been brown, was streaked now with blond like an animal's stripes.

"It seems strange and sad, nobody lives in your house now. Why did you all move away?"

Again Helen laughed. But there was no mirth or happiness in her face. Slowly she said, creasing her young forehead so that it resembled my grandmother's forehead, a shocking succession of deep wrinkles, as if she'd come to a conclusion to a puzzle that had long vexed her, "They all just—went away."

I wanted to ask where. But the look in Helen's face, the agitation with which she scratched at her forearms, dissuaded me.

Another time, after pausing to sit with Helen at a cafeteria table at which a scattering of special ed. students were sitting, who stared at me with faint, hopeful smiles, I left a plastic change purse with a few coins in it on the table; and when I returned, only a few minutes later, Helen was gone, and the change purse was gone. I asked the others at the table if they'd seen it and vehemently they shook their heads *no*.

Helen had stolen from me—had she? Or had this been a cruel test, and Helen had failed it?

Just one more time, I suggested that Helen Judd come to visit us, riding home with me on the school bus to Millersport to have supper with me and stay the night; and in the morning, we would both take the bus to school. It was a bizarre suggestion for my mother would have been horrified and would have forced me to cancel the date; our upstairs living quarters were so small, we had scarcely room for our family; and the presence of any Judd would have alarmed and upset my grandmother. Helen seemed to comprehend this. All that I could not say, Helen seemed to hear. She was looking at me with a faint, wistful smile as if wanting to say *yes*, for such an invitation would have been an extraordinary event in the life of any Judd, but finally saying, firmly—"No. Guess not."

"WHERE HAS GOD GONE"

1.

THE FIRST TIME I saw an adult man cry.

The shock of it! *A man does not cry. A man does not behave like this.*

The Methodist minister Reverend Bender was addressing the small congregation in his usually impassioned voice, at the pulpit of the Pendleton Methodist Church in Pendleton, New York, in the spring of 1950. His subject may have been the abiding nature of Jesus Christ's love, or the mysteries of God's harsher and more demanding love, or the temptations of the material world, or the grim choice we must make between Heaven and Hell—these were topics about which Reverend Bender often spoke, and to which I only half-listened, though turning to the man a rapt, attentive face; but suddenly, Reverend Bender had begun to cry, and was choking back sobs. His face was flushed and streaked with bright tears and appeared contorted like a crying infant's. His eyes that were usually so alert and kindly had lost their focus and seemed to have gone inward. Out of surprise and sympathy, and unease, many in the congregation began to weep with him; others, like me, were too shocked to react, and sat in stunned and baffled silence. A sensation of faintness came over me, almost terror. I had not seemed to know that a man could cry and the realization was a profound shock, as if our minister had shouted obscenities at us, or torn at his clothing.

Afterward I would learn that Reverend Bender was disappointed and agitated, that his efforts during the past week in the community to bring more people to our church had been "a failure." For what seemed like long minutes, though probably it was less than a single minute, Reverend Bender had been unable to continue, wiping his face with a handkerchief, while the congregation stared at him. Reverend Bender's wife and young children, seated in the first row in front of the pulpit, must have been mortified and frightened.

(I was not seated among the congregation but at a small footpump organ near the front of the church; on the bench, I had to twist about to see Reverend Bender at the pulpit. It is one of the curious facts of my life that, at twelve, and very new to the Pendleton Methodist Church, I had been asked by Reverend Bender to be their "organist" though I had only been taking piano lessons for a few years and had no training at all on the organ.)

Each Sunday I came to church in Pendleton with a friend from school named Jean Grady, who lived in Pendleton and whose mother my mother had known when they were girls. Jean was slightly older than I was, in eighth grade when I was in seventh grade; we sat together on the rowdy school bus that brought thirty students from the "north country" into Lockport, and had become friends of a kind. (Oddly, both Jean and I were outstanding badminton players at the junior high: when we played together, Jean beat me perhaps three times out of five, but each of us could beat any other girl opponent in the school.)

Unlike Helen Judd, Jean Grady was not from a disgraced family, or even from a "poor" family; she appeared to be from a family not unlike mine, except perhaps more prosperous than mine since Mr. Grady owned a small grocery store in Pendleton with a riveting sign above the door that contained the red-scripted word *Sealtest*. To all who knew her, stout plain-stern-faced Jean Grady was enviable; we could scarcely imagine the privilege of entering the grim little Pendleton store to select a Mars bar, a Coke from the refrigerator, an orange Sealtest Creamsicle from a freezer unit, without paying.

Most wonderfully, it sometimes happened that Jean Grady could select treats for a friend, too.

So it had happened, one afternoon on the school bus Jean Grady invited me to come with her to church the following Sunday, at the small white clapboard Methodist church our school bus routinely passed, and somehow, I seem to have said *yes*.

In fact I was eager to say *yes*. Any invitation put to me at that time in my life was welcome, and flattering; I was always eager to be included in virtually anything, if I didn't think that my parents would disapprove; if indeed, I would tell my parents. Like Alice, I was tirelessly *curious*.

(Yet, as a corollary to this eagerness, which is a kind of impulsiveness, or heedlessness, it should also be noted that after my acceptance I was usually repentant, and filled with doubt; I was ambivalent about nearly everything that had initially excited me. My childish eagerness to *say yes* was in refutation of my fear that *saying no* would be a terrible mistake.)

Jean Grady told me that she'd been going to Sunday and Wednesday evening services at the Methodist church for almost a year. In a thrilled voice she boasted that she'd been asked to help the minister's wife Mrs. Bender teach Sunday school. No one else in the Grady family went to church—"Mrs. Bender says I will be an example for them." She had an "extra Bible" for me, which I was grateful to be given for any book was of value to me, and there was no Bible in our household. Jean told me that she thought I would like the church very much and that it would "make a big change" in my life.

A *big change in my life* was a very exciting prospect. I could not imagine what this *big change* might be.

It had long seemed strange to me, though not particularly upsetting or significant, that no one in my family seemed to be "religious"—at all. Not my parents, and not my grandparents. (Though I knew that my Hungarian grandparents had once been Roman Catholic, in Budapest, Hungary; crossing the Atlantic to the new world they seemed to have sloughed off their old religion.) Later I would learn that my mother had been baptized Catholic in a church in Black Rock, and that my father's father Joseph Carleton Oates had also been baptized Catholic. The word for such Catholics was *lapsed*—an intriguing word I would not know for some years.

It was curious to me, I'd become a "Protestant" by joining the Methodist church—whatever that meant.

Soon after I'd joined the church with Jean Grady as my sponsor, I realized, from Reverend Bender's remarks in the pulpit, that Jean had invited me to join as part of a general campaign by the church to acquire new members; there were extra Bibles for this purpose, to be given away. I felt somewhat chagrined but told myself it was still flattering, that of the numerous other girls she knew Jean had invited *me*.

The congregation was small, probably less than one hundred people. Less than eighty people? When I shut my eyes I can't seem to see much of anything of the interior of the plain, white-walled church except the pulpit, the five-foot wooden cross at the front of the room, the pump-organ against the wall, the narrow windows and pinewood floor; I have no idea how many pews there were, or how many people could fit comfortably into a pew. But I remember the urgency of Reverend Bender's remarks—the need to bring more visitors to the church, to introduce more people to the church, to fill the pews and to "bring souls to Jesus." I remember Reverend Bender's claim that God wanted him to know—" 'You have not worked hard enough last week.' "

These words, uttered passionately at the pulpit, in front of the hushed and discomforted congregation, made a strong impression on me. I did not think—*But what delusion, to think that God cares about him!* What impressed me most were the condemning words—*You have not worked hard enough.*

As Reverend Bender continued to speak, wiping at his eyes with his handkerchief, coughing, clearing his throat, it became clear that there was a pressing need also in the church for money—"Funds for the upkeep of our beloved church."

Just before I'd joined the congregation, a team of volunteers (male) had repainted the church, which had become badly weatherworn. On a bulletin board in the church foyer were snapshots of this team effort, with a broadly smiling Reverend Bender himself in work clothes wielding a paintbrush dipped in white paint. And now, it seemed that the shingle-board roof needed repair.

You do not normally think of a church as an organization desperately requiring money—you do not think of a church as a property, a building, that has to be paid for, and has to be maintained, as a house or a barn is maintained; at least, I did not think of "church" in such a material way. (Naively I must have thought that churches simply *existed*. You should not have to pay to worship God—should you?) And so it was a surprise to me, a true revelation, to hear Reverend Bender speak frankly of the need of "our church" for money, like the need for new members; it was painful to hear how Reverend Bender came close to pleading, begging. Each Sunday service when the wicker collection basket was passed from hand to hand along the pews I was deeply embarrassed to leave such small change—a quarter, a few dimes, nickels—amid bills.

Weekly I was given some money by my mother as an "allowance"—payment for the numerous chores I did. I don't even want to think how modest this allowance must have been—possibly, a single dollar.

Yet, giving most of my money, or all of my money, to the collection basket seemed necessary. I could not reasonably expect Jesus to come into my heart if I held back. Jean Grady did not give much more than I did, or so it seemed to my (sharp, envious) eye.

What has this to do with God—I asked myself.

Also, when I was alone and not with others, such questions haunted me—*Where is God? Does God see us?*

An eye distant and large as the sun. An eye that would never close. An eye without an eyelid.

He sees you wherever you go. Nowhere to hide.

Yet, I did not really believe this. If there was a God—if there was Reverend Bender's "God"—why would He care about me? It was common to discover, in fields, in the woods, the shrunken and desiccated bodies of animals, from which life had departed; our flock of Rhode Island Reds was always being stricken with illness, mutilation, sudden death. It was not likely, I had to think, that any eye, any invisible presence, took note of such small deaths. You learned from trespassing into abandoned places and the silence of such places that no one took note of anything—fundamentally. Wasn't this the implicit lesson of war, those terrible photographs in *Life* at which I could not look, yet found myself looking, staring—memorizing . . .

There was the problem too of where God *was*. The Methodists believed in Heaven—(and in Hell)—as actual, literal places; even at twelve, I could not think that this was likely.

Yet, at the same time, with no sense of how contradictory such thinking was, I would have identified myself as *religious*; more importantly, *spiritual*. I was a new member of the congregation, who had not yet been "baptized." (That would come later, though soon.) It was natural to suppose that I would become more like the others, in time. It had not escaped me as a twelve-year-old who avidly read adult books (which I could now withdraw from the Lockport Public Library) that there was an intense consciousness of "religion" and "spirituality" that imbued the world beyond Millersport; in any library, there were shelves of books on the very subject of God, Jesus Christ, "Christianity." If I could not quite comprehend this consciousness, let alone believe in it, yet I could certainly appear to believe in it, I could emulate the behavior of those who believed. I did not want to be a shallow person, but a person of *depth*.

Waiting for God to take notice of me. Waiting for Jesus to *come into my heart*.

In his sermons Reverend Bender posed questions which he then answered. As if he were speaking for those of us who could not speak for ourselves.

How are our prayers answered?

In ways we can't always know.

It was not possible, following this logic, to know that prayer *did not work*; even when prayer seemed futile, as many of Reverend Bender's passionate prayers evidently did, the prayers might well be answered in some oblique, elliptical way—in the future.

My feeling for "religion" was not unlike my father's feeling for flying. Though I certainly would not have considered this at the time, it seems likely now, in retrospect. To fly, to be borne aloft, to *transcend*—this is the motive, and the goal. As Lear tersely remarks, "Reason not the need."

But my religious yearnings were wayward and indefinable. Like those creatures who take on the protective camouflage of their surroundings in order not to be devoured by predators, instinctively I adapted to whatever was around me, and to whatever was told me;

though I might not believe what I was told, I would give the impression that I did. My fear was that I had not a deep enough soul for Jesus to acknowledge. My efforts at prayer seemed to me self-evidently insincere, like one who is pretending to be swimming but is only flailing her arms about, in shallow water; praying was too much like begging, and could arouse only contempt. At school I was an ardent student, and rarely received any grade lower than A; quizzes and tests, anathema to other students, were thrilling to me, like playing badminton, indeed any activity in gym class where I was excited by competing with the other girls; in church, I was an ardent worshipper, or gave that impression, for badly I *wanted to believe—something*. I wanted to be perceived by the others as one of them, *blessed*. I did not want to be perceived as an outsider. I did not want to be perceived as *damned*.

To the Methodists in the little church "Jesus Christ" was not a distant historic or mythic figure but a living presence. It seemed to be believed by them—(by us, for I was now one of them)—that Jesus was close beside us at all times. Jesus was our companion, and our closest friend. Jesus was our brother who knew much more about us than we knew or would acknowledge about ourselves, and Jesus had forgiven us for what he knew of us, for Jesus loved us. Though Jesus was the Son of God, yet the Son of God could be "hurt" by us, His heart broken if and when we failed to live up to His ideals. The essence of Jesus was love and we had only to love Him without question, as He bade us: "Except as ye become as little children, ye shall not enter into the kingdom of heaven." God, who was Jesus's father, was a living presence too, though invisible as the wind, and never illustrated in Bible pictures (except as a fiercely burning bush, appearing to Moses in the Book of Exodus) as Jesus was many times illustrated; God the Father was unpredictable and wrathful, devoted to punishing the enemies of the Israelites, and less inclined to forgive than Jesus, perhaps because God knew us more thoroughly than

Jesus did. Never having been human, still less crucified, God had little patience with human weakness and hypocrisy. Reverend Bender spoke with grim satisfaction of God, though with warmth and affection of Jesus; God was a "jealous" God while Jesus was "forgiving"; Jesus was needed to intercede between God and man, bringing salvation to mankind after our first parents Adam and Eve committed "sin." Of course, just accepting this wasn't enough—prayer, good works, a constant welcoming of Jesus Christ in our hearts and a resistance to sin were also required.

Resistance to sin was "Saying *no!* to Satan."

It was amazing to me that Reverend Bender spoke of Satan with as much conviction as he spoke of God and Jesus Christ. Years of comic strips and comic books had habituated me to Satan—"the Devil"—as a cartoon demon clad in red tights with a scaly tail and a pitchfork.

Amazing too, to realize that for the seriously religious individual like Reverend Bender "religion" wasn't just a matter of Sunday morning but a matter of every day, every hour—every minute. *God is with us at all times awake and asleep.*

How exhausting this was! I could feel something of the pressure of such faith, a vise tightening about a skull. For even if you ran away to be alone, you would never escape the eye of God. You would never escape being judged wanting.

It was clear to Reverend Bender that if church attendance was low at Sunday service, this was a sign of God's displeasure with him for not having worked hard enough to bring more people to Jesus. If there wasn't much money in the collection basket, this was God's displeasure also. Was there any shame, any hurt, any catastrophe, that wasn't a sign of God's displeasure? You had not only the catastrophe to contend with but also the graver knowledge that the catastrophe was a sign of God's displeasure with *you.*

So Reverend Bender broke down in tears at the pulpit, and caused others to weep as well, as if emotion should be allowed to run wild as a burning bush, no matter that we were all flammable.

(How different, my irreverent father! Fred Oates would have stared at Reverend Bender in contempt for behaving in a way no man should behave in public or in private.)

Yet, I was eager to tell people that I belonged to the Methodist church in Pendleton, and that I went to services with Jean Grady. I was eager to tell people that I played the organ at church—in fact, I was the "organist" there. Of course I had never played anything like a pump organ, which is a crude, wheezing instrument compared to the far more rarefied and beautiful pipe organ; when I first began practicing, I had very little idea how to "pump" the organ with my feet to give volume to the notes I was playing on the keyboard, though I more or less figured out the mechanism as I struggled along. Each week I took home the heavy hymnal to practice assiduously—"Onward, Christian Soldiers"—"A Mighty Fortress Is Our God"—"Rock of Ages"—"The Old Rugged Cross"—along with my (secular) piano études by Czerny and Hanon. These were strangely beautiful hymns, pleas of unabashed yearning and abnegation, suffused with a militant righteousness that could cause the hairs on the nape of your neck to stir—

Onward, Christian soldiers, marching as to war,
With the cross of Jesus going on before.
Christ, the royal Master, leads against the foe;
Forward into battle see his banners go!

Onward, Christian soldiers, marching as to war,
With the cross of Jesus going on before.

There was a wild sort of happiness in playing such a hymn, and hearing the raw, untrained yet jubilant voices of the congregation behind me. Almost, you might think—*I believe! I believe all that you believe. I am one of you.*

THE FIRST TIME I'D seen a man cry, I would not easily forget. And now I remember that, at the Methodist prayer meetings, other individuals sometimes cried, though not usually men.

Vividly I recall a woman—a middle-aged woman with short, bluntly cut red-brown hair—removing her glasses in a paroxysm of weeping. (Because Jesus had entered her heart?) Amid the spirited singing of hymns, and Reverend Bender's impassioned words, there was the expectation that at any moment the miracle might occur: Jesus Christ might enter one's heart.

I'd become anxious that this miracle might happen, and that it would never happen. I'd become resigned, that it would never happen; yet childishly hopeful, that it would. At the same time, I had no idea what it could possibly mean—*Jesus will enter your heart.*

Jean Grady and I were too shy to speak of such things to each other. It would have required an excruciating effort for me to have asked my friend what it actually meant that "Jesus had come into her heart"—or indeed, whether "Jesus had come into her heart" at all.

At home, I could not bring up the subject of God. I could not imagine speaking of God, Jesus Christ, "Satan" in the familiar way in which Reverend Bender spoke of these beings, taking for granted that you knew exactly what he meant, and that what he meant actually existed.

I could not know at the time, but would realize later, how, for most people, certainly for people like my parents who have not had the benefit of much formal education, it is not an easy matter to speak of abstractions. Acquiring an education means, in part, acquiring a vocabulary in which to speak of such matters in a manner that suggests familiarity—(as an academic philosopher may speak casually and with a presumption of authority of "justice"—"infinity"—"the One"—"being"—"nothingness"—as if these were actual entities that existed, and not rather merely bits of language he has picked up in the course of his education)—if not mastery. In the long-ago world of Millersport, which is to say rural, minimally educated and minimally prosperous America, it would have been astonishing for anyone to speak in such a way; pretentious, if not laughable; you would be met with derision, or a blank uncomprehending stare.

It should not have been so difficult to ask my parents if they believed in God, or in Jesus Christ, but I never did. My mother would probably have frowned thoughtfully and said *Yes, I guess so*; my father would probably have laughed and said *Hell, no*. Neither would have elaborated and the subject would have been quickly changed.

(My father disliked and distrusted all figures of authority whether politicians, religious leaders, UAW officers. Though I think he admired Franklin Delano Roosevelt, his general attitude toward politics ranged from bemused disgust to vehement disgust and grew more pronounced with the passage of time.)

My grandmother Blanche Morgenstern, the avid reader among the adults in the family, who read and reread all the biographies, histories, and novels on the shelves of the Lockport Public Library about Abraham Lincoln, held the opinion that all religions are more or less alike—"They tell you how to live, and how to be good. But not everyone needs to be told."

It was my grandmother's conviction that Abraham Lincoln was not only a great man but that Abraham Lincoln was also a very wise man who believed in a non-denominational God. If Lincoln appeared to be a Christian, this was just an appearance; in fact, Lincoln believed in something like a God-principle, not in a "savior." But my grand-mother had no interest in discussing religion otherwise, and so far as we knew she never went to church. (Certainly not a synagogue: there were no synagogues in Lockport, or anywhere near Lockport.)

Trying to feel the presence of God, that "surrounded" me. Trying to feel Jesus Christ "in my heart."

Practicing hymns on our piano at home. Playing the wheezing pump-organ at church.

If I am a good girl, it will happen to me. Whatever it is, that others feel—God will love me. Jesus will come into my heart.

AND YET, FOR ALL my effort and my hope, my life as a Methodist came to an abrupt end within a year.

Bizarrely, as I'd been conscripted by Reverend Bender to play the organ at church, so I was conscripted by Reverend Bender to memorize approximately one hundred verses of the Gospel according to Saint John in a regional competition among young Methodists, to determine who could recite the most Bible verses without error.

I was not the only young adult in the Pendleton Methodist Church to enter the competition, but I was the only one who performed well enough to be passed on to the next level of competition, and to the next. In the finals, held in a church hall in Batavia, I was named one of three winners, all girls, to be awarded a free week at the Methodist Bible camp at Olcott Beach that summer.

A week at camp! No one in my family had ever seen a summer camp, let alone gone to one. A (cardboard, but sturdy) suitcase was purchased for me from Sears, which I began to pack at once, weeks beforehand. I had never been away from home except for a night or two at the Lockport City Hospital to have my tonsils and adenoids removed, like many children of my generation.

Of the miserable week at Bible camp I have only vague memories of acute homesickness and of crying myself to sleep in a musty-smelling bunk bed; more vividly I remember another girl in the cabin to which I was assigned, Nedra Fischer, a girl from Depew, as like myself as if she were a twin, wan and tearful, so stricken with homesickness she could not eat the awful food and finally had to be taken home by her parents, to the envy of the rest of us. Pitched in a desolate scrub-acre miles from Lake Ontario, a squalid nest of weatherworn cabins lacking electricity and indoor plumbing, Bible camp had twice-daily prayer meetings, Bible study hours each afternoon, singing of hymns each evening—activities of stupefying dullness which I remember as if they had happened to another person. I was filled with regret for having failed to bring library books with me, in which I might have taken solace when I had some free time; in my naïve excitement about Bible camp I had not even thought of bringing books other than the Bible my friend Jean had given me.

Strange that so much about that week at Olcott Beach has faded but the verses of Saint John remain, if but in fragments. As there is a kind of memory in a pianist's fingers after decades, so too anything that has been memorized in childhood is retained somewhere in the brain, awaiting rediscovery and retrieval. The Gospel according to Saint John remains stirring and incantatory—it is what I could not have identified, at the time, as "beautiful prose" with the power of beautiful music. Especially the opening lines, before the narrative of Jesus Christ begins, seem to have entered my imagination on a deep, primal level exclusive of mere meaning and comprehension—

In the beginning was the Word, and the Word was with God, and
the Word was God.

The same was in the beginning with God.

All things were made by him; and without him was not any thing made that was made.

In him was life; and the life was the light of men.

And the light shineth in darkness; and the darkness comprehended it not.

There was a man sent from God, whose name was John.

The same came for a witness to bear witness of the Light, that all men through him might believe.

He was not that Light, but was sent to bear witness of that Light.

That was the true Light, which lighteth every man that cometh into the world.

He was in the world, and the world was made by him, and the world knew him not . . .

IN THE BEGINNING WAS *the Word. And the Word was with God.* To be a writer is to understand that the Word is primary, even before meaning; and, whatever is meant by "God," it is the Word that coexists with God.

"YOU THINK YOU'RE SO *smart.*"

My friend Jean Grady, encouraged by Reverend Bender, had hoped to memorize one hundred verses of the Gospel according to Saint John too, but had failed in her effort, and would never entirely forgive me. We'd studied together for a period of weeks and it was clear from the outset that Jean could not memorize the poetic lines of the Gospel, that became confused in her mouth like snarled string. Abruptly, we were not such good friends though we continued to sit together on the school bus making its lumbering way along country roads in the direction of Lockport, and of course I sat beside Jean at church. (It was touching to us, at least to me, that some in the congregation mistook us as sisters.)

And now what a shock, that Jean Grady seemed to hate me. *You think you're so smart.*

Or did Jean say, mouth twisted in resentment—*Think you're so goddamned smart.*

How do you respond to such an accusation? How can you respond, seeing such dislike in a friend's eyes?

It seemed unfair of Jean to blame me for having succeeded in memorizing the Bible verses, and being chosen as a "winner," for this had brought luster to Pendleton Methodist Church, and had certainly pleased Reverend Bender and his beaming wife.

Nor was it true that I thought that I was *so smart*—others had chosen to depict me in this way, and these others were adults possessed of power. (At North Park Junior High in Lockport, to which we were "bused," I'd been recognized by my teachers as a student who obviously cared much for reading, and for school; out of the miseries of the one-room schoolhouse on the Tonawanda Creek Road I'd arrived in what was a dazzling *city school* with not one overworked and harassed teacher for five grades but a number of teachers for each grade, and each teacher specialized in a "subject"—arrived, in the eyes of these teachers, not unlike a missile shot from a cannon. A word for me, in those years, might have been *zealous*. In every course in the public school there was offered "extra credit" for "extra homework" and not once in my life as a schoolgirl did I ever pass up the possibility of "extra homework"—no more than a starving animal would fail to overeat. It did not escape my school-bus companions like Jean Grady that I'd been singled out for attention, but Jean had not seemed to hold it against me until now. Jean was always the better, because the stronger, badminton player; from now on she would be merciless when we played together, and unrepentant at winning every match.)

After Bible camp, my interest in the Methodist church quickly waned. I had come too close to Methodists, living with girls of my age who were very unlike myself, and did not seem at all "spiritual"—hardly. Jesus's admonition to love one's neighbor as oneself had not seemed to impress itself upon these girls and would prove too great a challenge for me, who was not sure that I could love myself.

2.

OF BLEEDING LUNGS MY grandfather John Bush died six months later. Of emphysema related to his longtime work at the steel foundry in Lackawanna, that did not pay its employees well but paid better than work elsewhere including blacksmithing and farming.

To placate my devastated grandmother, in return for the privilege of being allowed to bury John Bush in the Good Shepherd Catholic Cemetery in Pendleton, my parents promised the Good Shepherd priest that they and their children (Joyce, Fred Jr.) would become members of the parish.

My father would recall decades later being humbled by the priest, or humiliated—"I had to make out a check right then and there to give the s.o.b."

S.o.b., bastard— such language, that grates the ear in middle-class and academic settings, was commonplace in my father's world where it registers as mild profanity and does not signal extreme hostility.

Soon, my brother and I were taking catechism lessons from the priest who was called, oddly to our ears, Father O'Malley.

How strange, this purse-lipped stranger was *Father!*—a word we never uttered, for our father was *Daddy* and could not be addressed by any other name, by us.

Strange too, we were attending not "church services" but "mass" Sunday mornings at 10:00 A.M. in the somber dark-red-brick church in Pendleton.

It was "low mass" we attended whenever possible. For "high mass" was a longer and more elaborate service. In those days, a recitation by the Catholic priest in Latin, translated in our prayer books into English plain and devoid of romance as a lashless eye.

What a curious episode this was in the life of my family! I have not ever attempted to explain it to anyone, for there was much that was shameful about it, as well as baffling. My father who disliked any sort of organized religion and who was by temperament skeptical and doubting, forced to bring his young family, and his Hungarian-born stepmother-in-law, to Catholic mass at the country church . . .

How could Fred Oates bear it! But soon, Daddy joined the church choir, with a hope of improving it; soon, Daddy was asked (by Father O'Malley) to be choir leader. Within a year or two Daddy became the church organist, and no longer sat with his family in our pew as he no longer had to wince at mangled notes on the organ.

Though I loved my parents, and would not have rebelled against their wishes, I could not help but resent them for bringing me to this new and unwanted church—this "religion." To force me to take catechism lessons like a grade school child. (*Q. Who made the world? A. God made the world. Q. What is the purpose of the life of man? A. The purpose of the life of man is to know and love God in this world and to dwell with Him in the next.* How I yearned to rebel against these prescribed words, with very different words of my own!) Especially I resented being trapped in a crowded pew between my mother and my heavyset Hungarian-born grandmother who knew little English and certainly no Latin, and who seemed often at mass to have but a very vague idea of what was going on; or, as my father would say bemusedly—*What the hell is going on.*

Perversely, though I had ceased to "believe" in the Methodist church teachings, I missed the crude foot-pump organ and my participation in the service. I missed the Protestant hymns that surprised you with their sudden swell of emotion. I missed the much-smaller congregation and my feeling of independence—I'd been a girl of twelve attending church services without her family. I missed the more emotionally engaged worshippers at the Methodist church who could not know, as worshippers at Good Shepherd knew, exactly what their spiritual leader would say as he led each service through its clockwork routine.

At Good Shepherd, worshippers at the Latin mass were like zombies: glaze-eyed, uninvolved, stunned with boredom. No doubt, as my mother once hinted, Sunday morning's mass was a time for wives and mothers to *rest*. Like sleeping with one's eyes open, somehow managing to remain upright in the hard wooden pews. (And the kneelers were hard wood, too.)

Daddy hadn't such boredom to contend with. Typically, Fred Oates had managed to ascend to a level of participation that allowed him to think and make decisions, and not merely to drift and daydream through the hour-long mass with the small herd of worshippers. Playing the organ in the choir loft above the congregation was a great pleasure to him; immersed in music, he didn't have to listen to Father O'Malley's curiously falsetto singsong voice at all.

The most inhumanly soporific of religious activities is the "saying" of the rosary, and this too we were compelled to do, or to go through the motions of doing. Shuffling to the communion railing, we "took" communion—"This is the Body and Blood of Christ; take ye and eat"—or such was the translation from Latin. No one seemed remotely aware or even interested in what it might mean—what it would mean—if the "body" and the "blood" of Jesus Christ were literally contained within a crisp white communion wafer designed to melt on the tongue.

Transubstantiation: quite a miracle!

In all the Catholic years no passion, no zeal, no authenticity.

No tears like those of Reverend Bender.

"BLESS ME, FATHER, FOR I have sinned."

Or was it rather, "Bless me, Father, for I have sinned."

Or, an artful variant, "Bless me, Father—for I have *sinned*."

From the age of thirteen to eighteen I would attend what seemed like many thousands of masses out of respect for my parents and their promise to Father O'Malley, that had been made out of respect for my grandmother's grief. Though it seems bizarre to me now, and would cause anyone who knows me well to laugh aloud, I also went to confession during those years, dutifully, doggedly; like any seemingly observant Catholic I slipped into the shadowy confessional that resembles a small kiosk, knelt on the rock-hard kneeler, and shut the little door; through a sort of chicken-wire grating I would see a vague outline of my confessor's face, and would imagine his shut eyes; for a long afternoon of droning confessions in the Good Shepherd Catholic Church of Pendleton, New York* could not have failed to stupefy any sentient individual, even Father O'Malley. In the confessional one was not supposed to "recognize" the priest, nor was the priest supposed to "recognize" the penitent. In an abashed voice I would murmur *Bless me Father, for I have sinned. It has been _____ since my last confession.*

No doubt, it had rarely been more than *one week* since my last

---

* The most famous, or infamous, parishioner of the Good Shepherd Church was to be Timothy McVeigh, whose boyhood attendance at mass with his father, William McVeigh, overlapped with my parents' attendance in the 1970s.

confession, in those years when I was a captive at home, under the (benign) surveillance of my parents. Though there were rumors of penitents who returned to the confessional after years, even decades, of having been "lapsed."

Mortal sins, venial sins. Very few penitents in the Pendleton parish, I would guess, were capable of *mortal sins* (except those involving church law like eating meat on Friday, inexplicably as serious a sin as homicide); rather, it must have been a flood of *venial sins* cascading about the priest's head, trivial scrapings from ordinary life—*I was inattentive during mass, I did not attend mass. I did not obey my parents, I had "impure" thoughts, I told lies.*

Extreme embarrassment attended the admission—*I had "impure" thoughts.* Fortunately, Father O'Malley had no evident interest in these "impure" thoughts—(at least not mine)—and did not interrogate me further.

As for *lies*—the number of *lies* uttered by most people, certainly by me, partial-lies, trivial lies, inconsequential lies, rarely significant lies, had to be enormous. Some of us, particularly if we are born female, must cultivate an artful sort of dishonesty virtually from birth: we smile, we smile happily, we smile very happily, to assure others that we are fine, indeed we are happy; we smile to assure others that we have no criticism of them, no quarrel, in fact no contrary thoughts of our own. But perhaps such smiles are not precisely *lies* since they don't involve words.

It may have been that, in other parishes, under the watchful eyes of other priests, the penitent was expected to report sins in detail; but Father O'Malley, who may have been hard of hearing in one or both ears, did not often make inquiries. Whatever Father O'Malley's limitations he was not a voyeur, or a sadist—(at least not with me. But perhaps he had no interest in me). In the prayer book for young people there was a helpful appendix listing categories of sins, which appendix I would skim before each confession, that I might dredge up a reasonable amount of sins to offer to the priest. (One sin I never had to confess was *profanity*. This was, to me, the easiest sin of all to avoid. One sin I admitted repeatedly—*I was inattentive during mass*.)

After a suitable interim, when no more sins were forthcoming from the penitent, Father O'Malley would seem to rouse himself and grant absolution with a murmured *Say one Our Father, five Hail Marys* or an equivalent penance and the ordeal would be concluded until the next time.

Father O'Malley was a bald fattish middle-aged man who seemed often to lose his way in his rambling sermons, that were geared, in vocabulary and syntax, to parishioners of the mental age of elementary schoolchildren. I did not yet know the word for his glowingly flushed cheeks and nose netted with capillaries—*rubefacient*. His hard round beer-belly strained against the black fabric of his priest's clothing; with each week of Lent this belly would shrink until by Easter Sunday it was perceptibly reduced. But following Easter, and the end of Lenten fasting, the belly would make its inexorable return. (I am not sure that I would have noticed this eccentric detail except that others commented on it, with some mirth.) In Father O'Malley, who was probably a totally representative parish priest of his era, Christianity had been reduced to the particular strictures, rituals, pieties and dogma of the Holy Roman Catholic Church which was irrefutably *the only true church*; the political leanings of this parish priest, reflecting the general anti-Communist/anti-liberal bias of the era, were evident in sermons castigating a "modern" way of living, synonymous with "sin." (This was the era of the Catholic League of Decency which sternly rated "objectionable" movies with *X*'s connotating *condemned*. These films, like Otto Preminger's *The Moon Is Blue* [1953], Catholics were forbidden to see under penalty of mortal sin.)

Decades later when it was revealed how pervasive sexual molestation and pedophilia have been in the Catholic Church, how many parish priests not unlike Father O'Malley were involved in sexual coercion and its cover-up, I was astonished—how could this be possible? The priests we'd known at Good Shepherd seemed rather more like automatons or sleepwalkers than men of passion, or even emotion; it was difficult to imagine them behaving licentiously except with alcohol and food. How likely was it, such utterly bored and boring persons could commit such cruel sins?

So it is, former Catholics often exclaim to one another *But we had no idea—did you?* Not one Catholic of my acquaintance, practicing or non- , has ever remarked that he or she had any direct, or even indirect, knowledge of pedophilia in the Church. Yet, if the media is to be believed, such terrible things were raging about us, in parishes other than our own.

The experience of a Roman Catholic who is born into the religion, and who attends parochial school taught by priests or nuns, is typically very different from the experience I am describing here. I was spared the extremes of the catechism-religion of which so many writers have written so compellingly—the paragon being James Joyce; I came to the religion late, too skeptical already at twelve to take its elaborate cosmology seriously, and filled with resentment and incredulity at having to pretend otherwise. I found it very difficult to believe in "sin"—I found it very difficult to believe that there was a God who cared in the slightest if I'd eaten meat on Friday, or inadvertently licked a raindrop from my lips, before taking communion—I found it very difficult to believe that there was a God involved in the world of humankind at all. (What was the evidence? Earthquakes, hurricanes? Polio? My grandfather's terrible racking cough, that seemed to be tearing out his lungs?) The figure of Jesus the Savior, so immediate in Methodism, seemed to have retreated in Catholicism and was represented by grisly statues in the church with bloody heads and exposed, bloody hearts. This Jesus was not a *friend*.

If I had not cared so much for my parents, and had not wanted to upset them, I would have walked out of mass during one of Father O'Malley's droning sermons, and never returned. But I knew what my father would say—*We gave our word*.

How much is religion the honoring of one's parents?—the wish not to upset, not to offend, not to disappoint?

The *good girl* is one whose smile is assuring, though it is not to be trusted.

I could not disappoint my parents, who meant so well by their new, adopted religion. I could not upset them, still less humiliate them in the eyes of others. Our religion seemed to me a sort of family charade in which each individual tacitly agreed not to question the integrity of the others while divulging no crack in his or her own. Dutifully I went to mass with them, Sunday following Sunday, for years; even when I was a student at Syracuse University I continued to attend mass, perhaps not every Sunday but frequently, so that, even at a distance, I wasn't violating the promise my parents had made in their hour of desperation.

One day, in my early twenties when I was independent of my parents, I would cease attending mass entirely. No more abashed, faltering confessions! No more pretense! Even when I was composing my most Catholic novel *What I Lived For*, in 1993, I could not bring myself to attend a mass, by this time a mass said in English— I'd tried, but I could not.

Yet, ironically, it was in my mid-twenties, when I was teaching English at the University of Detroit, a Jesuit-run university, that I discovered a sort of Catholicism—intellectual, philosophical and literary-minded—that bore virtually no resemblance to the parochial religion of my childhood; among my colleagues and friends at the

University of Detroit were several Jesuits, men of surpassing intelligence, wit, warmth, and personal charisma, with whom I became friends. How astonishing these individuals seemed to me, dedicated Catholics who'd earned Ph.D.'s and had written excellent books! I would wonder—where had such priests been, when I'd been a Catholic? Would I have cherished the Roman Catholic Church, if just one of these priests had been assigned to the Good Shepherd Church in Pendleton? (But Jesuits are not parish priests, of course. The soldiers of the Society of Jesus aim higher than weekly sermons.)

By this time of this revelation, I had long ceased to believe.

What I most vividly recall was the stultifying nature of dogmatic belief, thrust upon a young and naturally inquisitive mind. A nightmare for a young person, trapped in the repetitive din of the Latin mass! Yet, in those years I had been a dutiful Catholic girl I could take refuge each Sunday for an hour in daydreaming; in the most intense, oneiric daydreaming, to be recorded in a notebook afterward, or typed on the (manual) Remington portable typewriter my grandmother Blanche Morgenstern gave me for my fourteenth birthday. *Out of the boredom of the pew, how many stories and poems have sprung! In desperation the Catholic writer learns young how to harvest the imagination where she/he can, in very defiance of those who would trap us in their nets and hold us captive.*

HEADLIGHTS: THE FIRST DEATH

WHY WOULD YOU DO *such a thing? That is not a good idea.*

But no one knows, and so no one asks.

Why in the night I slip from the rear of the darkened house. Why making my way along the graveled drive to the highway where in the shadows of evergreens I stand watching for headlights on Transit Road.

Sometimes there is a light rain. Overhead, a mottled sky and a fierce glowering moon-face behind clouds.

Like a sleepwalker who has wakened. In the night, past midnight, in this place in which such behavior would be perceived (by adults) to be aberrant, in a way rebellious.

It is disturbing to the adults of a household, when we are not in bed at the proper time. Our sleep, they can't control or monitor; how far we wander in our dreams, they have no idea. But it is an audacious gesture to leave the sleeping house and to venture outside, alone.

Insomnia begins in early adolescence. The swarming brain, the fast pulse. Excitement in realizing—*Something is about to happen!*

Out of nowhere has come this strange fascination that will endure for years, until I move out of the house on Transit Road forever.

A fascination with prowling in the night—standing at the end of the gravel driveway—watching for headlights of strangers' vehicles as they first appear beyond the V-intersection of Transit Road and Millersport Highway (to the south) and beyond the bridge over the Tonawanda Creek in the direction of Lockport (to the north). Lights that are scarcely visible at first, like faint stars, gradually growing larger, and then more swiftly larger, as if the vehicles were accelerating, and the headlights near-blinding—until abruptly the vehicle has passed, and now it is red taillights that are visible, receding.

Of all vehicles, Greyhound buses at night seem most fraught with romance. For I am often a passenger on these buses, riding to Lockport and back to Millersport, but mostly by day; rarely by night. (The bus station in Lockport, on a back street that runs parallel with Main Street, is not a place of safety or comfort for a girl or indeed a woman traveling alone after dark.)

Why am I entranced by headlights on Transit Road? Is it the contemplation of sheer randomness, chance? The intersection of lives—by chance? The life of the mind is essentially a life of control; if you are a writer, it is control which you bring to your work, by way of the selection of language, the arrangement of "scenes," the achievement of an "ending" . . . But life is likely to be that which lies beyond our control, and is unfathomable. And so I am entranced by the phenomenon of strangers' vehicles speeding past our house, that would elicit scarcely a glance by day.

There is something melancholy about this memory. The girl is a figure in a Hopper painting that Hopper never painted. The girl is in disguise as a (young, mere) girl—that is the explanation.

It is at such times that I feel my aloneness most strongly—which is very different from loneliness.

Loneliness weakens. Aloneness empowers.

Aloneness makes of us something so much more than we are in the midst of others whose claim is that they know us.

If they have named us, it is reasonable for them to believe not only that they know us but that *they own us*.

It is a peculiar fact of my young life, that I am under the spell of the Other; mesmerized by the prospect of mysterious lives that may surround me, to which I have no (actual, literal) access. The phantasmagoria of what is called "personality"—why we are, but also why we are so very different from each other.

When I am alone I think of such things. Especially when I am alone at night. Restless in my room, which is now, after my grandfather's death, a bedroom on the first floor of the farmhouse, with a single small window overlooking a small patch of outdoors. To see the night sky, I have to kneel at this window and crane my neck to look sharply up. Often there is nothing to see for the sky is opaque with clouds.

IT IS POSSIBLE THAT my wandering outside at night has begun in reaction to my grandfather's death. For this is *the first death*.

It is possible that this early insomnia, a restlessness of the brain, a sudden and profound wish not to be *in bed*, with bedclothes weighing down my legs and feet, has something to do with *the first death*.

A death in the family is an abrupt and awful absence. A presence as familiar to you as your own face in the mirror is suddenly gone.

Like stepping through a doorway, and there is no floor, nothing awaiting—you will fall, and fall.

The first death is a realization you cannot accept, as a child: that it is but *the first*, and there will be others.

The farmhouse, the farm buildings, the blacksmith's forge in the barn—all are linked so closely with my grandfather John Bush, it is scarcely possible to imagine these without him.

Yet, these will remain. The smithy's equipment, layered with soot; in a corner of the old barn, a pile of broken horseshoes.

Long after my grandfather is buried in the Good Shepherd Catholic Church cemetery, these will remain.

It was his time it was said.

John Bush died mysteriously—so it seemed to me. Suddenly my Hungarian grandfather was coughing more frequently, and more terribly, than before; his brash, bullying manner faded, and even his physical bulk seemed to diminish. My grandmother was no longer dominated by her forceful husband but rather terrified of what was happening to him, that took her, too, by surprise.

Emphysema, it was said. Ruined lungs, bleeding from tiny particles of iron, polluted and corrupted air breathed for years at Lackawanna Steel.

Nothing to be done, it was his time.

I am too young and too frightened of my grandfather's absence to wonder at this death. Far too young, to wonder why John Bush who was so canny and obstinate yet had to work in such conditions. Why he felt he'd had to work in such circumstances. Decades later such a death would be designated *work-related*.

But for now the peasant fatalism—*His time.*

I am too young to be angry on the behalf of my grandfather. In time, perhaps. But not now.

For now, it is enough to make my way through the darkened sleeping house, very quietly open the back door, and step outside into the night . . . Sometimes, one of the cats will approach me. There is that curious way in which a cat will approach you when you appear outdoors at an unexpected time, with a kind of animated intensity, and an inquiring *mew*. As if for a moment there is some confusion of categories, and the cat must determine if you are (still) a person, or in some way a cat. *Is this one of me?*

It is the headlights that captivate, on the road. The mystery of how vehicles seem to arise out of nowhere in the night and pass by me oblivious of me. I am hidden, and invisible. Yet I am here—and why? What has drawn me? Is it important somehow that I am here, and not in my bed?

Most of the nighttime vehicles are cars. Mostly, there is but a single person visible in them—the driver.

But sometimes I catch a glimpse of a second person in the passenger's seat and I feel a sudden pang of envy—*Who are you? Why are you driving together late at night? Do you love each other? Is that why you would be together late at night—because you love each other? And why are you driving along Transit Road? What do you look like, what are you thinking, where do you live, where are you going* . . .

In the next instant, red taillights receding.

"THE BRUSH"

ONCE, BEFORE I WAS born, he'd belonged to the IWW—Industrial Workers of the World. Though he'd had to shift his allegiance sometime in the 1920s from the Wobblies to the AFL (American Federation of Labor) in order to work at Lackawanna Steel, never did my Hungarian step-grandfather swerve from his vehement and profane conviction that workers—(by which he meant men, and men like himself)—should manage and profit from the "means of production."

That my swaggering barely literate grandfather John Bush could imagine that steel foundries might be managed by someone like himself, or indeed John Bush himself, was ever a source of amusement to my realistic-minded father (who belonged to the UAW—United Auto Workers); but my father did not "argue politics" with my grandfather who was profane, short-tempered, and derisive.

He was called by my father, not exactly to his face, "the Brush"— for Grandpa's steel-colored whiskers did suggest a stiff brush that stood out from his jaws. You would not want to disagree with this man whose grin of bared, badly stained teeth was a terror to behold. It was told of him that as a blacksmith John Bush had routinely struck resisting horses on their noses with his fists to subdue them, when he was shoeing them; he was that strong, and seemed to have no idea of the limits of his strength. He was graceless, obtuse, obstinate; he was a serious drinker (whiskey, hard cider drunk from a jug slung over his shoulder); he chewed (Mail Pouch) tobacco, and smoked cigarettes which he rolled himself with a crude device that left tobacco-crumbs scattered in his wake, always underfoot in my grandparents' kitchen; he swung a sledgehammer in a mighty arc with a grunt and a just-perceptible swelling of the veins and arteries in his neck. Beneath bib overalls stiffened with dirt he wore long underwear of a gunmetal-gray color, that showed filthy at his wrists. You did not want to think how filthy, how stained, the rest of that long underwear was. He washed his (filthy) hands with a special grainy gray soap, 20 Mule Team Borax. (My mother cautioned me never to wash my hands with this soap, that contained tiny bits of grit—"It isn't for a girl's hands.") He smelled powerfully—his tobacco-breath, with a smell of rotted teeth; his unwashed body, a palimpsest of sweats. Yet, unexpectedly, John Bush was a handsome man. He had dark, thick, tufted eyebrows and thick wiry hair. His eyes were very black "gypsy" eyes. His thick mustache drooped over his lips, his beard flared to mid-chest. His torso resembled a barrel filled with something heavy and unwieldy, like spikes. He spoke heavily accented broken English with a particular sort of vehemence as if speech, the very effort of speech, were a sort of ridiculous joke. And he could be playful; he could joke. His laughter mimicked the bellows of his smithy—sudden, expansive, loud. Though he seemed too blustering to be much aware of anyone or anything else he had a way of noticing a child who has been holding back, or hiding; for you could not hide from Grandpa Bush, ultimately. The Brush would find you.

Many times my grandfather dragged his calloused fingers through my curly hair, and laughed at my fear of him. He tickled my sides—a sensation indistinguishable from pain. How funny, to make little Joyce run away whimpering!

My grandfather was not an abuser of children. Rather, he was indifferent to a child's feelings. He did not take notice of a child as he did not take notice of an animal; at the most, he was angered by an animal's obstinate behavior, as by the behavior of horses he'd been hired to shoe; or, he was amused by animals, as by the strutting of Mr. Rooster.

Do I remember my grandfather twisting off the head of a red-feathered chicken? One of the panicked clucking hens? If I shut my eyes I can see this hellish scene and so, it is better not to shut my eyes. It is wisest to look away, into the distance.

There is relief, that the rough fingers are gone. And yet, there is a sick sort of fear, that the rough fingers are gone forever.

AN UNSOLVED MYSTERY: THE LOST FRIEND

1.

AN UNSOLVED MYSTERY IS a thorn in the heart.

It has been fifty-seven years since her death! Yet I still think of my friend with a stir of anticipation and dread.

As if Cynthia had not died, yet. As if there might be something I could do to prevent her dying.

We were each newly eighteen, the final time we saw each other in the late summer of 1956. It has been that long.

Joyce, what has happened to you! You are so much—changed. . .

Tell me what has happened, all these years I've been gone.

2.

TU ES MON AMIE.

In this way Cynthia spoke to me, elliptically. In our French class, scribbled on a sheet of paper.

Et tu es mon amie. Daringly, with a flourish, I replied on the same sheet of paper.

We were such good-girl students, ever prepared and ever reliable, our teacher Madame Henri would not notice us passing notes.

In our own language we could not have spoken so openly. In French, it wasn't clear what we'd said, still less what we meant.

After her death it would seem to me that Cynthia had been my closest friend but that (this was typical of Cynthia) she had not known it at the time. It would seem to me that Cynthia's death, her sudden and irrevocable dying, the angry self-loathing that had precipitated her death, even the choice of a particularly hideous and spiteful way to die—had been in some way my fault, or should have been my fault.

Or was it just that, in my grief, which was suffused with anger too, badly I wanted it to have been my fault.

Why did you kill yourself, Cynthia? Who else did you hope to hurt?

3.

"MY MOTHER SAYS . . ."

Obliquely, with a shy smile, Cynthia would approach me with these words.

My mother says if you want to, you can come for dinner anytime this week and stay for the night.

So that, if Cynthia's invitation were to be rebuffed, however unlikely this possibility, it would not be her invitation in fact but her mother's that was rebuffed.

Staying the night at a high school classmate's house was for me an experience fraught with awkwardness, yet one that could not be declined. It was with a tremulous sort of pride that I told my mother of such invitations for I knew that she would be happy for me, if perhaps apprehensive as well. When I'd been invited to a birthday party at the home of another girl friend whose affable father owned a small parts manufacturing company in Buffalo, my normally good-natured father had said, with a frown, "They sound like money people."

Money people. I had never heard this expression before, nor have I heard it since. How callow it sounded, how mean-spirited! Though I loved my father I felt a twinge of embarrassment that he should think in such terms, crudely and cruelly reducing the complexity of my several close friendships with girls who, despite the financial status of their parents, were not unlike myself in crucial ways.

Yet it was always evident to me, as to my parents, that the distance between Millersport and the suburb of Buffalo to which I was bussed for high school was far greater than eighteen miles could suggest.

My life had been altered irrevocably when the Niagara County school district made a decision after my ninth grade year at North Park Junior High not to continue bussing a half-dozen students from northern Erie County to Lockport public schools, though we all lived much closer to Lockport than to Buffalo. At once, by fiat, this *quirk of fate,* that had seemed devastating to me at the time, brought me from a mediocre public school district to a superior one in an affluent Buffalo suburb in which high school students were prepared for major universities and colleges. In Lockport, high school dropouts were common and virtually no one went to college; there, my fate would have been to hope for a scholarship to Buffalo Teachers' College where I could prepare to teach high school in a public school district not unlike that of Lockport. Without having been transferred to this superior school district I could not have made my way to Syracuse University on a New York State Regents scholarship, and from there to the University of Wisconsin at Madison, where I met Raymond Smith whom I would marry in 1961; I could never have made my circuitous way to Princeton University, still less to a writing career of substance; it is highly unlikely that I would be writing this memoir now.

Thinking of Cynthia Heike who died so young, at eighteen, I am thinking of that other life. For each of us, a succession of *other lives*, unlived.

For Cynthia the unlived life would very likely have involved medicine, medical science. For me, the more circumscribed life, the less ambitious career, probably confined to Niagara County and public school teaching, would have seemed nonetheless ambitious enough and rewarding enough to one from a family in which no one had (yet) gone beyond eight years of schooling.

Quirk of fate—turning the doorknob of a door you'd presumed to be locked. But it opens, and you step through.

4.

"I HATE MY BODY. I wish there was a way to get out of my damn body like a snake shedding its skin."

In the darkness of her bedroom Cynthia spoke suddenly, vehemently. Wide-awake I'd pretended to be asleep for this seemed the safest course.

5.

"RESEARCH BIOLOGIST. I THINK. Or maybe—a clinician like my father."

It was the first time I'd heard the term "clinician." Puzzling to me, that Cynthia Heike didn't describe her father as a "doctor."

Scientific American came into the Heikes' household, addressed to A. Emmet Heike, MD. Cynthia brought the magazine with its striking glossy covers—(many-times-magnified photographs of microbes, for instance, dazzling-beautiful photographs of distant galaxies)—to pass along to me.

When I was reading long, somber, antiquated-sounding tragedies by Eugene O'Neill, Cynthia gamely tried reading one or two— *The Hairy Ape, Mourning Becomes Electra.*

Did we discuss the articles in *Scientific American?* Did we discuss the O'Neill plays?

For me, the enchantment with O'Neill began with the playwright's titles. *Anna Christie. The Iceman Cometh. The Emperor Jones. Desire Under the Elms. Strange Interlude. Long Day's Journey Into Night.* The hardcover collection was enormous, at least eight hundred densely printed pages; when I'd withdrawn it from our school library, I saw that the card was blank—my name would be the first. Stubbornly I read even when I had only a vague idea of what I was reading. I certainly had no conception of how such unwieldy-seeming plays could be performed onstage.

The Hairy Ape was the O'Neill play I'd read with most fascination, for it reminded me painfully of my Hungarian (step)grandfather John Bush.

Reading *The Hairy Ape*, it was "the Brush" I was seeing. Brute animal vanity and pride and sudden physical collapse. Defeat and despair. My eyes welled with tears. I had not ever known my Hungarian grandfather, and had not really cried when he'd died; the spectacle of my wildly grieving grandmother and my suddenly agitated mother had badly shaken me.

Of one of the plays she'd read Cynthia said coolly, "It's about sex."

Sex? I had not grasped this.

"All these speeches that go on forever, whoever these people are if it's a man and a woman, that's what it's about."

I was shocked by Cynthia's matter-of-fact remark. In our girls' world, one did not utter the word *sex* so candidly—one did not utter the word *sex* at all.

Such simplicity in great literature didn't seem plausible—the O'Neill plays were so complicated, it would require much conscientious thinking just to figure out who the characters were, how they were related to one another; what had happened between them, to which they allude, at times heavy-handedly, yet not clearly . . .

Bluntly Cynthia interrupted, "In biology, everything is sex. Reproducing the species. Men and women are 'biology.' "

6.

THE FIRST PERSON I *knew to commit suicide.*

The first person my own age, of my acquaintance, to die.

7.

HERE IS THE PARADOX of the memoir: its retrospective vision, which is its strength, is also its weakness.

For the shadow of what's-to-come falls over the subject.

Like cloud-shadows, rushing across the earth. The shadow of the premature death-to-come falls over Cynthia Heike.

And now how hard it is, to envision Cynthia smiling! But when we knew her as our high school friend of course Cynthia was often smiling. No one would have predicted *suicide, so young*—the possibility would have left us incredulous.

In our classes Cynthia's hand was often raised. Teachers respected and admired her and in some cases were wary of her sharp tongue, her drawling remarks that evoked smirks and giggles in the classroom. Her intelligence was a kind of armor not easily penetrated. (Did I think—*Of course, she is a doctor's daughter.* Did I think—*That is the confidence of money. You have no idea.*)

Yet, Cynthia Heike did not give the impression of taking herself too seriously.

Taking yourself too seriously—no one wanted to be so accused.

Full of yourself—this was no ideal.

Cynthia Heike laughed often—at herself. Her caricature-cartoons did not spare the cartoonist who exaggerated the size of her nose and its flaring nostrils, the "wandering" left eye, the frizzy brush of hair—(other physical impairments were left unacknowledged). Rapidly executed in her spiral notebook, in the school cafeteria, in classes, these little drawings were remarkably mature to our eyes—as good, we'd thought, as professional cartoons or comics like "Pogo" and "Dick Tracy." It was revealing (if humbling) to see myself in a deft caricature by Cynthia Heike, in the school newspaper—deep shadows beneath owl-eyes, beak-like nose, simpering smile and a big dimple in one cheek—"Oatsie."

(The first caricature you see of yourself is indeed a revelation: all those facial flaws and idiosyncrasies you'd imagined you had hidden, and had learned not to see in mirrors, are publicly exposed for all to laugh at—"Looks just like you!")

(How strange it is, to type that name—"Oatsie"! No one before—no one since—my high school classmates has ever called me this name that suggests a comical sort of affection, and makes tears come into my eyes. I have not glanced into my high school yearbook in a long time but I would guess that "Oatsie" is the caption beneath my picture. And beneath Cynthia's more dignified and stern-smiling picture, just the name—"Cynthia Heike.")

In fact, just possibly Cynthia Heike was very slightly—justifiably—arrogant about her intelligence, as about her high grades in science and math; as a doctor's daughter Cynthia dared to consider herself the equal of anyone—any boy—in our class.

It was an era in which, on the whole, boys were naturally presumed to be smarter than girls. Yet it was simultaneously an era in which unusually smart and talented girls—Cynthia Heike, Lee Ann Krauser, a few others in our class—were accorded "exceptional" status as if they/ we were honorary boys.

In spring of our senior year Cynthia Heike was awarded a scholarship to the University of Rochester where she intended to study biology and prepare for medical school; I was awarded a scholarship to Syracuse, where I intended to study American literature and journalism. So close were the Rochester and Syracuse campuses, it seemed certain that Cynthia and I would visit each other often.

We would attend concerts, we promised. We would see foreign films.

8.

BACH SONATA FOR VIOLIN *Solo with Piano Accompaniment by Robert Schumann No. 1 in G minor. Cynthia Heike, violin. Lee Ann Krauser, piano.*

In the second row of the school auditorium I sat alone. In the second row of the school auditorium I sat alone scarcely daring to breathe.

As if my head were clamped in a vise I could not look away from my friend Cynthia Heike so exposed on the bright-lit stage in a black jersey dress that fell to her ankles, right shoulder raised, head bent and forehead creased as deftly she drew her bow across the strings of the gleaming violin; through a haze of beating blood I heard the clear, fluent notes, flawlessly executed, though rather rapidly, as if the violinist were breathless and her blood quick-beating too. And in the background at the piano the girl accompanist who seemed barely tall enough to reach the pedals with her feet, also in black, but a crisp taffeta-black, with a black bow at her waist, thin shoulders hunched and small blond head bent, striking quieter notes, near-inaudible notes, so familiar my fingers twitched involuntarily.

It is always a mild shock when music ends—abruptly. That beat of anxious silence before applause begins, and swells.

9.

JEALOUSY. NOT-JEALOUSY.

It is likely that if I tried I could count the times Cynthia Heike invited me to her home for dinner and to stay the night. (Because the Heikes' house was so far from my house in the "north country" it was not reasonable, in those days at least, to make so long a drive at night.) But I can't force myself to undertake this melancholy count, my memory begins to break into pieces like a distant radio station.

Even the first time at the Heikes' house is blurred. Experience is lived under a microscope, but recalled through a telescope.

Their house was a large stately red-brick colonial with white shutters and a steep shingled roof, set back from the road amid a scattering of evergreens. When I'd first seen it, from the rear seat of Mrs. Heike's car as she'd turned into the driveway, I had stared in disbelief.

"I hate living here. On the silly suburban *golf course*." From the passenger's seat Cynthia addressed me with an air of disgust.

Was I jealous of Cynthia's girl friends who lived in the Village (as it was called) as she did, and with whom she'd gone to school since kindergarten? Was I particularly jealous of her friend Lee Ann Krauser who lived near her in a prestigious residential neighborhood and who was, like Cynthia, a straight-A student and a serious young musician? (Cynthia had taken violin lessons since the age of six, Lee Ann had been taking clarinet lessons for nearly as long. Each girl played piano better than I did though in theory at least I was one of the designated "pianists" at school, and neither Cynthia nor Lee Ann would have considered herself a pianist—neither had had formal piano lessons.)

Both Cynthia and Lee Ann were friends of mine. We gave one another little gifts at birthdays, sent one another valentines and Christmas cards, sat together at assemblies and belonged to the same after-school clubs—French Club, Quill & Scroll, Girls Chorus, Yearbook. (Cynthia and Lee Ann were also in the orchestra. I was in girls' sports.) We published articles, short stories, and poetry in the school literary magazine quaintly called *Will o' the Wisp*. But Lee Ann was never so close to me as Cynthia was, for not once in three years of high school did Lee Ann Krauser invite me to her home for dinner and to stay the night; and (I could not help but presume) Cynthia liked Lee Ann more than she did me since (for one thing) she'd known her much longer.

Cynthia liked Lee Ann more than she did me. Here is the very blood-jet of jealousy, never more devastating than among adolescent girls.

It was a certainty that each girl was the other's *best friend* while Oatsie was *second-best*.

(Mostly, I did not mind being *second-best*. I took for granted that, in my suburban high school, I could not ever be other than *second-*

best. I had only to shut my eyes to recall the drab interior of the one-room rural schoolhouse on the Tonawanda Creek Road and the older, crude farm boys for whom profanities and obscenities were normal usage, and who so tormented me when I was a young child—I had only to shut my eyes to summon this painful vision and to feel that, at *second-best,* I was yet in a magical realm.)

Since fifth grade, Cynthia and Lee Ann had been serious music students. They frequently performed in recitals and each was likely to accompany the other on the piano.

Often I would hear on Monday morning that Cynthia and Lee Ann had attended a musical event over the weekend—concerts by the Buffalo Philharmonic at Kleinhans Music Hall, Bach's *The Messiah* at St. Paul's Cathedral. There were string quartets at the University of Buffalo, piano recitals, choral evenings. Belatedly I would hear of these wonderful occasions and would wish that I could have accompanied my friends; it was fascinating to me to determine, not by direct inquiry but by an accruing of incidental information, who had taken whom—Mrs. Heike had taken the girls; or, Dr. and Mrs. Heike had taken them; or, Mr. and Mrs. Krauser had taken them; or, both families had gone, in separate vehicles, but had had dinner together beforehand at the Buffalo Athletic Club to which the men belonged.

My interest was such, one or the other of my friends would say adamantly: "Next time you can come with us, Joyce. We'll plan for that."

Yes. I would like that. Thank you!

The Heikes owned a beautiful Steinway grand piano. Just the sight of such a piano, close-up, was intimidating. To depress the (perfect, ivory) keys, to hear the immediate sonorous sound, brought tears to my eyes as I thought of how my father would have loved to it down at such a piano . . .

Except, maybe not. *Money people* he'd have said.

My Lockport piano teacher, a retired church organist with floating snowy-white hair like Einstein, a creased melancholy face and
hands covered in liver spots, owned a much less impressive quasi-
grand Knabe piano with yellowed keys that stuck. A sensation of
giddy elation came over me, as of utter recklessness, when Cynthia's
father Dr. Heike insisted that I play something on his piano, since
Cynthia had told him that I was a piano student; and so I'd played for
the Heikes several of my meticulously memorized pieces—a Mozart
rondo, Beethoven's "Für Elise," and the first two movements of
Beethoven's Sonata no. 14 in C-sharp Minor, the so-called *Moonlight
Sonata*. (The first, dreamy movement of the sonata was my grandmother Blanche's favorite piano music which I'd played for her each
time she visited us, for years, rarely less than once a week; so totally
had I memorized this famous piece of music, my fingers could play
the notes without interference from my brain—even the demanding
stretches, which my hands were too small to execute smoothly, were
factored into my memory so that without thinking I steeled myself
for the tiny spasms of hand-pain without flinching and without quite
missing a chord.)

Playing the piano for this small audience was so stressful for me,
I could scarcely breathe as I played; when I could not hold my breath
any longer, my fingers faltered against the keyboard—just perceptibly, as only another pianist might have noticed. By the time I struck
the final chords of the Beethoven sonata's second movement I could
feel perspiration trickling down my back, and I was exhausted. But
Cynthia's father had been surprised by the bravura of my performance, it seemed, and clapped loudly. "Great! That's great, Joyce.
I really like that—*Moonlight Sonata*. Yes. A piano always sounds
good, a damn violin can squeak and hurt your ears." Cynthia laughed
wincingly as if Dr. Heike had reached over and pinched her.

At first I'd thought that Dr. Heike might be applauding me out of playful mockery, but it appeared that he was serious. Blushing badly, I thanked him.

I was sorry that, to compliment me, Dr. Heike had felt it necessary to take a swipe at his daughter. Soon you sensed in Dr. Heike's presence that he was an energetic man who looked upon life—even social life, domestic life—as rivalry, competition; it would not mean much to compliment one young person without suggesting a critique of another young person. Also, he seemed determined to "like" me—as if there might have been a history of his having been impolite to Cynthia's friends and so he meant, emphatically, to be friendly to me, that his daughter could have no complaint to make of him that night. Feathery-haired Mrs. Heike praised me also, and Cynthia made one of her terse comments: "Not bad. Lighten up the pedal."

But it seemed that Cynthia did think I played piano well—for a sixth-year student. (Cynthia had been taking violin lessons for more than ten years.) She'd been taken in by my canny, calculated performance of memorized pieces, my entire repertoire. Casually she asked if I'd ever accompanied another music student, a violinist for instance, and I said not yet, but I would certainly like to try.

Here was an impulsive and heedless statement like so many I have made in my lifetime—*I would certainly like to try.*

For our spring music recital at school, Cynthia was going to play a Bach sonata for solo violin with piano accompaniment composed by Robert Schumann. Now more pointedly she asked—maybe I could play the accompaniment?

Cynthia appeared to be sincere. I saw that I could not say no to my strong-willed friend.

It was a flattering request. It was an opportunity for me to partly pay back Cynthia's generosity. Yet, nothing could fill me with more dread than the prospect of accompanying a violinist as accomplished as Cynthia Heike on the high school stage before an audience of students, teachers, relatives. For this would be a musically sophisticated audience, at least in part; nothing like the warmly uncritical Methodist congregation in Pendleton who never failed to praise my "organ-playing" to which, as they loudly sang their beloved hymns, they barely listened. The horror presented itself to me as something akin to appearing naked in public— worse, having to remove my own clothes in the effort; like most less-than-gifted musicians I knew how poorly I actually played and how desperate were my stratagems to sound as if I did in fact know how to play.

(One of the comical nightmares of my young life had occurred in sixth grade when I allowed myself to be coerced by a well-intentioned teacher into playing piano in the school auditorium as students tramped into our weekly assembly; while I was playing one or another memorized piece with such a title as "Song of the Volga Boatmen" or "The Smithy's Anvil" my mind went blank as I approached the end, and I could not remember the final bar—so that in a state of commingled panic and paralysis I simply kept playing, repeating passages multiple times until at last in desperation I struck a chord—any chord—and dropped my hands from the keyboard in chagrin and shame. No one had noticed.)

"Are you sure you want me, Cynthia? What about Lee Ann . . ."

"Lee Ann! No. I want you."

Cynthia was incensed, that I should seem to be doubting her judgment. It was like her to speak vehemently, even angrily, when she sensed even mild opposition.

Cynthia's left eye, that was a weak-muscled "wandering" eye, did not engage me like her right eye, fierce, shining, fixed upon my face so that I could not look away.

I'd noticed that she and Lee Ann were not together so much lately at school. In the cafeteria I saw Lee Ann sitting with other friends, including boys; several times, I'd seen Lee Ann walking with a tall lanky-limbed boy whom I knew slightly from math class. If Lee Ann passed by Cynthia and me she would greet us warmly while Cynthia looked stonily away.

Lee Ann Krauser was a petite girl, scarcely five feet tall, with transparent pink plastic-framed glasses, pale bangs that fell to her eyebrows, the small sweetly naïve face of a precocious child. She wore her shoulder-length hair fixed with barrettes. She wore plaid jumpers with white long-sleeved blouses. She wore cashmere sweater sets in eggshell pastels, and white-and-brown saddle shoes with white woolen socks. From Cynthia's teasing remarks to her I gathered that the Krausers were well-to-do: indeed, "Krauser" was the name of a Buffalo manufacturer. In every class there is at least one girl like Lee Ann: child-sized, rather plain, very smart, but so innocent-seeming she is likely to be the favorite of her teachers, and attractive to a particular sort of brainy, socially maladroit boy who will fall in love with her and trail her about if she allows him.

In disgust Cynthia said of Lee Ann: "She's getting boy crazy. Which is to say—just plain crazy."

I thought this was unfair. It was not Lee Ann's fault that boys were attracted to her when, Cynthia would have to concede, girls were attracted to Lee Ann, too.

More obscurely Cynthia said, "She twists everything she touches and ruins it. I hate her."

This was a preposterous accusation. Cynthia was so vehement, I knew better than to ask what she meant.

Thinking—*Now I am her closest friend. Now there is no one else.*

10.

SHE SAID, "*YOU'RE* THE writer."

Tearing up stories, poems she'd written. The clever little caricature-cartoons that never seemed to please her the way they pleased others, for Cynthia discounted what came easily to her and the cruelty of satire came easily to her.

It was a time when I'd fallen under the spell of Hemingway. In a succession of stories set in a fictitious Millersport in imitation of the terse sculpted prose of *in our time*. For Hemingway is the great artist of the unsaid, the withheld. Hemingway is the great artist of silence, in the early stories most poignantly. (And how had I found my way to the esoteric *in our time?* The previous year in Mr. Stein's junior English class we'd read stories in the paperback *Great American Short Story Masterpieces* and in this wonderful collection I discovered not only Hemingway's "Soldier's Home" but stories by Ambrose Bierce, Ring Lardner, Sherwood Anderson, Katherine Anne Porter, William Faulkner, Conrad Aiken ("Silent Snow, Secret Snow"), and Eudora Welty that would be imprinted nearly as deep in my memory as the *Alice* books and *The Secret Garden*.) Some of my stories in the mode of *in our time* I showed to Mr. Stein, and some to Mrs. Ordway, another of my high school English teachers; some I showed to Cynthia Heike. (None I showed to my parents or my grandmother. Secrecy has always seemed most precious to me, among those with whom we are closest.) Eventually there came to be a manuscript of about two hundred pages of these stories, each neatly typed on the wonderful Remington typewriter my grandmother had given me for my fourteenth birthday, each ending irresolute and dramatically poised in the cool Hemingway manner, and this manuscript I would give to Mrs. Ordway to read, at her request; and though Mrs. Ordway promised that she would return the manuscript, weeks and eventually months passed and by graduation in June 1956 she had not returned it.

To recall the frustration and (even) despair of having lost this schoolgirl manuscript is to recall the way the ground could shift beneath your feet at any time, in adolescence; the way you lived under the (wayward, capricious) authority of adults who did what they wanted to do because they had the power to do it. Just as one teacher (Mr. Stein) could be encouraging, kind, thoughtful, "devoted to his students"—so another teacher (Mrs. Ordway) could be subtly discouraging, impatient, secretive and willful, given to provoking rivalries among students. To recall childhood and girlhood is to recall that sense of the unpredictable when any adult had the power to uplift, or to undermine; to reward, or to punish; to praise, or to withhold praise for his or her mysterious purposes.

Why did Mrs. Ordway behave so strangely?—I would never know.

When I mentioned to my friends that Mrs. Ordway seemed unwilling to return my manuscript even as she continued to promise to return it they were indignant on my behalf—like good high school friends!—but seemed not to comprehend why on earth I hadn't made a carbon copy of it. (That a flat box of twelve sheets of carbon paper was "expensive" could not have occurred to them.) They speculated that Mrs. Ordway had not (yet) read the manuscript, or had lost it.

Meanly, or perhaps funnily, Cynthia said: "Maybe she's waiting for you to become famous, Joyce."

11.

"I HATE MY BODY. Sometimes I think—I'm being led out into a prison yard, to be shot by a firing squad. Because when you are *so ugly*, you don't deserve to live."

In the darkness when I'd thought Cynthia was asleep she began suddenly to speak of the most private things.

She was a freak, her spine was twisted. And her eye—her pathetic eye—that made people think she was cross-eyed but *she was not.*

People looked at her with pity and scorn. Boys whistled at her out of meanness. Boys said terrible things to her which she would never repeat. She hated boys, and had a plan to one day carry a concealed gun, and shoot them in their jeering faces.

Or, maybe: she'd get some acid. From chem lab. Toss it in their hateful faces so they'd know what it was like to be *freaky* afterward.

Everything about her body was hateful except her hands. Her fingers. These allowed her to play the violin, that made her so happy.

"But that's almost all. Sometimes school, some of my courses— biology, chemistry. It's fun in French conversation—*avec mon amie très rusée.* But school itself—*c'est de la merde.* Seeing how people look at me and feel sorry for me."

It was astonishing to me that a girl of Cynthia Heike's reputation could feel like this about herself. A doctor's daughter, who lived in a beautiful house. Whose sarcasm could be withering, even as a sudden smile from her could be thrilling.

"Cynthia, nobody feels sorry for you! People admire you . . ."

"Adults maybe. Some adults. But nobody would want to *be me.*"

"That's ridiculous."

"Is it? Would you want to *be me?*"

The question was vehement, childish. I had no idea how to respond.

In the twin bed beside Cynthia's bed in the glimmering dark of her peppermint-striped girl's room as inappropriate for Cynthia's fierce spirit as a pink satin bow would have been in her thick unruly hair I could only murmur feebly protestations—she couldn't possibly mean what she was saying . . .

Joyce in the backyard
of the Millersport house,
aged three or four.
(Fred Oates)

(Fred Oates)

(Fred Oates)

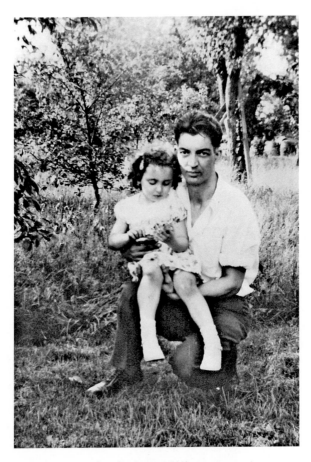

Joyce and Frederick Oates, 1943. *(Carolina Oates)*

Joyce with baby brother
Robin (Fred, Jr.), 1943.
(Fred Oates)

June high school
graduation, 1956,
age eighteen.
(Fred Oates)

Easter, April 17, 1949.
(Fred Oates)

Mademoiselle fiction
contest co-winner,
Syracuse, 1959,
age twenty.
(Dorothea Palmer)

Frederick Oates, 1935, age twenty-one.

Joyce's parents, Fred and Carolina Oates, on the wing of an open cocktail airplane, Lee's Airfield, Swormville, New York, 1940s.

Fred Oates with a Waco single-prop plane.

Fred Oates,
age mid-seventies.
(Ray Smith)

Carolina Oates,
age mid-seventies.
(Ray Smith)

"I do! It began back in grade school, being stared-at, laughed-at—called a freak."

"Nobody has called you a *freak*."

"Yes! I have been called a *freak*."

"I—I don't believe that."

Of course, I believed what Cynthia was saying. The crude, cruel, stupid and unvarying insults of boys were not unfamiliar to me, though I'd never been called a *freak*—I had been spared that at least.

Now I was led into confiding in Cynthia as I had confided in no one else how I'd been "teased" pitilessly at the one-room country school when the school had had eight grades; after my third year the school district transferred older students elsewhere, and the teasing stopped. Cynthia listened intently and asked if any of these boys had "done things" to me and I told her no—not exactly.

I explained to Cynthia that in the country school the oldest boys were fifteen, still in eighth grade, because New York State law did not allow anyone to quit school until his sixteenth birthday. These were farm boys deeply resentful of being kept in school who took out their antagonism on anyone weaker than they were.

I thought of their jeering eyes—the stupidity in those eyes, and the cruelty—for cruelty is a kind of stupidity: I knew that. I thought of how they had tormented me but I did not want to think that they had tormented *me*—that is, not exclusively me. For their meanness and brutality were indiscriminate, directed against several of us, because we were younger, and hadn't older brothers or sisters to protect us at the school. It is true, by contemporary standards some of this abuse would be categorized as *sexual*, but in fact it had seemed just roughness—physical roughness—not unlike the tormenting these same boys inflicted upon helpless animals (cats, rabbits, raccoons, snakes) they managed sometimes to catch. Much of the time they threw things at us—stones, mudballs, snowballs. Decades later reading of the horrific stonings of Muslim women and men condemned as "adulterers" I would feel sick at the memory of being harassed by these boys, my friend Helen Judd and me running, breathless and running for our lives (as we'd thought) along an over-grown path by the Tonawanda Creek, behind the schoolhouse where the teacher never went.

In desperation running ahead of Helen, who could not keep pace with me. Leaving Helen behind, abandoning Helen.

I told Cynthia that the most dangerous abuse hadn't been directed toward me or the other young girls but toward a boy a few years older named Hendrik who had weak eyes and wore glasses: they'd rolled him in the leaves so that the leaves would get in his eyes. I told her that because I could run faster than the other girls, the boys sometimes chased me in particular—"But it was more like 'teasing' then. I think you would call it that."

How pathetic this sounded. *More like teasing. I think you would call it that.*

My voice was trembling. I had never told anyone these things before and seemed unable to stop as if my words were a way of helpless sobbing. As I spoke in the darkness of this unfamiliar bed-room—to a girl whom I did not really know, and could not really trust—I realized how astonished I was that this harassment of my childhood, protracted over months and even years, had actually hap-pened to me, and that in some way I had learned to accept it, with the fatalism of a child who sees no way to alter things and so must alter her perception.

Cynthia was indignant on my behalf. She asked what on earth the teacher had been doing—or had not been doing—to allow such bullying and abuse in the school yard, and I said that the boys attacked us along the road, on the way home from school mostly, not usually in the school yard within view of the windows. She asked if I'd told my parents and I said yes. And my parents came to speak with our teacher Mrs. Dietz. And possibly, following that meeting, the harassment abated—for a while. But the problem was that Mrs. Dietz herself was intimidated by the older boys who were essentially unteachable. And several were taller than she, heavier, and physically threatening. How the poor woman had managed to confront such antagonism in the classroom, week following week, for years, I have no idea. By the time I'd enrolled in the school, Mrs. Dietz had been teaching there for at least fifteen years. I can shut my eyes and see her tall sturdy figure, flushed face and disheveled hair, but when I try to hear her voice there is only a muffled murmur.

Forgive me but I tried. I tried to do my best. Tried to be the best teacher in those terrible circumstances that I could be.

When the harassment began again, and became more physical and threatening, I could not bring myself to tell my parents a second time. Instead, I lingered inside the schoolhouse with Mrs. Dietz, until (sometimes) the danger was past. (For the older boys could not linger after school long, they were expected to return home to work.) I learned to run—very fast. I learned to run faster than other children like Helen Judd, who could not so easily escape our tormentors. I learned to run and to feel the intense excitement of such running which may become identical with exhilaration. Nor was the bullying constant, rather only intermittent. You learned to rejoice that another, more vulnerable and more accessible victim might appear. There are stratagems of survival we discover young that become so second-nature to us it is possible to forget that they are stratagems of survival at all.

Cynthia marveled that I'd gone to a one-room schoolhouse at all—"Like something on the frontier. Eight grades in one room!"

I told Cynthia of other girls in the school. Of Helen Judd and her sisters whose father had (allegedly) abused them. And possibly others had abused them—the older brothers, the father's friends. I told Cynthia of the house fire, the arson. I did not tell Cynthia that Helen Judd had once been my friend but referred to her as a "neighbor girl." (I no longer saw Helen, for she lived in Lockport and must have attended Lockport High School.) Helen Judd had never "told"—not anyone. As her mother had never told police of what her husband had done to her and the children. No one could accuse Helen Judd of trying to get anyone in trouble, blaming others, snitching on others for something that had happened to *her*.

"Was she pregnant? The girl? Did they—*make her pregnant*?"

This was an unexpected question. I had not ever thought of the possibility of Helen Judd pregnant.

"N-No."

"No? But how would you know—absolutely?"

Absolutely? I had no idea what Cynthia meant.

Later I would surmise that she was referring to an abortion, or a miscarriage. The neighbor-girl might have been pregnant and the pregnancy ended and I could not have known, for how could I have known.

"Things like that could be reported to the police," Cynthia said, thoughtfully. "If they happened to someone here . . ."

She was thinking of how, in the rural north country, different and cruder standards prevailed. In her genteel suburban village no girl could be so badly treated.

"What did she look like—'Helen Judd'?"

"I don't know . . ."

"What do you mean, you don't know? Why do you say you don't know?"

Cynthia was becoming impatient with me. It was inevitable, Cynthia often became impatient with her girl friends—even Lee

Ann Krauser whose way of contending with Cynthia's ill humor was to laugh at her and call her *Heik-ee* with a pronounced Germanic accent. But I could not laugh at Cynthia. I had not that power.

I could not think how to reply. It did not seem relevant to me what Helen Judd looked like, only what Helen Judd had endured. But I could not tell Cynthia this, for Cynthia seemed angry with me.

My hesitancy, my indecisiveness—others interpreted as obstinacy. My occasional shyness, others misinterpreted as aloofness.

Cynthia persisted: "She wasn't freaky-looking, was she? Like me?"

"No! She was not."

"And me? What about me?"

"For God's sake, Cynthia. You are not 'freaky-looking.' "

In the darkness Cynthia laughed loudly. She was making no attempt to keep her voice down. I was in dread of her parents hearing her through the walls, in their bedroom at the end of the hall.

Mrs. Heike would come to the door, and knock softly. Mrs. Heike would murmur through the door—*Cynthia? Joyce? Is something wrong?*

Or rather, she would not come to the door. Cynthia's mother was wary of Cynthia, I'd noticed. A tense veiled gaze, a hesitant smile— Mrs. Heike was conditioned not to press her high-strung daughter too far.

Before I'd known Cynthia Heike well, when I'd seen her from a little distance I had wondered if her back were somehow misshapen; one of her shoulders appeared to be higher than the other, and she walked just slightly oddly, dragging one of her feet. And her left eye seemed not quite in focus so that you looked from one eye to the other, disoriented, uncertain where to look. In gym class Cynthia was one of those girls last-chosen for teams for she lacked what is called hand-eye coordination: where another girl might snatch a basketball out of the air, or strike a volleyball with just enough force to propel it across the net at a shrewd angle, Cynthia would fumble the ball hopelessly, as a young child might do, biting at her lower lip and flushing with embarrassment and frustration.

But when I'd come to know Cynthia better, I seemed scarcely aware of her "twisted" spine. When I spoke to Cynthia I knew to look into her right eye, not her left eye. Her strong personality, her presence among others, her quicksilver wit and sardonic smile so dominated, you would not think—*That poor girl! There is something wrong with her.*

It is true that in gym class as in the school swimming pool I managed to avoid Cynthia Heike. This was not difficult, for Cynthia herself held back, reluctant to be involved, resentful. Often she did not attend swim classes at all, with an excuse from her mother. In such circumstances there is invariably a small cadre of girls for whom athletics is anathema as there is a small cadre of girls for whom athletics is a great pleasure, and competition exciting and not fraught with anxiety, and these cadres rarely overlap.

I tried to convince Cynthia that she was mistaken about herself, and should not say such things. And Cynthia said, in a voice heavy with sarcasm, "Would you change places with me, then?"

The possibility filled me with anxiety. *Of course not! No.*

"I—I would change places with you—of course. Your life, your parents—your musical talent . . ."

"But you'd have to be in my *body*. What about that?"

It was a rude unanswerable question. I was too young and too intimidated by Cynthia to think of a witty rejoinder, as Lee Ann Krauser might have in my place.

Cynthia could not know that the fantasy often came to me, that I might change places with another girl my approximate age: the next girl who came into my line of vision, the next girl who turned a corner. If I entered a room at school—if I hurried up a flight of stairs. If, closing my locker, I turned to see . . .

Of course, I didn't mean it. The thought of losing my parents and my grandmother whom I loved, and who loved me, filled me with horror.

And yet. The fantasy of *becoming another* was fascinating to me at this uncertain time in my life.

By the time I managed to stammer a reply to Cynthia's accusation I had waited too long. She said, "Thank you for not lying to me, Joyce. You're the only damn one who doesn't."

With a snort of derision Cynthia turned over in her bed.

12.

IT WAS TRUE, CYNTHIA Heike was afflicted with a curvature of the upper spine severe enough to require (as she told me, with a bitter laugh) a brace. She'd worn a "goddamned brace like a harness" prescribed by a Buffalo orthopedist, intermittently for years, for part of each day; it had been her father who'd insisted, and who had taken her to a number of specialists; for a while, he'd considered the possibility of surgery.

"*He* knows a freak when he sees one. 'A. Emmet Heike, M.D.' "

Once, I'd had a glimpse of Cynthia's naked back. It looked as if the upper spine had melted beneath the skin and fallen back upon itself. Cynthia had learned to compensate for the deformity by favoring her right side and by wearing oversized, boxy clothing that hid too her flat chest, thick waist and thighs. Her arms and legs were covered in coarse dark hairs. On her upper lip was a faint dark mustache. Her left eye was weak-muscled and "wandering." Her eyelids were prominent, giving her a languorous, sleepy look at odds with her sharp eye and sharper tongue; in the proper lighting, Cynthia was very handsome. Her mouth was small, perfectly chiseled. Her nose was wide at the tip, and her nostrils flared. Memorably Cynthia said, with a mock pout to make us laugh: "If I were a guy I'd be good-looking. But I'm not a guy. I guess."

One day in swim class something terrible happened. A silly girl swam beside Cynthia in the shallower end of the pool and tried to "ride" her—pulling herself onto Cynthia's twisted back in a foolish prank that precipitated a panic attack in Cynthia causing her to swallow water, choke, nearly drown.

Why would anyone do such a thing, it was asked. Not in malice, not to be cruel, just "playful"—mistaking Cynthia Heike for a girl without a handicap, as Cynthia Heike took such pains to disguise her condition. (Cynthia could not swim except by placing her feet on the bottom of the pool and pushing off for brief, fluttering seconds when her strong arms flailed like windmills and her legs kicked frantically. Almost you would think, witnessing this, that Cynthia was "swimming.")

Was I there that day? I think that I was, in the deeper end of the pool. I was one of the tireless divers in my high school swim classes for I'd learned young to swim and dive, at Olcott Beach. To *keep in motion* has always been an ideal. The commotion in the shallow end of the pool had been distracting but it hadn't been until afterward that I learned what had happened. My first reaction had been resentment, that that girl (who was not a friend of Cynthia Heike) could have presumed such familiarity with my friend.

13.

ASSIDUOUSLY WE PRACTICED THE Bach/Schumann piece for the spring recital. Each alone, and at Cynthia's house after school. Weeks in succession.

At home on our dull-toned upright piano that made me impatient, its tones were so dull and shallow. Several keys stuck. I complained that the piano needed tuning and my father said affably that that was so, the piano needed tuning.

The implication being *So much else in our lives need tuning. And—so what?*

Mrs. Heike sometimes listened to Cynthia and me practicing, for a few minutes at least; Dr. Heike, rarely. For Dr. Heike came home late, sometimes missing dinner. (That is, dinner at home. Obviously Dr. Heike was not missing dinner elsewhere.) Cynthia played the violin with a kind of anxious ferocity, biting her lower lip. She was impatient with me when I faltered at the keyboard striking a note too hard or too softly or hesitating, missing the beat. A true musician never "misses a beat"—an essentially untrainable musician has but a blind (or deaf) notion of what a "beat" is. Under the pressure of such practice, I'd begun to sweat inside my clothes. I had come to dread the practice sessions with my friend even as I yearned to please her. For Cynthia could be generous with praise—"That was perfect! Just the right tone, and volume. *Thank you.*"

Impulsively Cynthia hugged me. Her grip was hard, her breath against my face. I could not embrace her in turn, I was too taken by surprise. Yet I recall her twisted spine against my hands, so strangely. I am sure, I recall this.

Both my parents and my grandmother Blanche Morgenstern planned to attend the recital. My grandmother would take the Greyhound bus to our house in Millersport, and from there my father would drive us to the high school. Grandma, who was a skilled seamstress, was sewing a navy blue jumper and a white silk blouse for me from a Butterick pattern.

In anticipation of the audacity of what I was undertaking to do, playing piano *in front of an audience*, I had begun to sleep poorly. I would wake in the middle of the night and lie with my eyelids shut tight and trembling. My fingers ached for I'd been playing the Schumann composition in my sleep like a frenzied automaton, unable to stop. My fingers were claws, cramped with pain. Just the other side of an assiduously executed piano piece by any young person lies madness.

At the piano, a mist came over my brain. I had difficulty focusing my eyes. My fingers were damp and numb; desperately I rubbed them together to restore heat and agility. The cruel thought haunted me—*You will make the same mistake you made in sixth grade. You will forget the ending and will just play and play like a robot. And they will all laugh at you.*

I tried to take solace in the fact (many times told me) that an accompanist need only be adequate—"No one will hear if you make a mistake, Joyce."

A mistake! In the singular?

"HEL-LO! IS IT—JANICE?"

"Joyce, Daddy! You've met."

"Yes! Yes indeed, we have met."

Merrily Dr. Heike extended his hand to shake mine. His grip was hard, punishing. He seemed to take pleasure in making me uncomfortable as a way of teasing his daughter.

Dr. Heike was the first person with whom I'd shaken hands. The first adult. The handshake had been unavoidable.

Tonight Dr. Heike came to the dinner table a half-hour late. He had been expected at seven o'clock, now it was seven-thirty. He was a large man, jolly, hearty, but absentminded, smiling and indifferent. When he was in a good mood, he laughed. But when he was annoyed and irritated, he also laughed. A gold pin of some kind, small, sword-shaped, glittered in his left lapel.

A money person. What would he want with you?

There appeared to be some tension between Dr. Heike and Mrs. Heike which no one wished to acknowledge for when Dr. Heike stooped to kiss the cheek of his wife, who was seated, Mrs. Heike turned her head away with pained pursed lips; but Dr. Heike merely laughed, and rubbed his hands together. Cynthia had said that her father was an oncologist: cancer? Those eyes gleaming with merriment, those fat hands—*cancer?* How was this possible? Invariably when Dr. Heike entered a room the air was stirred and roused as with many small whirlwinds. You understood that Dr. Heike was the father of the family and much adored. You had always to acknowledge the father at the center of the room for even when you avoided his moist merry staring eye, you were acknowledging him. And there was a woman helper in the Heike household with whom Dr. Heike was on teasing terms that made her blush and stammer in confusion: "Jad-wiga, please say hello to our guest, too! In English, please— 'Hel-*lo.*'" A Polish girl, thick-thighed, about twenty-nine years old, Jadwiga was the first household servant I'd seen in actual life though servants were commonplace in Hollywood movies where they were invariably black.

I had not told my parents that the Heikes had a *servant*. I knew that my father would make a cutting remark about this and that my mother would recall how before I'd been born she'd done housework for a well-to-do family on Washburn Street, Lockport.

"Jad-wiga" was a name that seemed to amuse Dr. Heike for he

used it several times, always enunciating it carefully. You would think that Jadwiga had no last name.

This was the evening when Dr. Heike asked me what was happening in the "north country" and when I told him that not much was happening he'd shocked me, and others at the table, by saying, "Hell, no. That is not true, my girl. There is much going on in your part of the county. In the *Buffalo Evening News* I read an article about a fire in Clarence, and two small children killed. And arson is suspected."

I was so surprised by Dr. Heike's hostile tone that I sat unmoving at the dinner table, unable to reply.

Out of nowhere had come this attack. As soon as Dr. Heike had settled into his dinner, conversation had seemed ordinary, even dull; the Heikes had been talking together about some domestic incident, and I had scarcely listened. But now, I was stricken to the heart.

I should have protested—*But Clarence isn't Millersport! It's miles away . . .*

Still, Dr. Heike was essentially correct about my evasiveness. If the fire had been in Millersport, I would have told Dr. Heike that nothing much had happened there, to avoid speaking to him. Instinctively Dr. Heike knew this.

The Heikes—Mrs. Heike, Cynthia, eleven-year-old Albert—were embarrassed by their father's tone, as by the fierce look in his face, as if he'd been personally insulted. Adroitly Cynthia intervened telling her father that we had so much homework in just chemistry alone, we didn't have time to read the silly newspaper. *He* had time for that.

Dr. Heike chuckled at this riposte. Mrs. Heike tried also to be playful telling me that her husband was accustomed to commanding the nursing staff at Buffalo General, who could never live up to his high expectations. "There are too many females in the doctor's life, he says. It's not your fault, Joyce." Mrs. Heike laughed as if she'd said something both witty and embittered.

A few minutes later Cynthia became the brunt of Dr. Heike's irritation when she (evidently) replied to a question of his with her mouth partially full. "Excuse me. Please do not speak with your mouth full, Cynthia. You are not an infant."

Cynthia's face darkened with embarrassment. Then boldly, bravely she countered, "Infants don't talk, Daddy. With or without their mouths full."

Dr. Heike surprised us by laughing at this lame joke. You could see that Dr. Heike was a man who had to be approached from an unexpected angle, to make him laugh; if you approached him head-on, and he saw you coming, he would be contemptuous.

"And what does your father do, Joyce?"

"My father is a tool and die designer."

Carefully I answered Dr. Heike's question. There would be no ambiguity now.

"A 'tool and die designer'—is he? Where?"

I told him: Harrison Radiator, in Lockport.

"In Lockport! That's a corrupt little canal city, did you know?" Dr. Heike laughed genially.

To this I had no reply. I had no idea what Dr. Heike meant by *corrupt little canal city*, in such satisfied terms.

"Your mayor has been indicted. Not for the first time. I mean— not the first time that a *mayor of Lockport* has been indicted."

Dr. Heike spoke with vague amusement. I had not reacted except to smile faintly and perhaps now he felt sorry for me. The doctor was accustomed to his more spirited daughter resisting him. Even a sadist may be disappointed when a victim fails to fight back.

" 'A tool and die designer'—in a factory? Is that where?"

I thought so, yes. Harrison Radiator was a *factory*.

"Where did your father train?"

Where—train? The use of the term "train" was unfamiliar to me.

I was sure that I'd never heard my father use it in regard to his work. I felt that Dr. Heike was teasing me—tormenting me—hoping to make me cry, like the boys at the rural school. They had not stopped when a victim cried.

Young I had learned that there is really no way to placate the cruel except by escaping them. If you resist, or if you acquiesce—they will not show mercy in either case.

Quietly I spoke, so that the man should not know how miserable I was at his elegant dinner table, in his elegant home, and how I hated him. "I guess I don't know, Dr. Heike."

"Don't know? Probably in Buffalo, at the vocational school. It's said to be among the best of its kind."

My father had not "trained" at any vocational school in Buffalo or elsewhere. My father had probably been an apprentice to an older worker at Harrison's.

A wave of faintness had come over me. I had set down my fork on my plate, I could not eat. My heart beat dangerously fast. It was only an exchange at a dinner table—it was, essentially, *nothing*—yet I felt threatened, disgraced. I felt that I had betrayed my father whom I loved. I had betrayed both my parents. Just being here, at the rich doctor's table, was a betrayal of my parents.

Next, Dr. Heike interrogated Cynthia about our chemistry course.

He fired questions at her involving "combustible" chemicals to which Cynthia knew the answers but did not speak clearly. Her tongue seemed too large for her mouth. Chuckling, Dr. Heike said that, next year at Rochester, when she was taking organic chemistry, his "brainy daughter" would need to know a little more than she was getting away with in high school. Impudently I said, "Cynthia gets the highest grades in our class."

It was not exactly true that Cynthia Heike got the very highest grades in the class. There was a boy who, like Cynthia, had a doctor-father and intended to be a doctor, who often got higher grades than she did, scoring 100 percent in quizzes and tests.

By saying this I was also saying *Leave your daughter alone. Your daughter is plenty smart.*

Cynthia glanced toward me startled as if she had no idea who I was. Her left, weak-muscled eye seemed to be swinging loose. Dr. Heike seemed pleased by my remark but could not resist saying, " 'Highest grades' doesn't mean much in itself. Grades are relative. What sort of grades do you get, Joyce?"

In fact, I get high grades too. So go to hell.

"Not so high as Cynthia."

Nor was this true, overall. But it was the right move, as slamming a volleyball across a net, at the level of an opponent's face, and "accidentally" into the face, can be the right move for the moment.

Soon then, Mrs. Heike intervened with a query about the progress of Bach/Schumann and the conversation swerved, like a blind bull, in another direction.

14.

A WEEK BEFORE THE recital Cynthia told me suddenly that she'd changed her mind —"Lee Ann is going to accompany me, after all. It just seemed easier."

I was stunned by this information. *It just seemed easier*—what did that mean?

Obviously it must mean that I wasn't playing well enough, after all our practicing. I was not a "real" musician like Cynthia and Lee Ann—I could not be trusted with Cynthia Heike's violin solo.

Yet I stood mute staring at Cynthia as if I had not entirely heard. Or if, in another moment, there would be another phrase from her, that refuted the first. Seeing the look of shock in my face (which perhaps she had not anticipated) Cynthia murmured an apology of sorts, not very convincingly; for Cynthia could not lie convincingly. An individual of pride and dignity *cannot lie*.

"It just seemed easier," Cynthia said, evasively. "Lee Ann knows the piece pretty well. She can play by ear, you know . . . "

I went away shaken. I did not hear Cynthia calling after me. We were at school, in the corridor outside our homeroom, a tunnel of slamming lockers, contorted faces. Yet soon, when I was alone, and calmer, I understood, and did not blame Cynthia. For one with my musical limitations, a "perfect" performance could only be a fluke. I could not play a composition identically each time; each time, I played differently; I could not "keep time"; I had not a sense of pitch; I could memorize notes, and repeat passages until I'd seemed to master them; essentially, I was untrainable and no amount of practice could remedy that. The fact that I'd had inferior piano teachers in Lockport (whose modest weekly fees my grandmother had paid, happily for years) could not be disguised, for fatally they had allowed me to play piano badly, as they had praised me irresponsibly, and a sharp-eared music student like Cynthia Heike or Lee Ann Krauser could detect such deficits, she had but to listen closely.

THEY WERE FRIENDS AGAIN. Cynthia Heike, Lee Ann Krauser.

They would perform the Bach/Schumann piece beautifully at the recital. And I would wear the navy blue jumper and the white silk blouse that my grandmother had lovingly sewed for me, seated in the audience, and it would not seem evident to anyone who knew the circumstances, even Cynthia herself, that I was disappointed to be seated not onstage at the piano, but in the audience.

Long I would ponder the Zen koan—*It just seemed easier.*

15.

"WE'LL GO TO KLEINHANS. At Christmastime."

Yet, soon after she went away to college, Cynthia Heike ceased to behave like a friend to me.

If I wrote several letters and cards, Cynthia might be provoked into writing a letter—a lengthy, handwritten letter brimming with sardonic insights and witty observations of her sorority/fraternity classmates at the University of Rochester whom she seemed both to despise and envy. Her stationery was adorned with tiny caricature-cartoons in the borders, some of them so small I could not decipher their meaning. Often, she wrote of the "surreal" size of the Rochester campus; she complained of the "vast" lecture courses she was taking, and the "claustrophobic" science labs. If I'd asked questions of her in my letter, she rarely replied to these questions as if she had not read the letter closely but was simply writing to someone to whom she could write intimately, yet not personally.

I hate it here. I think it was a mistake to come here. I don't have any friends here. Just because Daddy got his medical degree here. My silly roommates whisper & laugh among themselves & when I come back late from the library, they roll their eyes and get very quiet. Everyone cheats! In the pre-med courses especially—the profs must know but don't give a damn or don't know how to stop it. C'est de la merde!

Vaguely we'd made plans for mutual visits to our campuses but neither of us seemed to have time. My visit to Rochester, a bus trip of an hour from downtown Syracuse, was several times postponed, then forgotten. At Thanksgiving, when we were both back home, we spoke over the phone briefly; over the long Christmas break, when we might have seen each other, Cynthia didn't call, and when I called her I was hurt by her affected coolness—"*Who* is calling?"—as if she didn't recognize my voice. Half-accusingly Cynthia said that I didn't sound "like myself" somehow. After the new year we stopped calling and writing each other. With the childish spite born of hurt I thought—*If she does write to me, I won't write back.*

From mutual friends whose parents were neighbors of the Heikes came rumors that Cynthia was having "emotional problems" away from home for the first time. Her classmate/rivals in pre-med at Rochester represented a very different sort of competition than our high school classmates; organic chemistry was a particularly challenging course in which Cynthia received the first C's of her life. Even an advanced French course was challenging, to one who'd been so fluent in Madame Henri's low-stress class. And there was the shock of Cynthia's closest friend Lee Ann Krauser, a freshman at Wells College, engaged to be married to a young law student at SUNY Buffalo Law School whom she'd met only the previous summer.

Not just why Cynthia Heike took her own life in February 1957 in her dormitory room at the University of Rochester but, for some time, how—this was part of the terrible mystery. Sleeping pills, slashed wrists, poison?—none of us knew, for the Heikes kept such information confidential. Rumors raged, but no one *knew*. This was an era when universities suppressed news of student suicides; newspapers and TV did not report such deaths unless the suicide was famous and press coverage unavoidable; obituaries were circumspect, and did not include such details. There was a private funeral for Cynthia at her church to which only family members, relatives, and the closest family friends were invited, which did not include me. From a distance I mourned my lost friend, but I made no attempt to get in contact with her family. *It just seemed easier.*

SOME TIME AFTER HER death I would learn that Cynthia had swallowed a corrosive chemical taken from her chemistry laboratory, with the property of a powerful cleanser like *Drano*.

There it is: I have typed that word at last, after fifty-seven years: *Drano*.

"START YOUR OWN BUSINESS!"

A PREVAILING NEED TO *make money*. For never was there *enough money*.

Always the fear that we would lose the farm. This was a fear no less audible for being unarticulated.

It was because the small farm in Millersport did not prosper, that my grandfather John Bush and my father Fred Oates worked in factories in Lackawanna and Lockport respectively. As John Bush died fairly young of emphysema, so my father too would be stricken by emphysema in middle age, but advanced medical treatments allowed him to live well into his mid-eighties—"Half a lung is damn better than no lung."

Clear-minded and cheerfully stoic to the end of his life. My dear father who lived in the country in his in-laws' house initially to save money, and finally because he'd come to love the solitude of Millersport which was—indeed, is—no actual place but rather a mere intersection of Transit Road with Tonawanda Creek Road.

In Millersport, farmland surrounded by a no-man's-land of open fields and forests. And the wide creek (that is actually a small river) snaking through the countryside to join with the Erie Barge Canal and the Niagara River some miles away.

It was no idle fantasy, to fear losing your house and property. For others whom my parents and grandparents knew had lost their land, and finally their houses; no one who'd lived through the Depression ever quite overcame the fear that everything can be lost virtually overnight and even minimal prosperity was a chimera in which one scarcely dared believe. To possess something is to be vulnerable to losing it: possession is audacity in the face of imminent loss.

It was sometime in the late 1950s when my father was inspired to invest in pigs—to start his own business "on a small scale at first." Very likely, Fred Oates had been talked into this adventure by a friend for, being city-born, knowing little of farm life and having little aptitude or enthusiasm for it, he would not have thought of so desperate a measure by himself. Whatever our farm had once yielded by the time I was in high school its primary products were chickens, eggs, corn and Bartlett pears; we also sold apples, cherries, strawberries, cranberries, and such common vegetables as peppers, tomatoes, and cucumbers, in small quantities. We had never owned cows, sheep, or pigs. (Long ago, my grandfather had owned a team of horses but these had passed into oblivion by the time I was born; only their badly weathered wagon remained, abandoned at the rear of the barn.) The saga of the pigs was not a happy one. Though decades later my father would fashion it into an entertaining anecdote there was nothing amusing at the time about raising pigs to butcher and sell their meat.

Not only do pigs stink to a degree that makes the smell of chickens—droppings, wet feathers—seem quaintly "rural" but perversely, pigs are much smarter than chickens and try to resist their destinies as chickens do not; my father was no match for the sagacity of alert young pigs especially, who burrowed beneath the fence he'd built to contain them, and escaped into the countryside. Vividly I can recall my father chasing after pigs along the highway, shouting and cursing and trying to catch them by hand. (Though possibly I never saw this but only heard it described.) Perhaps some of the pigs were never captured. As my Hungarian grandmother had learned to cannily hide wounded or dying pheasants that had fluttered onto our property, shot by hunters in the woods adjacent to our property in the fever of hunting season, so surely our neighbors hid Fred Oates's escaped pigs for their own purposes.

Yet more ironically, after the pigs were slaughtered—not by my father but by a butcher in Lockport—their meat unaccountably spoiled and could not be sold or eaten, for evidently it had been inadequately cured. Fred Oates's entire pig-project, a considerable expenditure of money, time, and spirit was a loss.

Years later my father would transform this humiliating episode in his life into a bittersweet/funny anecdote like a scene in a comic movie, to make people laugh. "Better laugh than cry"—this came to be Fred Oates's belief.

And it was so: we never saw Daddy cry.

ON A FARM EVERYONE works. Farmwork is seasonal and accelerates to a fever pitch in the autumn, at *harvesttime*.

Harvesttime is the time of reaping what you have sown. Or, it is the tragic time when what you have sown fails to be reaped for it has atrophied, or died. Perversely, as if to spite the very persons who labored so hard to bring what has been sown to fruition, it has *failed to thrive*.

Through the summer and well into September we had a small roadside stand fronting Transit Road. Mostly it was Bartlett pears we sold, in season. I helped my mother at the stand, for my father had no interest or perhaps no wish to present himself as a merchant hoping to sell his produce to wayward and unpredictable customers among whom might be people whom we knew; it was Daddy's more difficult, far more frustrating and occasionally dangerous task to pick the pears, climbing a ladder to reach into the higher branches of the trees.

Bartlett pears! On the trees, the pears were greeny-hard as rocks for weeks as if reluctant to ripen; then, overnight, the pears were "ripe"—very soon "over-ripe"—fallen to the ground, buzzing with flies and bees. Apples are hardy and resistant to rotting, apples can be stored in a cool place for months, but pears seem no sooner pale yellow than they are bruised and softening, of no worth. Why did my grandfather John Bush buy a farm with a pear orchard, and not an apple orchard? We had only a few (McIntosh) apple trees, and still fewer cherry trees, both sweet and sour. But rows upon rows of Bartlett trees stretching to the very rear of the property.

It is tempting to think that my grandfather John Bush didn't know that pears are more difficult to harvest than apples. Before moving to the "north country" from Black Rock, in Buffalo, he'd had no experience as a farmer; so far as we knew he'd had little experience as a farmer in Hungary. But perhaps Grandpa thought that his experience with pears would be exceptional.

In spring, the fruit orchard was ablaze with blossoms. Pearly-white pear blossoms, pale pink and white apple blossoms, rosier pink cherry blossoms. And out of these blossoms, fruits were to form, to be one day harvested; out of the luminous beauty of the field of blossoms, the practical matter of *pears, apples, cherries* to be translated into cash.

Often I helped my father pick pears. I could climb the stepladder while Daddy climbed the taller ladder. The rough, vertically-striated bark of a pear tree is permanently imprinted in my memory: its texture is harsh, not pleasant to touch with your fingertips, very different from the smooth skin-like bark of apple trees. There is not much romance in fruit-picking for to reach continually overhead is to soon feel dazed, dizzy; and if you are scouring the ground for fallen fruit that isn't obviously bruised, and so disqualified to be sold at the roadside, you are continually shrinking back from yellow jackets and other buzzing insects. How many bee stings! Filling bushel baskets, one after another. Your right hand begins to ache, then to cramp. Your right shoulder aches. In the heat of September, swarms of gnats, mosquitoes. Harvests of small young mosquitoes biting arms, legs, face.

As children, perversely we would count our mosquito bites. Six, eight, a dozen? But when you are picking pears, the itchy swellings of mosquito bites are not a childish diversion.

Often I've wondered if pear trees, for all their beauty, are among the least resilient of trees, or whether it was just our pear trees that seemed to rot easily, to be infested with bees or swarming ants; to fall apart, crumple from within, as soon as ladders were set against their trunks. At least, pear trees are among the shorter fruit-bearing trees; it is less difficult to pick pears than to pick apples.

Still I am haunted by these beautiful and mysteriously elegiac lines of Robert Frost's "After Apple-Picking"—

My instep arch not only keeps the ache,
It keeps the pressure of the ladder-round.
I feel the ladder sway as the boughs bend.
And I keep hearing from the cellar bin
The rumbling sound
Of load on load of apples coming in.

At the roadside stand I would sit reading. Scarcely aware of my surroundings which is the consolation of reading.

Comic books—*Tales from the Crypt*, *Superman*, *Classics Illustrated* (*Ivanhoe*, *The Last of the Mohicans*, *Moby Dick*, *Robin Hood*, *Sherlock Holmes*, *The Call of the Wild*, *Frankenstein*), *Mad Magazine*.

Or, books from the Lockport Public Library with their crisp plastic covers—Ellery Queen, H. P. Lovecraft, Isaac Asimov. Bram Stoker's *Dracula*. Jonathan Swift's *Gulliver's Travels*. Illustrated editions of *Iliad*, *Odyssey*, *Metamorphoses*, *Oliver Twist* and *David Copperfield*. *Great Dialogues of Plato*.

(Yes, it is bizarre: I was reading, trying to read, Plato as a young girl. More bizarre yet, I was writing my own "Platonic dialogues"— though perhaps Socratic irony was lost on me.)

(Often the librarians at the Lockport library would look at me doubtfully. Who is this girl? Is she really reading these books? *Trying* to read these books? Who is giving her such outsized ideas? But I'd been brought to the library by my grandmother Blanche Morgenstern whom the librarians knew as a loyal patron with an impassioned love of books; since my grandmother had arranged for me to have my first library card there, the librarians may have felt kindly disposed toward me.)

Difficult to concentrate on any kind of reading in such circumstances! At a roadside stand you are distracted by vehicles approaching on the highway, and passing; for the majority of the vehicles pass by without slowing. Only now and then a vehicle will slow, and park at the roadside, and a *customer* will emerge, usually a woman.

"Hello!"

"Hello . . ."

"Is it—Joyce?"

A hopeful smile. Or is it a craven smile. When you are *selling*, you are *smiling*.

Quart baskets, bushel baskets of pears. How much did my parents charge for a bushel basket of pears, I have no idea; surely not much; their prices had to be competitive with commercial vendors, if not lower. If you were a small-time farmer you could pitch your goods so low that you made virtually no profit and worked for nothing.

(All of the farms in our vicinity employed "child labor"—the farm owners' children. Hours of such employment are not negotiable.) Yet I remember the sting of embarrassment when a potential customer, frowning over our pears, or strawberries, or tomatoes, deftly turning back the tight leaves of our sweet corn to examine the kernels, decided that our produce wasn't priced low enough, or wasn't good enough in some way, returned to her car and drove off.

Sitting at a roadside, vulnerable as an exposed heart, you are liable to such rejections. As if, as a writer, you were obliged to sell your books in a nightmare of a public place, smiling until your face ached, until there were no more smiles remaining.

MAKE MONEY! START YOUR Own Business! Mail-order catalogues flooded our rural mailbox bearing the magical name *Joyce Oates*. For in a fever of inspiration I filled out and mailed coupons from Sunday supplements, magazines and comic books, cereal boxes. From the age of twelve onward I was a natural target for such ploys though wanting to think of myself—and thinking of myself, still—as smart, skeptical, suspicious, not-naïve like others my age and even older. My father quoted P. T. Barnum—*There's a sucker born every minute.* Neither my father nor I would have supposed that this insight might apply to anyone in the Oates family.

Like an actor bizarrely miscast for her role I bicycled from house to house for hours gamely trying to sell "beauty products" to neighbors who had little use for beauty, and especially for cosmetic beauty; the leading product was Noxzema, a night cream in a heavy midnight-blue jar with a powerful medicinal odor. (Unsold, these jars remained in the household for years.) For a season I dared to take orders for "costume jewelry" which I made myself with excruciating slowness, from a mail-order kit containing rhinestones, *faux* pearls, rubies, sapphires, tweezers and a tube of glue; for another season I dared to take orders for "artificial flowers"—bright red tulips, bright yellow daffodils, "waxed" lilies ingeniously fashioned from crepe paper and arranged in artistic bouquets. (My mother's female relatives were my most faithful customers, after my grandmother Blanche Morgenstern who bought everything I made as well as extra items as gifts for friends.) In the interstices of these enterprises I sold magazine subscriptions (*Reader's Digest, Pen Pal, Argosy, Collier's, Ladies' Home Journal*); somehow, I acquired a jigsaw and was soon making what were called "lawn ornaments" out of plywood—sheep, cows, flamingos, windmills, dwarves and elves, bonneted girls with sprinkling pails—even, following a popular design, a chocolate-skinned boy eating a very pink slice of watermelon. (These "lawn ornaments" were laid on sheets of newspaper in the grass so that when I painted them, I did not deface any surface indoors or out.) The gift (from my grandmother Blanche) of a "wood-burning" kit allowed me to engrave letters and designs into blocks of wood suitable (as it was advertised) for displaying atop a fireplace mantel. (I can smell still the pungent odor of burning wood as I can feel still that sense of panicked loss, when the wood-burner realizes that she has burnt too deeply or too ineptly, and that a block of wood has been ruined, and will be suitable only for "displaying" at home.) In 4-H crafts club girls made aprons, pot holders, kitchen towels; we braided plastic bracelets, belts, and whistle-holders to be worn around the neck. Some of us learned—to a degree—to knit mittens, caps, sweaters, even socks. We made plaster-of-Paris platters and bowls—a sickeningly cold, slimy sensation of congealing liquid on my fingers, and a strong stench as of raw sewage; these misbegotten, often subtly misshapen objects we painted bright cheerful colors, to be sold, or more likely given to our mothers as presents. (For years, well after I'd gone away to college, my mother continued to use one of my earliest

gifts—a Pepsi bottle ingeniously painted blue and fitted with a per-
forated rubber cap, used to sprinkle water onto clothes being ironed.
Of the many gifts I would give my mother through her lifetime, this
blue sprinkler-bottle was the most practical.) At 4-H sewing class I
undertook to make a skirt—for myself—a "gathered skirt" (essentially, a "gathered skirt" is just drawing threads tight through a wide
swath of cotton material, to constitute a kind of waistband); the hem
was criticized by our instructor for being "unevenly stitched." When
I explained that no one would see the hem the instructor countered,
with unassailable logic, "But, Joyce, you will know it's there."

Yet to my shame I did not tear out the offensive stitches and resew
the hem; probably, as I often did in those days, I gave up the project in childish despair. For it was typical of me to become intensely
involved with projects for a while—occasionally accruing praise in
the effort—only to lose interest abruptly and abandon them. Yet I
have always remembered the pious admonition—*But, Joyce, you will
know it's there.*

Once, 4-H chapters were everywhere in rural America, particularly in the West and Midwest. (For the record: western New York
State is "Midwestern.") The cloverleaf is the 4-H emblem; 4-H colors are white (for purity) and green (for growth). As I had eagerly
memorized Bible verses in order to attend Bible camp at Olcott
Beach, that had promised to be a great adventure, so too a scant year
later I eagerly signed up for numerous 4-H projects in the hope of
self-improvement and acquiring skills to make saleable items. My
major agricultural project was to grow a special kind of jumbo-sized
strawberry: though I set the plants carefully in rows, and was dili-
gent about watering and weeding initially, soon I became bored and
neglectful, and only with my mother's help on the eve of a county
inspector's visit did "Joyce Oates" qualify for some sort of citation
for having satisfactorily completed her 4-H project. (Did I win a blue

ribbon, ever? At least a red ribbon? Surely not at the New York State
Fair at Albany, but possibly at the Niagara County Fair for one of my
ingenious "crafts" or indeed for the jumbo-sized strawberries.) The
most thrilling 4-H competition was square dancing, at which I must
have been fairly capable, since eight of us (four boys, four girls) from
our 4-H chapter were selected to dance on a local Buffalo television
show—the most astonishing sort of celebrity for all of us teenaged
farm boys and girls, if short-lived.

Only vaguely can I remember my farm-boy square-dancing
partner, whose first name was Harvey. Or perhaps his last name was
Harvey. In the television studio, we were so tense, so frightened, so
reluctant even to breathe, our clutching hands were clammy-cold,
yet sweaty. The great achievement of our several minutes of local
fame on WBEN-TV was that not one of us fell down in the dance.

Many times I'd recited the 4-H pledge, with fellow 4-H'ers and
alone, as a kind of secular prayer. Years later the calm unquestioning
words float through my mind like petals on a slow stream:

> I pledge my head to clearer thinking,
> my heart to greater loyalty,
> my hands to larger service,
> and my health to
> better living for my club,
> my community, and my country.

(Reciting the pledge, the 4-H'er uses earnest hand gestures to
indicate head, heart, hands, and health; the hand comes to rest on the
heart, as in the Pledge of Allegiance to the United States of America.
Though religious piety left me restless and uneasy there was something thrilling to me about these words, that promised so much yet
did not seem to seriously commit the pledger to any course of action

and did not evoke any Savior toward whom one was obliged to feel gratitude or guilt. Indeed, it is surprising that the 4-H pledge conspicuously omits any reference to "God"—though in the early 1970s the closing line was expanded to include the words "and my world.")

To recount the tireless energy of my early teenaged years is to feel again something of the fervor of an era when peddling things door-to-door was as common as trick-or-treating at Hallowe'en, and involved the same cast of characters. Though I could not have made much money, I was allowed to save everything that I made, and to have a bank account of my own in a Lockport bank; one of the great pleasures of my life was to contemplate the bankbook and to note the accretion of "interest"—in pennies.

As a slightly older teenager I took on babysitting jobs, like most girls my age; babysitting was more lucrative, less unreliable, than making and trying to sell things. But this career came to an abrupt end when, one evening at the home of a couple who lived about two miles away, on the Tonawanda Creek Road halfway to Rapids, I found myself terrorized for hours by a (drunken?) male relative of the family for whom I was babysitting, who appeared at doors and windows, knocking, teasing and tormenting, insisting that I let him in. I was too frightened to call home—too frightened to pick up the telephone since he could see me; I believed that he might break into the house if I did. And afterward I never dared tell anyone what had happened, for nothing actual had happened; I knew that reporting to my parents would initiate consequences in which I would be made yet more unhappy, and I could not bear being interrogated. But I never babysat again.

It suggests the desperation, and the quixotic nature of such desperation, that I applied for a job in a canning factory in Lockport—indeed, the canning factory in which Helen Judd's mother worked; I applied for a job in the Niagara County Tuberculosis Sanitarium, a ghastly forbidding place on the outskirts of Lockport, set far back from the country highway that led to Olcott Beach. Neither of these applications, and others, resulted even in interviews, for I was too young, and had no experience. I did work—for a single day—at a food tent at the Swormville Volunteer Firemen's picnic, an exhausting and wholly unrewarding experience; other waitresses, my age and older, quit one by one during the interminable day until only a few of us remained, staggering on our feet. Yet my most humiliating experience was another single day as a "cleaning girl" for a woman who lived in a large house in Pendleton: here, under the instructions of the woman, I was obliged to dust, sweep, vacuum, scrub; clean and polish linoleum floors; wash some windows; polish silverware. It was not work for which I had any natural aptitude but I had thought I'd done fairly well and was surprised and hurt that I was never asked to work for the woman again. (Through a 4-H friend I inquired what was wrong and was told that the woman had said: "Joyce's attitude. She looked like she wanted to be somewhere else.")

THE MOST CONTINUOUSLY DESPERATE period of my life, financially speaking, was intermittent through my undergraduate years at Syracuse University. Here, I'd been awarded a New York State Regents scholarship, which enabled students whose parents could not afford the relatively high tuition of private universities to attend universities that, like Syracuse, matched the public scholarships. Still, there were myriad college expenses, not least room and board and books. My parents were very proud of my scholarship but must have felt the economic strain. Though I was the most conscientious of students, I lived in constant anxiety of doing poorly academically and losing my scholarship; any grade below an unambiguous A seemed to me a harbinger of loss to come, and utter defeat. (It should be noted that I was hardly alone in such fears. Virtually every undergraduate whom I knew on a scholarship like mine felt the same way, and some of these, despite their anxieties, did in fact have to drop out.)

At Syracuse, I was grateful to work as a "page" in the university library for as many hours a week as I could manage—for one dollar an hour. This was my first authentic job; I could consider myself now an adult. Alone, stationed on one of the upper floors of the library (that seemed immense to me, for whom a "library" was the Lockport Public Library), as I pushed a cart to reshelf books like an enthralled Alice in Wonderland I could explore the stacks—rows upon rows of stacks—*English Literature, American Literature, Philosophy*; there was an open reading area with a long wooden table that was usually deserted and here I could sit and read with fascination what are called "learned journals" and "literary magazines"—an entire category of magazine utterly unknown to me before college. Discovering these journals was the equivalent of my discovery at age nine of the wonderful *Alice* books. For here was *Poetry*—(in which I read Hayden Carruth's harrowing autobiographical poem "The Asylum")—*Epoch* (the first literary magazine in which a story of mine would appear, under the name "J. C. Oates," in 1960)—*Journal of Metaphysics* (which I read avidly, or tried to read, as if "metaphysics" were as firm and respectable a discipline as physics)—*Modern Fiction Studies* (the first academic literary journal of my life). Equally intriguing were *Philological Quarterly, PMLA, Romanticism, American Literature, American Scholar*. A treasure trove of original fiction, poetry, essays and reviews—*Kenyon Review, Virginia Quarterly Review, Southern Review, Southwest Review, Kenyon Review, Paris Review, Hudson Review, Partisan Review, Dalhousie Review, Prairie Schooner, Shenandoah, Georgia Review, The Literary Review, Transatlantic Review, Quarterly Review of Literature*—the very "little magazines" in which, over the next several decades of my life, my own work would appear.

(My first published story in a national magazine wasn't in one of these, but in *Mademoiselle*, in 1959. Like Sylvia Plath in a previous year's competition I'd received an award from this chic fashion magazine in which, in those days, writing by such distinguished contributors as Tennessee Williams, William Faulkner, Paul Bowles, Katherine Anne Porter, Flannery O'Connor, Jean Stafford, Truman Capote routinely appeared. How improbable this seems to us, by contemporary standards! Yet high-quality fiction appeared in many glossy magazines of the era, *Vogue*, *Harper's Bazaar*, *Cosmopolitan*, intermittently even in *Saturday Evening Post* and *Playboy*, as well as in the more likely *Atlantic*, *Harper's*, *Esquire*, and *New Yorker*. It did feel to me, at the age of nineteen, that my life had been magically touched, if not profoundly altered, by the *Mademoiselle* citation.)

One of the great reading moments in my lifetime—if it isn't more accurately described as a life-altering moment—occurred in the second semester of my freshman year when I entered a classroom in the Hall of Languages, and idly opened a book that had been left behind—a philosophy anthology in which there was an excerpt from the work of Friedrich Nietzsche. A sentence or two of this German philosopher of the nineteenth century, of whom I'd never heard, and immediately I felt excitement, and a kind of rapport; after class I ran to the campus bookstore where with reckless abandonment for one who had virtually no spending money I bought paperback copies of Nietzsche—*Thus Spake Zarathustra*, *The Genealogy of Morals*, *Beyond Good and Evil*—which I have on my bookshelves, heavily annotated, to this day.

For here was one who argued as if "with a hammer"—the very weapon to counter those years of enforced passivity as a quasi-Christian conscripted into an adult world of piety in which nothing was clearly explained, nothing was sincere, and all was obscured; my sense that, as a child, and as a young person, the elders of my world were conspiring to convince me of "beliefs" in which none of them believed, even as the pretense was *Ours is the way, the truth, the light. Only through our way shall you be saved.*

To counter such smug pieties, the devastating voice of the philosopher—*What is done out of love always happens beyond good and evil.*

AS A FRESHMAN I lived not in a dormitory but in a less costly "cottage" on Walker Avenue with approximately twenty other scholarship girls, all of us from upstate New York. (We were "girls" and not "young women"—in age, experience, appearance. This was an era when "girls" were under a kind of protective custody at universities, subject to curfews which male undergraduates did not have. It is an accurate description of the "scholarship girls" of Walker Cottage that none of us minded in the slightest that we had to be back in our residence by 11:00 P.M. weeknights—we had nowhere else we'd have preferred to be than in our rooms, studying.) My room was a single room, cell-like, sparely furnished, where I could work uninterrupted for long hours; for the first time in my life, I was free of the surveillance of my parents, however benevolent this surveillance might have been. And I could work in the university library, until curfew, at the long oak table that seemed magical to me, surrounded by shelves of "little magazines" I came to revere and even to love; I wrote by hand in a spiral notebook, sketches for fiction, outlines, impressions, which I then brought back to the residence to convert into typed pages. Stories, novels—even poetry, and plays—hundreds of pages of earnest undergraduate work which I would not have known to identify at the time as "apprentice work"—much of it discarded, some of it reworked and refined into the stories which I would submit to the writing workshops I took at Syracuse and which would eventually appear in my first book, a story collection titled *By the North Gate* (1963).

If I open that book, composed and assembled so long ago, it's as if I am catapulted back into that era—I can shut my eyes and see again the oak table in the library, the displayed magazines on both sides; I can see again the room in which I lived at the time, the plain table-desk facing a utilitarian blank wall.

As the Lockport Public Library had been a sanctuary for me as a child and young girl, and a hallowed source of happiness, so the library at Syracuse University would be its equivalent, if not more, in my undergraduate years. Overall, Syracuse was a young writer's paradise: my professors Donald A. Dike, Walter Sutton, Arthur Hoffman among esteemed others were brilliant, sympathetic, and unfailingly supportive. (Disclosure: not once was I made to feel, by any of my professors, that as a young woman I was in any way "inferior" to my male classmates. However, it did not escape my awareness that there was but a single woman professor in the English Department and no women at all in Philosophy.)

If the university library was a treasure trove to a word-besotted undergraduate like myself, it was also, I suppose, a little too much for me. My memory of my work-place is of a labyrinth so dimly lighted—for stacks not in use were darkened: you had to switch lights on as you entered the aisles—as to inspire hallucination; here was a universe of books, overwhelming and intimidating and seemingly infinite as a library in a Borges fiction. One could never begin to read so many books—it invited madness just to think that each had been catalogued and shelved. Each had been conscientiously *written*!

One day, I would convert some of these experiences into prose fiction—quasi-memoirist fiction, titled *I'll Take You There*. But not for decades.

"Seventy cents? *Seventy cents?*"—it was a shock to me to receive my weekly paycheck for the first time, to discover that I wasn't even earning a dollar an hour but, after taxes, considerably less. My pride in attending Syracuse University and working in the library was undermined by such reminders of how desperate I was, or how naïve.

When, after the first check, I expressed my dismay to one of the librarians for whom I worked, the woman said, curtly: "It's the same for all of us, Joyce."

Yet I had no choice but to continue at the library. It has been the mantra of my life—I have no choice but to continue.

I would work at the library until it closed at 11:00 P.M., then I would return to my room and study until 1:00 A.M. or 2:00 A.M. It is not uncommon for undergraduates to suffer sleep deprivation. To be chronically short of sleep is akin to being chronically short of money—you have a sense of something crucial missing from your life, that can scarcely be defined for it is not only material and actual, but spiritual. Not in my freshman cottage of scholarship girls but elsewhere, and generally, the student body of Syracuse University was affluent, if not showy. These were conspicuously well-to-do young men and women from New York City and environs, very different from the residents of upstate New York. To be poor amid affluence is to feel oneself both an outsider and yet oddly privileged: as a scholarship girl I was a spy in the house of mirth. I was not alone, yet I was of a distinct minority; on Saturday afternoons in my room in Walker Cottage or in the stacks of the university library I would hear the sound of crowds cheering in the football stadium some distance away, like the cries of another species. How happy they seemed, and how detached I was from their happiness! My aloneness was precious to me if it meant that I could accomplish something—anything. My concern about failing my courses must have inspired over-compensation for I was valedictorian of the Class of 1960.

Forty years later, going through my recently deceased father's papers, I would discover the amount of the New York State Regents scholarship that had made my parents so proud and had so changed my life: it was five hundred dollars a year.

THE LOST SISTER: AN ELEGY

1.

SHE WAS NOT A planned birth.

She was purely coincidental, accidental. A gift.

Born on June 16, 1956. My eighteenth birthday.

"Help us name your baby sister, Joyce."

WE WERE THRILLED, BUT we were also frightened.

Though my brother Robin and I had known for months that our mother was *pregnant*, somehow we had not quite wished to realize that our mother would be *having a baby*.

In the sense in which *having a baby* means a new presence in the household, an entirely new center of gravity. As if a radioactive substance had come to rest in our midst, deceptively small, even miniature, but casting off a powerful light.

At times, a blinding light.

And if light can be deafening, a deafening light.

"HELP US NAME YOUR baby sister, Joyce."

It was a great gift to me, who loved names. I took the responsibility very seriously.

As I was "Joyce Carol" so it was suggested that my baby sister have two names as well.

Names passing through my brain like an incantation.

Names that were fascinating to me, in themselves. Syllables of sound like poetry.

As a young child I had imagined that a name conferred a sort of significance. Power, importance. Mystery. Sometimes when my name was spoken—in certain voices, though not all—I shivered as if my very soul had been touched. I felt that "Joyce Carol" was a very special name for it sounded in my ears musical and lithesome; it did not sound heavy, harsh, dull.

I knew that my parents had named me, and that their naming of me was special to them. I think I recall that my mother had seen the name "Joyce" in a newspaper and had liked the name because it seemed to her a happy-sounding name. But both my parents had named me.

My father who loved music, who played the piano "by ear," often sang, hummed, whistled to himself when he was working or around the house. You could hear Daddy in another room, singing under his breath. The name "Carol" to my father suggested music, song. Somehow, this musical tendency in my father is bound up with my name.

Now, it was my responsibility to name my baby sister.

(DID I CONFER WITH my brother Robin? I want to think that I did.)

FAVORITE NAMES WERE *VALERIE*, *Cynthia*, *Sylvia*, *Abigail*, *Annette*, *Lynn*, *Margareta*, *Violet*, *Veronica*, *Rhoda*, *Rhea*, *Nedra*, *Charlotte*—names of girls who'd been or were classmates of mine in Lockport or in Williamsville; girls who were friends of mine, or might have been; girls I admired close-up, or at a distance; girls who were clearly special, and special to me.

The writer/poet knows that names confer magic. Or, names fail to confer magic. The older sister of the newborn baby knew that the baby's name would be crucial through her life. *She must not be named carelessly but very carefully. With love.*

MY HIGH SCHOOL FRIENDS were nothing short of astonished when I finally told them, as I'd been reluctant to tell them for months, that my mother was going to have a baby in June.

"But your mother is too old!"—one of my friends said tactlessly.

Was my mother even forty? I did not want to think that she was *old*.

Having to tell others of my mother's pregnancy made me painfully self-conscious. I felt my face burn unpleasantly as my girlfriends plied me with questions.

"When did you know?"

"Why didn't you tell anyone?"

"Isn't it going to be strange—a baby in the family? So much younger than you?"

With girlish enthusiasm, perhaps not altogether sincerely, my friends expressed the wish that there might come to be a baby in their households. In their midst I stood faintly smiling, hoping to change the subject.

Not wanting to think—*Why are you smiling? Why are you so happy on my behalf? The baby is my replacement. I will be forgotten now.*

WHEN MY PARENTS TOLD my brother Robin and me about the baby expected in June we'd been surprised, and embarrassed. We must have been somewhat dazed but true to our family reticence, we had not asked many questions. We'd been mildly, moderately happy about the news—I think. At least, we hadn't been unhappy.

Neither of us had exclaimed to the other—*Why are they doing such a thing!*

They don't need a baby in the family, when they have us.

(INDEED, IT SEEMED TO me not long ago when my parents had told me the astonishing news that I had a "new baby brother" whose name was Robin.)

A baby brother! A *baby*!

I'd been five years old. Five and a half. (Such fractions are crucial when you are a child.) I don't recall that I had known that my mother would be having a baby, or that I knew anything at all about human babies. Though I would have seen barn-cats heavily pregnant, that gave birth to litters of kittens, and it could not have been a total mystery to a sharp-eyed child like myself that the kittens had somehow *come out of the momma cat.*

My brother was born at a preposterously inconvenient time, I'd thought: Christmas Day! Was it the baby's *fault*? What could the baby be thinking? Interfering with a five-and-a-half-year-old's long-awaited Christmas Day—December 25, 1943.

His eyes had been robin's-egg blue. A beautiful baby with soft, silky fair-brown hair. How astonished I'd been, and how betrayed I had felt by my parents!

Soon afterward I came to adore my baby brother and was often photographed holding him or playing with him. There is a favorite photograph of us together and Robin is tugging at one of my long corkscrew curls while I gaze down at him with a kind of prim alarm. But when my father brought my mother home from the Lockport Public Hospital with the *new baby brother named Robin* wrapped in a blanket, my reaction was to run away and hide. In a drafty closet of the house I heard my name called—*Joyce? Joyce?*—but refused to answer. I was determined not to answer for a long time.

JUNE 16, 1956, WHICH happened to be, purely coincidentally, my eighteenth birthday.

But no one believes in the purely coincidental. There is a predilection in us to believe in symbolism, which is a kind of purposeful meaning.

What does it mean, my sister has been born on *my birthday*?

Apart from the coincidental date, it was natural to surmise that my parents had planned their third child to be born at about the time their oldest child would be leaving home.

So I found myself thinking, though I knew better. As in later years it would be presented to me as meaningful in some benevolent astrological way, that I'd been born on Bloomsday—I, who would grow up to admire James Joyce.

(And did my parents name me for the great Irish writer?)

(No, no, and *no*.)

But among the relatives, and among my friends, and among anyone who thought they knew my parents, it seemed to be taken for granted that my mother and father had calculated to have a third child to replace the one to be leaving home. *As if anyone could calculate a pregnancy with such precision!*

The fact was, as my (naturally reticent) parents would indicate, the pregnancy seemed to have been an accident. A surprise, possibly a shock to the middle-aged parents, but an accident with no hidden symbolic significance.

A not-unhappy accident.

As my parents would come to view it, a gift.

"It will be easy to remember your birthdays. We can celebrate them both together."

"HELP US NAME YOUR baby sister, Joyce."

But I was having difficulty choosing. Among so many beautiful names, how to select just two?

I understood, of course—asking me to name my baby sister was a kindly way of involving me in her presence in the family, so that I would not feel slighted, or cast away.

Or perhaps my parents sincerely believed that I was the one in the family who had a way with *words*, and was to be entrusted with this responsibility.

Did I love my baby sister? Yes. For I could not help myself seeing the baby in my mother's arms; seeing how happy my mother was, and my father; feeling my eyes fill with tears.

Was I ever so small? Did they ever love me so much?

It is claimed that the firstborn of a family will always feel, in an essential way, very special, "chosen." Yet it seems logical that the firstborn is the one to be displaced, whether graciously or rudely, by the secondborn; still more, by the thirdborn.

In a large family each sibling must feel not so very "chosen"— not likely to feel self-important. Yet, surrounded by brothers and sisters, wonderfully not-alone.

It seemed natural to me, the new baby must nullify the others in my parents' emotions: my brother, myself. The very vulnerability of a new baby is a displacement of the so much less vulnerable older children. This was something to be accepted as inevitable, and desirable.

As if my parents were nudging me to think, sensibly—*You are an adult now, or nearly. You are ready to leave home. And now, you will leave home.*

THE NAME I FINALLY chose for my baby sister was "Lynn Ann"— for the gliding *n*-sounds.

2.

No. I can't speak of her.
It is not possible. The words are not available.

As she has no speech, so I have no ready speech to present her.
I am not allowed to "imagine"—and so, I am helpless.
There is no way. There is no access.
There is only distance, as across a deep chasm.

If there is a way it is oblique, awkward.
It is the way of one foot in front of another, and another—
plodding, cautious of the steep fall.

It is not exactly cowardly—(I suppose: for if I were cowardly
I would never undertake such a hopeless task but flee from it)—
but it is cautious. It is not the sort of pain that becomes pleasurable.

Reckless to press forward when you know you will fail and yet—
you cannot go forward except by this route.

You cannot pretend: your sister was never born.

SPOKEN QUICKLY AND CARELESSLY, "autistic" can sound like "artistic."

IT WAS NOT REALLY true that I'd fled to college. More accurately, it was time for me to depart and so I departed.

And after I graduated from college, I went to graduate school at the University of Wisconsin at Madison, where I met, fell in love with, and married Raymond Smith. And so I never came home again to live in Millersport.

At the time it wasn't known—it was not yet suspected—that my sister would have severe "developmental disabilities." For such suspicions are slow to manifest themselves in even the most alert, responsible, and loving parents.

After five or six years, when my husband and I were living and teaching in Detroit, Michigan, I began to hear that my parents were taking my sister to doctors in the Buffalo area, having been referred by her Lockport pediatrician who understood that there was nothing he could do, nor even confidently name.

Lynn doesn't look at us. She doesn't talk, or try to talk.
She doesn't seem to recognize us. She will only eat certain foods.
She is getting to have a bad temper.

THE TERM "RETARDED" MIGHT have been suggested. But never did I hear "retarded" spoken in our household, nor did I ever speak this term in any way associated with my sister.

There may have been a taboo of sorts, against the articulation of this word with its associations of poverty, ignorance, dementia. A crude word sometimes used as an epithet of particular cruelty.

Eventually, the diagnosis "autistic" came to be spoken. (By my father, gravely. So far as I knew my mother would not ever utter this word which would have greatly pained her.) Not much was known of *autism* at this time (in the mid-1960s) but there was a distinction between *autism* and *mental retardation* that seemed crucial to maintain.

For *mental retardation* was not uncommon in the north country, in those years. I have not spoken in this memoir of the numerous examples of "retarded" persons I'd encountered in the vicinity of Millersport and in Lockport, mostly school-age; how there would seem to have been a disproportionate number, compared to my experience elsewhere, later in my life; so that, when I think of *mental retardation*, immediately I am thinking of certain rural families, and of their offspring, routed into "special education" classes in school, and generally shunned, avoided, or in some unhappy cases teased and tormented by the presumably normal.

In the Judd family, for instance, there was very likely *mental retardation*. But I did not want to dwell upon this likelihood in writing about my friend Helen Judd, for that was not my subject; that *mental retardation, sexual abuse of children and incest* were related in crucial ways seems to us obvious, but requiring of greater length and space to examine.

My grandmother Blanche Morgenstern did not seem to accept this diagnosis of "autism," in fact. It seemed to be her (implicit, unargued) conviction that there was nothing seriously wrong with her younger granddaughter. Year following year she took the Greyhound bus from Lockport to visit her son's family in Millersport and with each visit she brought a present for Lynn, as she'd once brought presents for me—coloring books, Crayolas, picture books; each present, as my brother dryly remarked, our sister destroyed within a few minutes, with varying degrees of fury.

What will become of Lynn, do you think?
What will become of Mom and Dad?

IT MAY BE DIFFICULT for others to understand, very little of this was ever discussed in our family, at least not among my parents and my brother and me. By degrees Lynn Ann became my parents' unique and in a way sacred responsibility, as it is said children afflicted with Down's syndrome are particularly loved by their parents; not as a "problem" but as a sort of "gift." You might ask after Lynn in the most casual and sunny of ways—"How's Lynn?"—and the answer was likely to be "Good." But the matter of Lynn Ann Oates was a private one, and such privacy was inviolable.

None of my friends from high school or college would ever meet my sister. My husband Raymond Smith would never meet my sister. For nearly fifteen years my parents lived in a kind of quarantine with my sister; few people visited them, for few would feel comfortable in a setting in which a seemingly deranged/retarded girl roamed freely, ran in and out of rooms. Or perhaps my parents simply didn't want anyone to visit, which is equally likely.

Until her final illness, my grandmother Blanche continued to visit Millersport bearing her symbolic gifts. My grandmother deeply loved her son and his family, for she had no family otherwise; what we knew of her remarriage, after her young, handsome Irish husband Carleton Oates had abandoned her decades before, did not seem happy, and did not bear examination. (Is it my family's reticence, or is this not-wishing-to-violate-another's-privacy commonplace?) Perhaps it was an expression of love, respect, dignity that you did not ever ask any question that would embarrass another, or suggest that a facade of domestic happiness was not altogether sincere.

Certainly, no one spoke of Lynn in any way other than casual. In my memory, any discussion of Lynn was not welcomed at all.

What will become of us! We are badly in need of help.

FOOLISH TO HAVE LEFT my paperback copy of Henry James's *The Golden Bowl* on a table in my parents' living room. I'd come home to visit for a few days and unthinking left some of my books where Lynn could find them. All of the books were destroyed but it's only *The Golden Bowl* I recall, the irony, the pathos, James's great web of words, printed words, as impenetrable to my sister as Sanskrit would be to me, and for that reason richly deserving of destruction.

Or, more plausibly: my rampaging sister destroyed the book not knowing it was a *book* or even that it was *Joyce's book* but only that it was an object new in the household, therefore out of place, offensive to her sense of decorum or order.

It is painful to recall: my sister would tear pages in her fists, she would tear at the pages with her teeth. She would make high-pitched strangulated cries, or she would grunt, in her misery, frustration, desperation. She would not ever—not once—so much as look at me, though she must have sensed my presence.

(Though she could not have known how uncannily she resembled me, and I resembled her. *Like twins separated by eighteen years.*)

It was inanimate objects my sister would attack, generally. She would never attack me.

(And yet—one day, she might have attacked me. As a pubescent child, older, taller, stronger, very likely Lynn would have attacked me, as she would one day attack my mother.)

How vivid it is still, the ravaged copy of *The Golden Bowl* with its eloquent, elaborate, and all but impenetrable introduction by R. P. Blackmur. Badly torn, and the lurid imprint of small sharp teeth on what remained of the pages.

"Oh, Lynn! What did you *do*."

I was acutely aware of my mother in the kitchen doorway a short distance away, who'd come to see what was wrong. If words were exchanged between my mother and me at this time I have forgotten those specific words.

Very likely my mother had suggested that it was my own fault for having left the books in that vulnerable place where Lynn would find them. And of course this was true. If there was *fault* here, it could only be my own.

In the kitchen my excited sister was on her feet but hunched and rocking from side to side making her strangulated *Nyah-nyah-nyah* sound. It was not laughter, and it was not derisive or taunting—it was purely sound, devoid of meaning. At this time Lynn might have been eight, nine, ten years old—a child who grew physically, but not mentally.

The confrontation with *The Golden Bowl* had been the child's triumph but it had left her dangerously over-excited, there was the danger that she might attack something else now, or someone.

Still, they kept Lynn at home until she was fifteen. And taller and heavier than my mother, and very excitable. And dangerous.

And that would be the last time I saw my sister, at about the age of fifteen.

IT WAS REPEATEDLY SAID of her—*But Lynn seemed perfectly normal as a baby. She was so beautiful! She gave no sign.*

Was it so, Lynn had given no sign? Who can recall, so many years later?

In retrospect, we see what we are hoping to see. We see what our most flattering narrative will allow us to see. But *in medias res* we scarcely know what we are seeing, for it happens too swiftly to be processed.

For it came to be a story told and retold—no doubt, recounted endlessly by my parents to doctors, therapists, nurses—of how when she'd been very young, two or three years old, Lynn had fallen and fractured or broken her left leg. For many weeks she had to wear a cast. She'd been walking, or trying to walk; now she reverted to crawling, or dragging her leg along the floor. She wept, she rocked her little body from side to side in the very emblem of child misery. Later it was speculated (by my parents, but also by others) that, at this crucial time in her development, whatever progress Lynn had been making—learning to walk, to speak, to communicate—was retarded.

It was said of the afflicted child—*She thinks she is being punished. How can we make the poor child understand, she is not being punished?*

How make her understand, she is loved?

Possibly, the heavy cast on Lynn's leg had something to do with her mental deficiencies, which grew more evident with time. Yet possibly, the cast on Lynn's leg had nothing at all to do with her mental development.

Some years later it would be suggested (by one of the numerous specialists to whom Lynn was eventually taken) that "autism" is a form of schizophrenia caused by bad mothering.

Bad mothering. It is very hard for me to spell out these cruel and ignorant words.

Carolina Oates, the warmest and most loving of mothers, made to feel by (male) "specialists" that she was to blame for her child's mental disability!

For years we were distressed by this crude "diagnosis." We knew that it was not true—my mother was not "cold and aloof" as the bad mother is charged; but this pseudo-science was confirmed by the general misogynist bias of Freudian psychoanalytic theory in which the mother (alone) is the fulcrum of harm—the mother who "causes" her son's homosexuality, for instance. (And what of the father's role in a child's development? Has the father no corresponding responsibility, or guilt?) The fraudulent diagnosis hurt my mother terribly, and surely entered her soul. You do not tell a woman who is already distressed by her child's disability that it is her fault.

So many years later I am upset on behalf of my gentle, soft-spoken and self-effacing mother who'd given as much as any mother might give in the effort of a futile and protracted maternal task. My mother was not so much upset as crushed, shamed. And this for years.

Blaming the mother for autism, indeed for schizophrenia or homosexuality, would seem no less reprehensible than the popular treatment of the 1940s and early 1950s for bad behavior of another kind, the lobotomy, now thoroughly discredited.

The misogyny of science, particularly psychology! Those many decades, indeed centuries, when the medical norm was the white male specimen and the female a sort of weak aberration from that norm, when not openly assailed condescended to, pitied, and scorned. Do you know that the much-revered "Father of Modern Gynecology" J. Marion Sims (1813–1884) was a doctor who experimented upon his African-American female slaves, without anesthetics, over a period of years; that he performed gynecological operations, without anesthetics, on Irish (i.e., non-"white") women who were too poor and uneducated to protest? By the by, the revered Dr. Sims also experimented on African-American infants. If you know these lurid facts, perhaps you also know that there is a statue of the Father of Modern Gynecology still in Central Park, New York City—indeed, Dr. Sims is the first American physician to have been honored with a statue. And so for me to lament the crude, careless mistreatment of my mother by "specialists" in child development in mid-twentieth-century America in western New York State is surely naïve.

Decades later in the twenty-first century a newer, neurophysiological examination of the phenomenon of autism suggests that the condition isn't caused by bad parenting of any kind but by congenital brain damage.

Neurochemistry, not "bad mothering."

Still, the old misogyny dies hard. You will still find plenty of people including presumably educated clinicians who will tend to blame the mother for a pathology of the child.

In recent years there has been a populist, anti-scientific movement against vaccinations, based upon the (erroneous) belief that vaccinations cause autism in young children; more widely, and more convincingly, neuroscientists believe that the causes of autism are manifold: genetics, environment. No single factor will "cause" autism but there are conditions that are likely to increase the possibility of autism. Yet unaccountably, at the time of this writing, incidents of autism seem to be on the rise in the United States.

Those of us who know autism intimately have long been baffled by high-profile cases of "autism" in the public eye. Dustin Hoffman in *Rain Man*, Temple Grandin as author, speaker, animal theorist. Such individuals seem very mildly autistic compared to my mute, wholly disengaged sister who was never to utter a single coherent word let alone give public lectures and write best-selling books. (But Temple Grandin's ingenious invention of a "hug-box" to hold her, who shrank from human touch and contact, might have been an excellent device to contain my sister's fits of excitement and distress.)

It is even being proposed, in some quarters, that autism might be celebrated as a kind of "neurodiversity." Just as a considerable number of deaf persons do not wish to be made to hear, but prefer the silence of sign language to oral speech, so there are those, among them Temple Grandin, who believe that autism should not be eradicated, if any cures might ever be developed.

This is a romantic position, but it is not a very convincing position, for one who knows firsthand what severe autism is. Even if autism could speak, from its claustrophobic chambers, could we believe what autism might say? And how responsible would we be, to act upon that belief?

3.

IN 1971, WHEN LYNN was fifteen years old, my father at last arranged for her to be committed to a therapeutic care facility in the Buffalo area for mentally disabled individuals like herself, who had become too difficult to be kept at home. This was a decision very hard for my parents to make though it would seem, to others in the family, belated by years—long overdue.

One day, my sister had "turned on" my mother in the kitchen of my parents' house. Since neither of my parents wished to speak in any way negative or critical about Lynn, and did not willingly respond to queries about their safety in continuing to keep her at home, I never learned details of the attack. But I had long worried that something like this might happen, and that my mother, who spent virtually all of her waking hours caring for my sister, might be badly injured; at the very least, my mother would be exhausted and demoralized.

You could not simply say to such devoted parents—*But you have to put Lynn in a home! You are not equipped to take care of her.*

My normally reasonable father was not reasonable when it came to discussing this domestic crisis. It was not advised to bring the subject up, for Daddy would quickly become defensive and incensed. To speak in even a hushed and apologetic voice was to risk being disloyal, intrusive. The strain on my mother, who was Lynn's primary caretaker, day following day and week following week for years, was overwhelming; eventually her health was undermined. I would one day learn that my mother was taking prescription tranquillizers to deal with the stress of taking care of Lynn, and this with my father's approval. My father, of course, spent most of his time at work—out of the house.

By this time my parents were living in a small ranch house they'd had built on the original farm property; the old farmhouse and the farm buildings had been demolished. My Hungarian grandmother Lena Bush had died. My brother Robin—that is, Fred, Jr.—was in his late twenties, married, and living some miles away in Clarence, New York. The old life of the farm, the life of my childhood, was irrevocably lost and in its place, it sometimes seemed, a surreal nightmare of domesticity: my beloved parents, no longer young, in a single-storey clapboard ranch house like so many others on Transit Road, obsessively tending to their mentally ravaged daughter who so uncannily resembled the elder daughter whose place she had taken.

It must have been a relief for my parents, particularly my mother, when Lynn was at last committed to a therapeutic facility—yet at the same time, a kind of defeat. They had tried so hard to keep their daughter at home; they had not wished to concede that something was wrong with her, and that she might be a danger to others as to herself. *They had loved Lynn no less than they'd loved their older daughter and their son Fred and this love for Lynn would never abate.*

In this facility near Buffalo, which specialized in the care of autistic and other brain-damaged young people, my sister would receive excellent professional care. Eventually she was placed in a group home with five other patients; all were taken by van to a school for the disabled, five days a week, six hours a day. In these highly structured communities it is said that the mentally disabled are happiest.

It is the exterior world that distresses them, the world inhabited by their "normal" brothers and sisters. For in their confined world they are safe and at peace.

I would think she has a horrible life but she does not seem sad—so my brother has said.

THE SHINY HELMET LOOKS heavy and unwieldy but in fact it is made of a very light plastic. The interior is padded and is (said to be) comfortable, like the interior of a bicycle helmet. The chin straps are easily adjustable and (it is said) not likely to cause strangulation or injury except in the most freakish of circumstances when the afflicted individual is bent upon injuring himself.

At some point in adolescence Lynn began to suffer seizures that resemble epileptic seizures. Though these are controlled to a degree by medication, she is obliged to wear a safety helmet at all times except when she is secure in her bed.

Doctors have said—*She isn't angry. As we understand anger.*

Carefully they have said—*Your sister does become frustrated. It is typical of those with her condition, to become frustrated. Her face is sometimes contorted in what appears to be a look of rage or anguish but it is not a psychological or emotional expression of the kind one of us might feel. It is an expression caused by a muscular strain or spasm in the face.*

Do not think that it is hostility directed toward you.

Do not think that she is aware of, or in any way responding to, you.

ACROSS THIS ABYSS, THERE is no possibility of contact.

It is romantic to think so. It is consoling to think so. And so my parents never gave up hoping, and perhaps (they imagined) they were able to bridge that abyss. Certainly they brought Lynn home with them every Sunday without fail until they were too ill and too elderly to do so, even after she began to have seizures occasionally, and had to wear her safety helmet at all times during the day; even when it was clear that she did not "know" them and that, after a while in their house, always kept clean and tidy before her arrival, she began to fret with discomfort, wanting badly to be returned to the facility which was now more familiar to her, and more, if she'd had a word for such a place, her "home."

No one would have wished to contest my parents' conviction that they could communicate with their younger daughter. Nor did they speak of it. Their love for this daughter was intensely private even as it appeared to be, to others in the family, infinite in its patience, generosity, fortitude. This is what is meant by "unqualified love"— that does not diminish over time. It is heartrending to think that my parents loved my brother and me in this way also, not more than they loved our sister but surely not less, and not because of religious conviction, or even ethical principle, but because this was their nature.

A parental love as natural as breathing, or dreaming.

YOUR SISTER HAS NEVER once acknowledged you.

Your sister has never once looked at you.

Your sister has never once glanced at you.

Your sister has no idea who you are, what you are.

That you are, that you exist your sister has no idea.

No idea that anyone else exists, as she can have no idea that she herself exists.

If there is a riddle, your sister is the riddle.

Here is the *tough nut to crack*. The *koan*.

Disconcerting how with her dark brown eyes, wavy dark brown hair and pale skin, your younger sister so resembles *you*.

Anyone who sees her, and sees you—looks from one to the other—feels this *frisson* of recognition: how your sister who is eighteen years younger than you and who has never uttered a word in her entire lifetime so strikingly resembles *you*.

She will not meet your eye no matter how patiently, or impatiently, you wait. For she is not like *you*.

She is an individual without language. It is not possible for you to imagine what this must be, to be without language.

For nearly sixty years she has lived in silence. She does not hear the voices of others as we hear voices; but she has learned to hear in her therapeutic classes at the facility. Her own speech is grunts, groans, moans, whimpers and cries of frustration and dismay. She does not laugh, she has not ever learned to laugh.

In the presence of the brain-damaged we find ourselves in the Uncanny Valley. It is we who are made to feel unease, even terror. I am made to feel guilt—for I have had access to language, to spoken and to written speech, and she has not. And this, by an accident of birth.

Not what we deserve, but what is given us.

Not what we are, but what we are made to be.

I HAVE NOT SEEN my afflicted sister since 1971, when she was fifteen years old. Tall for her age, wiry-thin, gangling, with pale skin, an expression in her face of anger, anguish—or as easily vacancy and obstinacy. *A mirror-self, just subtly distorted. Sister-twin, separated by eighteen years*. Though I have thought of Lynn often in the intervening years, I have not seen her; initially, because my parents would not have wished this, and eventually, because such a visit would be upsetting to her, as to me. And futile. *She would not know me, nor even glance at me. What I would know of her, I could not bear.*

It is difficult to imagine a mouth that has never uttered a single word, and has never smiled.

Eyes that have never lifted to any face, still less "locked" with another's gaze.

All literature—all art—springs from the hope of communicating with others. And yet, there are others for whom the effort of communication is not possible, or desirable.

Seems like she doesn't know we're here.

What do you think she is thinking?

PERHAPS THIS IS THE unanswerable question: does the brain *think*?

If the brain is sufficiently injured, or undeveloped: can the brain *think*?

In itself, perhaps the brain does not *think*; it is the human agent within the brain, which some have called the soul, that *thinks*. And yet—can a soul, or a mind, be differentiated from its brain? We speak of "our" brain as if we owned it, in a way; as we might speak of "our" ankle, "our" eyes. But such common usage is misguided, perhaps. *We are nothing apart from our brains, thus it is our brains that think. Or fail to think.*

Obviously, our brains generate consciousness—but this is an unconscious process. We are habituated to believe, at least in our Western tradition, that "we" are located somewhere inside our brains, behind our eyes; for it is our eyes "we" see through. When we look into the eyes of others, as we speak to them, we are looking "into" the brain, that is the core of personality—or so we think. (It is unnerving to think that just as our personalities reside in an organic, perishable brain, in some infinitely vast network of neurons beyond all efforts of tracking, the personalities of others reside in a similar place.) Except, of course, in some individuals, there is no "eye contact"—the brain refuses to function in accord with our expectations.

In April 2014, fourteen years after our father's death, in response to a query, my brother brings me up-to-date on our sister's condition, which seems unchanged:

Lynn is totally non-verbal and does not talk at all. She has frequent seizures and wears a helmet at all times to protect her when she falls . . . She does not recognize me nor do I think she recognizes anyone at all. She is shy, and does not like it when her routine is changed.

"HELP US NAME YOUR baby sister, Joyce."

It was a festive time. It was in fact my birthday: my eighteenth birthday. I had not been forgotten after all.

My parents smiled with happiness. It was their hope that if I helped to name my sister that I would love her, too.

This was long ago. Yes, it was a happy time.

For so much lay ahead, unanticipated. No reason to anticipate the wholly unexpected of years to come.

After days of deliberation I presented my parents with the name that seemed to me the ideal name—*Lynn Ann Oates.*

A very nice name, they said. "Thank you, Joyce."

NIGHTHAWK: RECOLLECTIONS OF
A LOST TIME

WHERE WE FIND OURSELVES is often not where we've sent ourselves. One day it happens we are awakened to the thought *Here. Here I am. Why?*

Madison, Wisconsin. September 1960. For the first time in my (relatively) young life, I'd flown alone—I arrived at the small airport in Madison breathless with anticipation. No doubt, I had not slept the night before in anticipation of the *flight into the unknown*. For I was leaving home after a brief summer in Millersport, after graduating from Syracuse University; this time, enrolled in graduate school at the University of Wisconsin with the intention of earning a master's degree in American literature and, if all went well, eventually a Ph.D.—it seemed clear to me, as to my parents, that I was leaving home permanently.

I was twenty-two years old. Though it seems preposterous to me now, at the time twenty-two did seem somewhat *old*.

At Syracuse, a special aura could be perceived about certain girls—(in the parlance of contemporary twenty-first-century usage, "young women")—who, though possibly not distinguished academically, and with no plans to attend a prestigious graduate school to earn an advanced degree, nonetheless basked in their great good luck: engaged to be married.

This was a particular category of girl, the *fiancée*. The *fiancée* was one who'd been given an engagement ring, and this ring on the third finger of the left hand conferred a blessing of such value, it could hardly be described. As one who had no hope, though perhaps also no great wish, to be a *fiancée*, or to wear an *engagement ring*, I stood at a little distance from my companions in that social world, in a kind of penumbra. Any girl who graduated from college in 1960 who was not a *fiancée*, and did not have an engagement ring, was made to feel, however foolishly, *old*. You might joke about it, and if you were literary- or artistic-minded you would certainly feel superior to such conventional prejudices, and yet—you could no more escape that atmosphere than you could cease breathing toxic air. If you were there, you breathed it.

Vividly I recall one of my classmates lifting her ring hand so that we could admire the minuscule yet unmistakable diamond— "At least, I'm engaged before graduation." An intelligent and mature girl, yet Diane spoke without irony.

Unknowingly, by enrolling in graduate school, I was escaping this atmosphere almost entirely. Never again would I live in any social environment in which *being engaged* was so crucial; never again, in any environment in which *to be married* was so high a priority. (Nor did I live in a social environment in which having children was a high priority.) Yet, I'd never anticipated this escape, for I had not really known what graduate school would or might be. Naively, I had imagined it as essentially an extension of undergraduate life and not, as it would turn out in Madison, an entirely different experience.

Though in years I was an adult, in experience I was still very much an adolescent. I did not look twenty-two—I scarcely looked twenty. In my classes and seminars at Syracuse I'd been one of the shy girls—it would astonish and embarrass me, years later, to read recollections about my undergraduate self from a selection of professors and classmates, about how intensely shy I was. (Even now I want to protest—*But I could not have been so shy! That is not possible—is it?*)

It is humbling to discover that our former selves, recollected by contemporaries, were so imperfect. And imperfect in ways we hadn't quite allowed ourselves to realize at the time. Though we may recall dramatic incidents clearly, we are not so likely to recall the daily, hourly texture of our lives with others.

Painfully shy. Would not speak in our fiction workshop so Professor Dike read her short stories to us.

At twenty-two I had not yet quite dared to think of myself as a *writer*—though I'd published some short stories by September 1960, and one of my professors, Donald A. Dike, had particularly encouraged me. (Professor Dike whose literary heroes were Faulkner and Conrad had strongly urged me not to go to graduate school but just to "write"—living anywhere except near a university campus.) I was naïve, romantic-minded, and vulnerable to hurt as if the outermost layer of my skin had been peeled away; the most wonderful thing about having been valedictorian of my graduating class at Syracuse was the fact that, at commencement, which was outdoors, a ferocious rainstorm had ended the ceremony abruptly, and I hadn't had to deliver my commencement speech to thousands of strangers spread out before me in a football stadium—a responsibility that had filled me with terror for weeks beforehand. (Yet I've never forgotten the excellent advice given to me by the faculty advisor for the valedictorian: "When you stand up to speak, they will be waiting for you to sit down.") Though generously praised by my professors, and a recipient of a Knapp Fellowship from the University of Wisconsin (which meant that I could complete a master's degree in a single year since unlike most graduate students in English I would not be required to teach), I was uncertain, insecure, as a newly licensed pilot on her first solo flight in a small plane—doubtful about the good judgment of my instructors who'd licensed me and encouraged me as about my own ability not to disintegrate mid-air and crash.

By romantic-minded I mean in terms of books, literature, a career of teaching. Since first grade at the one-room schoolhouse in Millersport, I had always wanted to be a teacher and indeed such a life seems magical to me even now after decades—*teacher*.

And what of my own writing? All summer I'd been working on a novel with the hopeful Joycean/Faulknerian title *Proserpina*—one of several novels I'd written as an undergraduate at Syracuse. These were "experimental" works of fiction undertaken for no clear purpose other than to lose myself in the discipline of novel-writing. It was my vague hope that, at Madison, I would continue with writing fiction in the interstices of graduate school work, though I understood that my graduate studies would be demanding. With the blithe disregard for the future of one who has not really thought through what the future might bring I seem to have assumed that my writing—my fiction writing—would always in some way assert itself, like tough, sinewy wildflowers bursting through cracks in concrete; I would not actually need to *make time for it*.

It had been an astonishing surprise, to learn that I'd received a Knapp Fellowship to Wisconsin; as great a surprise as learning that I'd been a co-winner of the *Mademoiselle* fiction contest in 1959. The sheer size of the university was daunting, for it was much larger than Syracuse, with twenty schools and somewhere beyond thirty thousand students; winters in Madison were reputed to be worse even than winters in Syracuse. Yet I felt vaguely encouraged to learn that the state of Wisconsin had a history of political "progressivism"; despite the notorious Senator Joseph McCarthy, there had been socialist politicians elected to office in the state for decades. When I thought of politics it was invariably my grandfather John Bush who came to mind—whose convictions were somewhere left of socialism though (so far as I knew) "the Brush" had never evinced the slightest interest in joining the Communist Party, or any party; nor was it possible to imagine any organization that would have wished him to join. My father had particularly loathed the duplicitous "red-baiting" Senator Joseph McCarthy (R, Wisconsin) but conceded that, overall, Wisconsin was an "enlightened" state, and that the University of Wisconsin at Madison appeared to be one of the great land-grant universities in the country. (When my father spoke of college, it was with a wistful air. He had taken an interest in my courses at Syracuse and had done some of the reading for my American literature classes. How Daddy would have loved to have been educated beyond the eighth grade! But he and my mother would never visit me in Madison during my single year there for there wasn't money for such non-urgent trips; nor could they have left my sister Lynn with any caretaker.)

Despite its excellence, the University of Wisconsin at Madison would not have been a first choice for me, for graduate school; it was too far away from Millersport, which meant that I might not be able to return home even over the long Christmas break. (In those days, at least for people like myself, air travel was enormously expensive, and seemed daunting; as one did not casually make long-distance telephone calls, unless after eleven o'clock at night, and then infrequently, so one did not fly casually.) It was at the urging of my Syracuse professors that I applied to the "outstanding" English department at the university, and obviously their letters of recommendation must have been strongly supportive. I had not considered that writing could be a self-sustaining life or any sort of career; writing sprang from my deepest, most private self and could have nothing to do with *earning a living*.

Later it would seem to me the most extraordinary sort of luck, the flimsiest sort of chance, that had brought me to this university at the age of twenty-two, and not to another university equally likely for a young student like myself intending to study English and American literature—Cornell, University of Michigan, University of Minnesota. For then, I would not have met my husband-to-be Raymond Smith: an alternative life, without Raymond, is not fathomable to me.

To be young is to be particularly vulnerable to the vagaries of luck; to tear open an envelope and discover that your life has been set upon a course you could not have predicted.

When you are young, each day can be the start of a great adventure. And the adventure one of growth, happiness, prosperity—or derailment, disintegration, despair.

For always at the back of my mind there hovered the spectral figure of my lost friend Cynthia. Rarely did I think of Cynthia by day, only by night. And in my dreams, Cynthia's identity had dissolved, even her facial features were blurred. *You are as much myself, as another. You are myself.*

IT SEEMS A FACT rarely acknowledged, that fantasies of self-hurt flourish when we are alone, and lonely; when homesickness fastens like a leech to an exposed artery. Though I was not ever "suicidal"— the very word is a kind of posturing, wrongly used by those who have never actually felt this way—it did seem to me, it had seemed to me for years, that my friend Cynthia had somehow "shown the way" for the rest of us, her friends; her friends who had not quite loved her enough, perhaps; or had not known her fully, that we might have loved her, and saved her. *The saddest fantasy, that we might save another from self-hurt. The wish, the yearning, to have been so meaningful in another's life.*

I had told no one, and I would tell no one, that my strongest motive for leaving New York State and journeying to Wisconsin—just far-enough away to make visits difficult—was an emotional quagmire which, naively, but as it turned out accurately, I hoped that sheer distance would resolve.

This great adventure! An intellectual adventure, as I was not equipped to deal with an emotional adventure. I'd fled the East because I had no wish to marry a young man, a chemistry major, with whom I'd become emotionally involved; and yet within five swift months in the Midwest I would fall in love, and marry; within ten months I would become profoundly and irremediably disillusioned with the Ph.D. academic-scholarly profession even as I was (grudgingly) granted a master's degree qualifying me to teach literature in a college or university (as it would happen I would do for decades, very happily).

The malaise of Madison, Wisconsin, was the more difficult to absorb because it was so enmeshed with happiness, as a tumorous growth is enmeshed with healthy veins and tissue and cannot be easily extricated. What was stunning to me, and could not have been predicted (by me), was that, in graduate school, I would be unable to write anything genuine, anything real, anything that "sprang from the heart," but only critical/scholarly papers; a development that would have seemed to me until this perilous time equivalent to ceasing to dream, or to breathe.

At Syracuse, our professors were scholars and critics to a degree, but they were also very good, very encouraging and lively instructors; at Madison, our professors were predominantly scholars, secondarily critics, and hardly instructors at all, if by "instructor" is meant an individual who is intellectually and emotionally engaged with his or her material and students. The mode of instruction at Madison was lecturing: the scholar-professor *lectured to*, the classroom or seminar room of students *listened*. (In one unsettling instance, a renowned American literature scholar simply read from his own book, on the subject of the New England Pilgrims; we graduate students listened, we took notes, we despaired and sighed with boredom, but we prevailed. Or most of us prevailed.) Our professors, most of them Harvard-educated, were at least a generation older than my Syracuse professors had been, and resisted, or were oblivious to, even the analytical/text-oriented New Critical approach to literature, that had become influential in the 1950s; to these conservative elders, with the (notable, wonderful) exception of the medievalist Helen C. White, for whom I wrote an inspired long paper on the English and Scottish popular ballads, canonical texts were never to be questioned, still less deconstructed, but rather approached as sacred/historical documents to be laden with footnotes as a centipede is outfitted with legs. When, in my idealism, or naïveté, I dared to write a seminar paper on Edmund Spenser and Franz Kafka, on the ways in which (it seemed to me excitingly) the allegorical and the surreal are related, my professor, Merritt Hughes, who knew nothing of Kafka and had not the slightest interest in correcting his ignorance, returned the paper to me with an expression of gentlemanly repugnance and suggested that I attempt the Spenser assignment again, from a "traditional" perspective.

My face burned with shame. Poor deluded Joyce, who'd been too frequently praised for such flights of fancy at Syracuse, and even previously in high school, now caught as in a net, and revealed as profoundly foolish in the eyes of fellow graduate students as in Professor Hughes's disdainful vision—a barbarian who stood before them naked, utterly exposed.

How many times in the weeks and months to come as a first-year graduate student, trailing remnants of literary idealism, I was made to feel in the entombed confines of venerable Bascom Hall, like the humiliated boy-narrator of James Joyce's "Araby"—a "creature driven and deluded by vanity." I saw myself, too, as the older sister of a child born autistic (for this was the diagnosis, in 1960) and doomed never to utter a single coherent sentence through her life, nor even a coherent word, as a creature of sheer chance, the consequence of a "normal" birth, and my parents "young" parents at the time of my birth; the biochemical nature of my brain, unlike those of my unlucky sister Lynn, in a benign equilibrium. I could not claim autonomy, or free will, as I could not claim credit for having created myself, yet I was obliged to play at autonomy, to assume free will, for what alternative is there? As William James has said—*My first act of freedom will be to believe in freedom.* Yet to be proud of one's intelligence, talent, looks, or achievement has always seemed to me misguided; to betray a misunderstanding of the shake of the dice that grants us, or fails to grant us, our humanity.

For some personalities, the stronger the conviction of fate, the more driven to assert "free will." How is such a contradiction possible? Perhaps it is as F. Scott Fitzgerald observed in his self-excoriating confession "The Crack-Up": *The test of a first-rate intelligence is the ability to hold two opposed ideas in the mind at the same time, and still retain the ability to function.*

"HOW STRANGE THIS IS! We're all together—here."

Not I but another young woman spoke, in a way of childlike wonder tinged with something like irony. But a very subtle irony, for "Marianna Mason Churchland" (a close approximation of her quaintly lovely name) was a very subtle person.

Marianna was from a small town near Raleigh, North Carolina; her melodic accent was enchanting, especially to one from the flat nasal terrain of western New York. The first glimpse I had of Marianna, I was struck by her prim schoolgirl beauty, ivory-pale skin, dark eyes and dark brows, very dark hair, and straight posture. Marianna was the quintessential "good girl"—but her lips curved in prankishness and irony. She wore crisp white blouses (which she ironed herself, lovingly, in her room in Barnard Hall with the door open so that neighbors could drop in and visit if they wished) and pencil skirts or perfectly pleated black woolen slacks; her hair was severely parted in the center of her head, and gathered in a chignon at the back; if Marianna wore makeup, it was as subtle as she, scarcely discernible. Here was a sister, as my own sister could never be; as my dear lost friend Cynthia Heike had not been, for I'd never gained access to Cynthia's heart, and Cynthia had not finally cared to gain access to mine. But Marianna was a girl essentially so like myself, we might have been gazing at each other through a glass mistaken as a mirror; like Milton's Eve gazing at her own reflection, enthralled, mesmerized, irresistibly moved to love. Like me Marianna was a first-year graduate student in English though her interest wasn't American literature but rather medieval English literature, which seemed suddenly to me so much more rarefied, so much more distinctive, than the nineteenth-century American works that were my major field of study. Like me, Marianna lived in a single room on the third floor of Barnard Hall, which was the graduate women's residence on campus, a solemn stony place to contemplate from the foot of the hill at University Avenue, but a more solemn place to enter. *In a place of stone, be secret and exult*—Yeats's vehement admonition came to me frequently as I ascended this hill, though I could not think that Yeats would have meant quite this. In deference to the rigors of graduate school, so very different from the more gregarious and lax atmosphere of undergraduate life, each of the rooms in Barnard Hall was a "single"—spartan, cell-like.

As an undergraduate I had once been fortunate enough to live in a "single" room, but I had also been paired with roommates; in my last semester, with two roommates. Fortunately, these were sympathetic friends, and serious students like myself, and in any case I had done most of my studying and writing elsewhere. Often I'd returned to our room after my roommates had gone to bed and so their presence hadn't been distracting, and I had not distracted them; I had liked these roommates very much, and I believe that they'd liked me. But Barnard Hall was not a place for girlish friendships. *All that* was behind me now.

Surreal and disquieting smells as of disinfectant, bandages, old books and (stale?) food pervade my memory of this graduate women's residence in which I lived for a single exhausting semester; Marianna was the one to first identify these odors, prankishly, with a crinkle of her delicate nose to suggest how strange all this was, a kind of reverse-miracle, that we'd all come from far-flung parts of the country to this place—"Bah-nard Hill" as she called it.

The pressure of graduate school, at least as first-year English graduate students experienced it, was unrelenting: hundreds of pages of reading each week, and these pages densely printed on tissue-thin paper—Old English *Beowulf, The Wanderer, The Dream of the Rood, Anglo-Saxon Chronicle,* works by Bede, Cynewulf, Caedmon; *Liturgical Plays of the Story of Christ, The Castle of Perseverance, Gammer Gurton's Needle, Damon and Pythias, Second Shepherd's Play, Everyman, Noah's Flood.* Chaucer's *Canterbury Tales* and *Troilus and Criseyde,* Spenser's *Faerie Queen,* witty John Skelton, Jacobean and Elizabethan and Restoration drama and more. Much more. We discovered Sir Thomas Wyatt, and committed to heart the mysterious gem "They Flee from Me" (1557)—

They flee from me, that sometime did me seek,
With naked foot stalking in my chamber,

I have seen them, gentle, tame, and meek,

That now are wild, and do not remember

That sometime they put themselves in danger

To take bread at my hand, and now they range,

Busily seeking with a continual change . . .

The great works of English literature were monuments to be approached with reverence. Unlike my Syracuse professors, these older, Harvard-trained professors at Wisconsin did not regard literature as an art but rather more as historical artifact, to be discussed in terms of its context; there was little or no discussion of a poem as a composition of carefully chosen words. History, not aesthetics. The thrilling emotional punch of great art—totally beyond the range of these earnest scholarly individuals. One might lecture on Latin influences in pre-Shakespearean drama, or "influences" in Shakespeare, but the white-hot dynamic of *Macbeth*, for instance, the brilliant and dazzling interplay of "personalities" that is Shakespearean essential drama was unknown to them. If they were explorers, they'd been becalmed in an inlet, while the great river rushed past a few miles away.

Yet, at Madison, I did read, reread, and immerse myself in the work of Herman Melville. For a course at Syracuse I'd read the early, relatively straightforward *White Jacket*, and the wonderfully enigmatic short stories—"Bartleby the Scrivener," "The Paradise of Bachelors and the Tartarus of Maids," "The Encantadas." While still in high school I'd read *Moby-Dick*—our greatest American novel, which one might read and reread through a lifetime, as one might read and reread the poetry of Emily Dickinson. At Madison, I became entranced by the very intransigence, one might say the *obstinate opacity* of the near-unreadable *Pierre; or, the Ambiguities*—a pseudo-romance written in mockery of its (potential, female) readers, as if by a (male) author who'd come to hate the effort of narrative prose fiction itself. (It isn't surprising that *Pierre* sold poorly, as its great predecessor *Moby Dick* sold poorly. Tragic Melville—"Dollars damn me!") After a few pages of its curiously stilted, self-regarding prose I fell under the spell of the slightly more accessible allegory *The Confidence-Man*, as well as *Billy Budd*. I wondered what to make of *Benito Cereno* with its perversely glacial-slow pace: in our racially sensitized era we expect that Melville will surely side with the slave uprising, and not with white oppressors like Captain Cereno, but Melville doesn't comply with our twenty-first-century expectations in this case in which "the shadow of the Negro" falls over everyone— including even the executed rebel Babo.

Writers who are enrolled in graduate programs soon feel the frustration, the ignominy, the pain of being immersed in reading the work of others—illustrious, renowned others—Chaucer, Shake-speare, Donne, Milton—Hawthorne, Poe, Melville, James—when they are themselves unable to write or even to fantasize writing. During these months of intense academic study when my head was crammed with great and not-so-great classic works, of course I had no time for fiction or poetry of my own (as I thought it) except des-perate fragments in a journal like cries for help.

Suffocated by books. Crushed by books. Library stacks, tall shelves of books, books, books overturning upon the young writer groping in the dark for the overhead light to switch on . . .

IT WAS THRILLING TO undertake such bouts of reading, as in a plunge into unfathomable depths of the ocean; it was thrilling and also terrifying, for at such depths one could not easily breathe, and the more desperate one was to concentrate one's thoughts, the more likely one's thoughts were to break and scatter like panicked birds from a tree. It was not fair to think of Barnard Hall in hospital terms. Its occupants, graduate women, were very different from the undergraduate girls with whom I'd lived for four years at Syracuse; they were not, obviously, patients or convalescents; most of them appeared to be older than I was, and exuded an air of determined bustle, grimly cheery energy like that of nuns in a convent who must brave the world outside the convent which is run by men, the *other*. (In fact there were two nuns on my floor, each from a different Catholic order, living in separate rooms. They were to be observed sitting together in the residence cafeteria quietly speaking together.) My convent-cell with its single window overlooking University Avenue was on the third floor of the residence and in that room already in the first weeks of my adventure at Madison I was stricken by intermittent insomnia as by a swarm of invisible mosquitoes lying in wait in the dark no matter how exhausted I was from hours of reading, note taking, research at the graduate library, an increased restlessness (walking, running) that has long characterized my life, no matter how I tried to calm my rampaging thoughts.

Insomnia! There is a sickly romance to the affliction—initially. To be awake while others are asleep, especially if you leave your room and wander the corridors, is to feel that you are moving through others' dreams. To be awake for long hours is to seem to possess more of the day, and of consciousness, than those others who merely sleep. But the romance is short-lived and soon you find yourself panting in fear lying in, or on, your narrow bed willing *sleep, sleep* like a hypnotist with fading powers. My particular insomnia-affliction in Madison was to see pass before my tight-shut eyelids careening shapes, bizarre forms, hallucinatory objects (dog-snouts, human limbs encumbered by braces, splintered vegetation like storm debris) and most persistently the faces of strangers vividly delineated as in photographic close-ups, their eyes locking with mine. I would wonder if I was losing my mind—if "my" mind was a singular entity, that I might "lose"—or rather, if my brain was suffering a kind of seismic stroke, or strokes, that would leave me whimpering and wordless like my poor sister. Or were such visions what had driven my friend Cynthia to suicide, swallowing a horrific chemical with the property of Drano—of which I did not allow myself to think.

Was I supposed to recognize the individuals in my hypnagogic dreams? Why did they stare at me so intently as if demanding *Don't you know who we are? The secret that connects us?*

I did not share my unhappiness with my neighbors in Barnard Hall, not even Marianna who seemed so like myself, at least as I presented myself to the world. (I did not want to jeopardize even these tentative friendships. I did not think that I could afford to be so utterly alone in this strange new place.) Madison, Wisconsin, was in those days a seemingly idyllic university town built on the south bank of Lake Mendota. The enormous sprawling campus inhabited woodland near the lake; the terrain was nearly as hilly as Syracuse, a landscape convulsed by glaciers in the Ice Age, and retaining still, even on sunny autumn days, a wintry Ice Age flavor. Warmth feels temporary, freezing-cold is permanent beneath. In Madison as in all new and unfamiliar places before habitude dulls or masks strangeness I realized how precarious is our hold on what we call *sanity*.

I was missing a part of my soul, it seemed. I was homesick—for Millersport, for my family, and for the part of my life I had never quite examined, that urged me to *write*.

I felt breathless, edgy. I could not sleep, for my brain could not shut down. Oxygen seemed to be draining out of any room in which I found myself. It was not good to be alone, and yet, with others, I yearned to be alone. I yearned to cry, and rid myself of unhappiness. But unhappiness is not so easily thrown off.

I can't fail, I must succeed. Like deranged Muzak this mantra ran through my head. *Can't fail. Must succeed. Can't. Must. How? Why?*

"I'M ASKING MYSELF—WHY ARE we *here?* Not one page I've read has come to mean a thing."

The student of literature is a soul-searcher in a way that, we can assume, the student of electrical engineering or economics is not. The student of literature is a pilgrim. We yearn to be suffused with holiness. But in graduate school, life had become for us a swift current bearing us onward, blindly, out of our control. *This is not what we'd wanted. This is not what we'd expected.*

Marianna began to speak often of home. Often, of her fiancé whose name was quaintly decorous as "Marianna Mason Churchland."

Marianna warned me to be cautious when I entered her room— "I've broken some glass in here. I tried to sweep it up but there may be some sharp pieces remaining."

Or, Marianna warned me that there was a "strange, choking-kind" of smell in her room, coming from a vent in the ceiling she wasn't able to shut.

Though her eyes were frightened behind her tortoiseshell glasses, Marianna laughed a beautiful wind chime sort of laugh. Beneath the sweetly mellifluous North Carolina accent was the breathlessness of dread.

The brilliant schoolgirl, the favorite daughter of her elders, the all-A student primed from kindergarten to succeed is not unlike a Thoroughbred horse trained to jump obstacles, and with each success the bar is raised; eventually, the horse must fail, or must fall and break one of her beautiful slender legs—so I thought, observing Marianna who seemed to be having the difficulties I was having in adjusting to graduate school as well as some sort of (unspecified) difficulty with her family or with her fiancé (for Marianna was often on the phone downstairs) and who was willing to speak of her disillusion with her courses and professors more readily than I was.

"I almost can't believe—I used to *love reading*. Now, I'm getting to *hate it*. Some nights I can *hardly sit still to concentrate*."

It's with a fond memory, or rather a bittersweet memory, that I recall our much-admired professor Helen White advising her seminar students that the way she'd dealt with the massive readings assigned in graduate school at Harvard was to "lay out on my bed all the books that had to be read or consulted"—and not go to bed until her work was completed.

Excellent advice? Not-so-excellent advice? For those of us inclined to insomnia in any case, it was at least heartfelt advice.

AMID THE PRESSURE OF academic work it happened that something unexpected and benevolent occurred in my beleaguered life: I, too, fairly suddenly acquired a fiancé.

A young Ph.D. candidate in English literature (field of research eighteenth century; from Milwaukee) and I met on October 23, 1960, in the Memorial Union at Madison, at a Sunday afternoon graduate students' reception. It was the only such social occasion I'd attended, overwhelmed with work as I was; a measure of my desperation, that I'd dared to detach myself from my cell of a room in Barnard Hall.

At this graduate reception, an "older man"—(Ray was twenty-nine)—approached me, and asked if anyone was sitting in the chair beside me.

Soon, it developed that this person, Ray Smith, was not only "older" but far more experienced in the labyrinthine ways of the English graduate program; and he was delighted to give me advice, and to speak with me at length about the remarkable, if also formidable literary-historical works I was obliged to read. That evening, following the reception, we had dinner together in the student union overlooking Lake Mendota—the first meal together of countless thousands in the more than four decades to come.

I have written of Ray elsewhere—at length, in *A Widow's Story*. A memoir of a death is an attempt to commemorate the living being, who has passed into "death." But it is not an attempt, usually, that succeeds in evoking anything of the fleeting, thrilling, elusive, essentially unsayable impressions that pass between individuals, rarely just words, but rather mannerisms—facial, expressive, part-conscious. There is the mystery of *touch*, *touching*. Impossible to convey.

I am sorry, but I am not able to write about Ray here. I have tried—but it is just too painful, and too difficult. Words are like wild birds—they will come when they wish, not when they are bidden.

Even if you hear their cries at a distance, you cannot summon them. You will only exhaust yourself in the effort, and the quixotic project of *writing a memoir decades after living the life* will come to an abrupt end.

Raymond Joseph Smith and I would become engaged on November 23, 1960; we would be married on January 23, 1961. (Ray's parents came from Milwaukee for the small wedding, for it was a short drive to Madison. My parents did not attend, perhaps because they didn't feel that they could afford plane travel, and certainly they could not have left my sister Lynn behind, or in anyone's care.)

I had not thought that I would ever be married. Vaguely I retained an ideal, or an image, of being a "teacher"—based upon Mrs. Dietz, of my old one-room school. And though Mrs. Dietz was obviously a married woman, she did not exude any wifely air, or even any clearly defined sexual air. She had always seemed, amid the schoolchildren, of whom a number were hardly "children" but precociously mature young adults, essentially alone, stalwart in her authority.

And yet, I had become married. I was deeply in love, and a little frightened of my new state, in which suddenly one "cares for" another as one "cares for" oneself—yet the other is not always predictable. (Is he?)

Soon you realize that your fears for yourself are now doubled—you will fear for the other, too. *His* happiness, *his* well-being. *His* career.

Nonetheless, it was certainly the case that I could be defined as *happy*.

In some quarters, observed by my Barnard Hall neighbors and friends, *very happy*.

And yet, inwardly, simultaneously, contrary to Aristotle's logic that one cannot be X and non-X at the same time, in the interstices of happiness, *very unhappy*.

Or rather, *distracted, distressed. Uncertain. Overwhelmed*.

In the decades following 1960 to 1961 the confessional mode has become a predominant literary genre. As a writer I have not been drawn to what is called memoirist prose because I have never felt that my life could be nearly as interesting as what my imagination could make of another's life; whatever my "story" is, it is not compelling set beside others' stories, including those of my parents and my grandparents and others of their generations who have lived, it had always seemed to me, a life closer to the bone than their children and grandchildren. (In my single novel that suggests memoirist fiction, *I'll Take You There*, only the setting, Syracuse University, is "real." The young woman undergraduate protagonist, unnamed, does not share the author's biography and is not the author but a means of writing about an intensely observed experience of a certain time and place. Yet she is obviously closer to me than any twin sister!) And I know that the "confessed" is a text; a text is language artfully arranged; language artfully arranged is not authentic; the not-authentic is not the aim of the serious confession. The vogue of seemingly sensational confessional poetry of the 1950s and 1960s was a dramatic reaction against the airless, stiffly impersonal, acrostics-poetry being written at that time, under the influence of (Anglican) T. S. Eliot who decreed that poetry should be impersonal, a matter of elite cultural allusions and symbols, never a *cri de coeur*. No Shelley, no Whitman, no D. H. Lawrence! Indeed, no Nobel laureate William Butler Yeats! With the eruption of the Beats into American culture at mid-century the old way of poetry was overcome as by rabble cheerfully beating down palace gates, and poetry would never be the same again. Fortunately! But the new, seemingly raw mode of self-expression imposes its own conventions on practitioners who may feel compelled to be radical, sensational, merciless, and unsparing in their exploitation of themselves and others. (Think of the preeminent Establishment poet of his time, Robert Lowell, appropriating the intimate, candid, pleading letters of his former wife Elizabeth Hardwick for his poetry: "Why not say what happened?" is Lowell's apologia.) When our experience doesn't match the high stakes of self-expression, ever ratcheted upward, experience has to be falsified; the remainder of life, the unsensational, the quotidian, the quiet, the sentimental and tender and obvious, has to be denied. For these reasons, as well as for reasons of personal/familial reticence, until *A Widow's Story* (2011), I did not write about my private life; my intensely personal life; I did not write "thinly disguised fiction" or outright memoir about my husband Raymond Smith, my marriage, the initial experience of *falling in love*; never have I attempted to record the minutiae, the daily-ness, of an intimate companionate life. It is enough to state that I met by chance, at a Sunday afternoon reception for graduate students in the student union at the University of Wisconsin—Madison, the individual who would so alter my life as to seem to revise my very history so that there is the *life leading up to* and the *life subsequent*.

Of our hurts and bafflements we create monuments to survival;

of our good choices, and our good luck, we are obliged to remain silent. We dare not speak for another, and it is always wrong to expose intimacy even in the celebration of intimacy.

AND THEN, AMID A time of happiness, my body began to break down.

A sudden attack of tachycardia in my room late one night when I was reading and annotating John Lyly's *Euphues: The Anatomy of Wit* (1578)—a Renaissance text of such Herculean dullness it must be read to be believed but who would wish to read it, except under duress? Suddenly, a kind of clamp shut over my heart, and opened again, propelling my heartbeat into a rapid hammering that made my chest vibrate visibly, and sucked away my breath. What had happened? Why? So swiftly, without warning? It was as if a switch had been pulled, and suddenly—I was helpless.

Tachycardia pulls blood from finger- and toe-tips so that you begin to feel the chill (of impending death?)—like Socrates observing the chill of death rising in his legs, in Plato's *Phaedo*. I was twenty-two—I was alone in my room in Barnard Hall—my first thought was that I did not want my fiancé to know about this attack—really, I did not want anyone to know. Though having difficulty breathing and in terror that I would die I was not able to lie down on my bed—the hammering heartbeat is unbearable in such a position—and even sitting still at my desk became unbearable; so in a kind of trance, shivering, trembling, very cold and yet beginning to sweat, I made my way slowly—very slowly—out into the corridor.

There was no one to witness. Some doors down was Marianna's room, and a light shone beneath her door; but I did not want to alarm Marianna who had health issues of her own, and I did not want to reveal my weakness to Marianna who thought of me as a "beacon of sanity" (Marianna's lightly ironic words). Other doors, shut, with no light shining beneath, held no appeal for me—I could not bring myself to knock, to beg for help.

(Isolated incidents of health crises occurred in Barnard Hall not infrequently. There was a young woman mathematician who'd fainted after returning from a meal, falling heavily just in front of her room; several of us had tried to help her but she'd begun sobbing hysterically, and had repelled our offers of comfort. Another young woman, a mutual friend of Marianna's and mine, a Ph.D. candidate in psychology, very thin, dangerously thin, who wore white short-sleeved blouses even in cold weather of a gauzy near-transparent material that allowed the pained observer to see how skeletal she'd become, had fainting spells, and spells of weeping; vividly I recall this young woman's pale freckled face, pale red very short hair, damp eyes as she spoke of her work as a lab assistant for an experimental cognitive psychologist who was also her advisor.)

In the corridor for some reason I made my way with painstaking slowness, a small step at a time, and leaning against the wall, and so to the stairs; and down two flights of stairs to check, bizarrely, my mailbox into which some flyers had been shoved. (I might have called my fiancé from the phone room off the foyer but I was determined not to worry him, as I was determined not to allow him to know that I was so stricken.) At the front door of the residence I stood and breathed in the freezing-cold air; I observed a few vehicles on University Avenue, and wondered wanly who was inside, who those strangers were, whose hearts did not threaten to explode inside their chests; I thought of my younger, lost self who'd slipped from her room in the old farmhouse on Transit Road, standing in a trance of oblivion at the side of the road, like a creature who has been drawn to a vision for which there is no name, no comprehension. I did not want to think that, in my secrecy, in my wish not to alarm or inconvenience others, I had (inadvertently, unhappily) caused a shock in my parents' lives: for I had telephoned home one night, calling collect, after 11:00 P.M., as instructed, to tell my parents that I was *engaged to be married*; I had not told them that I was seeing anyone, still less that I had *fallen in love*; for our family reticence would have forbidden the divulgence of such information, until it was absolutely necessary.

I even had an engagement ring of my own now. A very small diamond in a white-gold setting. My parents had been too surprised by my news to have thought to ask if I had an engagement ring, nor had I thought to tell them. But I wore the ring proudly, as if it were proof of—what? Normality?

How long I remained at the front door of the residence, I don't remember. I had hoped that fresh air would somehow revive me but it seemed to have had no effect at all except to make me colder, and tremble more violently.

After a while, I decided to return to my room, and not to knock on the door of the residence advisor whose quarters were close by. Sensibly I worried that the woman would immediately summon an ambulance to take me to the ER at the university hospital; such a plunge into the unknown terrified me as a prospect, and, practical like all of my family, I worried that I would be billed for such treatment, and I could not afford it.

Returning upstairs to my room was more arduous than descending, for I had virtually no breath; the slightest movement made me gasp for air; there was no elevator in the residence, or at least none that I can recall. Walking with severe tachycardia you feel as if you are walking on the thinnest of ice; at any moment it will break, and you will plunge through. (Did no one notice me? It was after midnight, and so the corridors must have been deserted. It is strange that I so dreaded being found out, and made to explain why my chest was visibly vibrating and my face was deathly pale; why I could have barely drawn breath to speak.) What would have required five minutes ordinarily required forty minutes now.

At Syracuse I'd had a similar but much less severe attack of tachycardia while playing basketball, in the fall of my freshman year; I'd been knocked down, violently, by a large, aggressive girl who'd sent me sprawling onto the hardwood floor and immediately my heartbeat had gone wild, and had not ceased its hammering for a half hour or more. (This was the first time I'd had such an attack, and it had greatly frightened me.) The gym instructor herself had nearly fainted with shock, at my condition; she'd helped me walk off the court, to a place where I could lie down; eventually, she'd taken me to the university infirmary where I was made to lie down also, and spent the remainder of the attack reading Wordsworth's *The Prelude* in my *Great British Writers* anthology.

It seems curious to me now, that no one called an ambulance. In our present hyper-anxious time, no university would wish to make itself vulnerable to a wrongful death lawsuit.

The medical term for my condition at the time was *paroxysmal atrial tachycardia*. It is believed to be triggered by stress and caffeine though in my case it seemed purely idiopathic, arising out of nowhere, provoked by nothing, a state of accelerated heartbeat that is associated with persons who have "heart murmurs." (I must have had a "heart murmur" since birth, undetected by any Lockport doctor.) Tachycardia can be eased by a powerful intravenous medication, and the most severe attacks require emergency medical treatment, but attacks frequently cease as abruptly and mysteriously as they begin, within an hour or, if you are very lucky, within a few minutes.

This attack, which was only the third or fourth such attack in my life, kept me incapacitated for more than an hour. And when it suddenly ceased, and I could breathe again, I nearly wept with relief and happiness; my mouth was so dry that it hurt, and my feet and hands were icy-cold, but I was happy suddenly, for I'd been spared; my way of celebrating was to continue with *Euphues* as if nothing had happened.

Telling myself—*See? You did the right thing. No one knows!*

(EVENTUALLY, MY FIANCÉ WOULD learn of my medical condition. That is, I would tell him. For I could not not tell him, if we were to be married.)

(We are all in dread that we will be loved less if we are revealed to be flawed—surely sometimes that dread is not misplaced.)

INSOMNIA ALLOWS YOU TO *see clearly—like seeing things when you aren't present, or after you have died.*

In this way, in my journal I tried to comfort myself.

More frequent than tachycardia, insomniac nights. Since the age of thirteen I'd had difficulty sleeping; my brain raced with a kind of exhilaration that was purely mental, and seemed impersonal. (Most of my dreams seem "impersonal"—that is, the dreamer is not me, nor anyone I know; it's as if I find myself in another's mind, or imagination, and not my own. Settings are rarely familiar, other figures are rarely anyone I know.) In Madison, in steam-heated Barnard Hall, my insomnia worsened, unsurprisingly.

There was too much to think about, that was the simple explanation. As if odd-sized objects were being crammed into an ordinary-sized head, distending the skull. What might have been—what should have been—the pleasurable excitement of reading major works of English and American literature under the guidance of distinguished professors was spoiled by so much that was certainly not "major" and by what seemed an insane excess of historical background with emphasis upon "sources." A play, for instance, was not likely to be considered as a distinctive work of literary art, but rather as a sort of hodgepodge of influences dating back to Roman theater; a Shakespearean tragedy was an occasion for lengthy footnotes and a barrage of "sources." That literature might be disturbing, mysterious, provocative, joyous, psychologically astute or in some way relevant to the reader was not an issue—as if no one had thought of it.

The major literary work was a sort of beached whale lying moribund or indeed dead on the sand, providing sustenance for myriad scavengers ("scholars"); it seemed to have no significance otherwise, certainly no relationship to anything approaching "entertainment."

(Though probably I am being unfair, and my professors at Madison did truly love their fields of study. As young people they'd surely read these major works of English literature with enjoyment and interest; with the passage of time, their relationship to them had become professional, with all that "professional" means.)

Insomniacs divide (unequally) into two types: night-insomniacs and morning-insomniacs. Night-insomnia can be defined as simply an extension of day-consciousness: the insomniac can't switch off her brain but remains awake until, if she is lucky, she falls asleep sometime in the night—usually by 4:00 A.M., in my case. If you are young and in reasonably good health you might not feel the effect the next morning as adrenaline kicks in and you are borne along as by a swift-running stream. *Morning! Sunshine! A new day!* The morning-insomniac, however, is one who falls asleep normally, perhaps out of exhaustion, but wakes suddenly and irrevocably soon after falling asleep—within two or three hours, miserably. At once, thoughts come stampeding through the brain like maddened horses . . .

There is the terror of lying awake until dawn, in either case. The terror of dawn itself.

I wondered if the rushing thoughts, the hypnagogic images of strangers' faces, were related to the fact that for the first time in my life I was not able to *write*—only just critical and scholarly papers, which don't seem to require the same sort of imagination. *Another world to live in is what we mean by religion*—so George Santayana remarked; but *another world* might also mean the particular solace of art, for the artist; *another world* is the place to which the writer takes herself, a thrilling journey into the unknown.

(When I have completed a novel, which requires enormous concentration and a focusing upon this *other world*, in the aftermath of completion I am flooded with new ideas, or rather these rushing, oneiric visions that exert a powerful spell, and make sleep all but impossible.)

In Madison, I wondered if I was losing my mind—whatever that means, to "lose" a mind.

Or was my distress just sleep deprivation, I didn't know.

Usually I gave up trying to sleep when stricken with morning-insomnia. Two or three hours of sleep is not so bad, for any dreams are better than no dreams.

Early-morning hours when the sky is still dark. From a window, streetlights on University Avenue. Few vehicles, and the red tail-lights receding—a vision that continues to haunt me, still.

And so I would walk in Barnard Hall, by night. Prowling the semi-darkened corridors as if (if someone were to see me) I was simply on my way to a communal bathroom.

Sometimes, silently, I ran. I loved to run, I have always loved to run, for only when I'm running does my body's metabolism feel normal. What is painful to me, deeply boring, is walking slowly—*sauntering* is the least attractive word in the English language.

My hope was to make myself physically exhausted so that I could return to my room and sleep, if only for an hour or two. The sweetness of oblivion! Insomniacs overvalue what eludes them, elevating sleep to a near-mystical experience. As a lanky, skittish teenager I'd been subtly reprimanded by our family doctor who'd called me "high-strung" when he'd tried with some difficulty to examine me; the implication being that someday when I was more mature I would become "normal." And so I had not told my future husband how often I suffered from insomnia, preferring to think that, once I was married, my insomnia might fade.

And so too, I did not want to present myself in any way as "weak"—even to one who loved me. As a young woman in an overwhelmingly masculine, patriarchal, and hierarchical world, studying in a field in which there were virtually no women professors, I understood that to require sympathy, protectiveness, pity might be a solace in the short run but in the long run, it would be a mistake for if I were to succeed in my profession, I would have to be perceived as an honorary male. There was no place in the academic world for the *female*.

(This was an instinct shared by other women graduate students of my acquaintance. We were not living in convents exactly, but the qualities of personality cultivated by the convent were desirable— docility, obedience, self-effacement, acquiescence to authority. For years I would publish critical/scholarly articles in academic journals under the gender-neutral names "J. C. Oates" and, my married name, "J. Oates-Smith.")

Sometimes wandering in Barnard Hall at night I would see a band of light beneath a door. Could this be a sister insomniac, or just a young woman working late? If I longed to knock gently at the door, and meet a sister-insomniac, or an individual as intensely engaged in her work as I was, of course I never dared. Nor did I seek out the room's occupant in the daytime.

By day the obsessions of the insomniac fade like screen images when the lights come on.

But in the night, you can hear, you can feel the very wings of madness beating near . . .

Downstairs in the twilit foyer with its sharp ammoniac smells of newly scrubbed floors and scoured ashtrays—(yes, this was an era in which even sensible, bright young women academics smoked, and sometimes chain-smoked)—I once found on a nubby old sofa the paperback *Notes of a Native Son* by James Baldwin. This was not a book I might have read ordinarily, concentrating as I was on early centuries of English literature; how it came to be in this place, at this time, would be a mystery to me. In heightened states of consciousness we become superstitious, and seek out "signs": I spent the remainder of the night avidly reading not about ecclesiastical controversies of England in the mid-1500s but a contemporary black American's eloquent and deeply disturbing memoir, the first of this great writer's work I would read, with the insomniac's rapt concentration and sense of fatedness.

All of my father's texts and songs, which I had decided
were meaningless, were arranged before me at his death
like empty bottles, waiting to hold the meaning which life
would give them for me.

(Baldwin was speaking of his estranged, emotionally unstable father who had been a Christian minister; he was mourning the man's death, and trying to comprehend his tragic life.) Though I was a young and inexperienced "white" woman whose skin had granted her privileges through her lifetime of which, like most "whites," I'd been unaware, I was thrilled by the beauty, calm, and certitude of these words, and by their prophetic truth as it might apply to me. *The meaning which life would give them for me.* I was filled with a sense of mission that had no immediate object, like one on the verge of mania.

I believed that my hateful insomnia had granted me this revelation for a reason and I would not have traded a full night of sleep for this revelation.

Next day I returned *Notes of a Native Son* to the lounge where I'd found it. For a while I lingered in the vicinity hoping that I would see who came to pick it up—but no one came while I was there, and when I returned later in the day the book had vanished.

SOMETIMES, I WENT OUTSIDE. My most thrilling bouts of insomnia were outside. If it wasn't bitterly cold, or freezing-rain, or snowing, or so windy it took my breath away. Most nights I would have an evening meal with my fiancé and he would walk me back to Barnard Hall at about 10:00 P.M. I would lie on my bed and work until midnight and then I would try to sleep and by 4:00 A.M. often I'd given up on sleep in dismay or disgust and decide to get up, to dress, and begin the day early as I'd begun many days in my life in Millersport, in darkness. If you live on a farm the darkness before dawn is a familiar darkness and seems to bleed into the darkness after sunset as if daylight itself were but an idle interruption. Rising early in the dark, in fiercely awful weather, was routine in Millersport. Before I'd been transferred to city schools, and was picked up a short distance from our house by a school bus, I would walk on foot to the one-room schoolhouse across the creek, and did not think this was a terrible hardship since everyone walked to school in any sort of weather. Twenty years before, my mother had walked to the school and would not have thought of complaining.

My breath steamed as I walked quickly on University Avenue, and on Park Street, to the foot of Bascom Hill; and up the steep, wind-whipped hill until my legs began to cramp. It seemed urgent to be *in motion*—to appear to have a destination.

Under the gradually lightening sky I would continue past Bascom Hill in the direction of the observatory; my destination was a State Street diner that opened early, but I forestalled arriving there too soon, before the front door was unlocked and the lights on. In these long-ago years a dense gathering of trees, both deciduous and evergreen, bordered the hill; beyond that was slate-dark Lake Mendota. Eventually I would return, down the long hill, passing the State Historical Library and the mammoth Memorial Union, not yet open; if it wasn't too cold or windy, I would walk along the lakefront; I would pause on the terrace, to stare at the lake; here, I was nearly always happy; freed from the confines of my over-heated room and from the rampage of my thoughts; I was both exhilarated and comforted by the lapping waves, and Lake Mendota was often a rough, churning lake; in the twilight of early morning it appeared vast as an inland sea, its farther shore obscured by mist. On such mornings, which were common in Madison, the lake's waves emerged out of an opacity of gunmetal gray like a scrim; there was no horizon, and there was no sky, and it would not have surprised me if when I glanced down at my feet there was no ground.

I was in no danger, I thought. My engagement to be married was like a safety-harness, I could not be swept into the water.

Then there were mornings of stark, eye-aching clarity. A moon, or a remnant of a moon overhead, and isolated mica-bits of light that must be "stars"; tattered clouds blown across the sky like shreds of thought. No sound except the waves of the lake and random cries of those curious nocturnal birds, common in urban areas, unknown in Millersport, called "nighthawks"; nighthawks must have nested beneath the eaves of the Union, or in trees nearby. I liked to feel that, at this hour, alone, anonymous, and unaccursed by gender, I was a nighthawk; a pair of eyes, a skein of brooding thoughts. How beyond mere happiness—or unhappiness—I believed myself. What rang in my head was Walt Whitman's poem of surpassing strangeness and beauty, "A Clear Midnight":

> This is thy hour O Soul, thy free flight into the wordless,
> Away from books, away from art, the day erased, the
>   lesson done,
> Thee fully forth emerging, silent, gazing, pondering the
>   themes thou lovest best,
> Night, sleep, death and the stars.

In my circuitous route to the State Street diner I would pass the still-darkened university library, which was one of my places of refuge during the day; I would walk along Langdon Street past fraternity houses with their stolid, impressive facades bearing cryptic Greek letters emerging out of the gloom, and invariably there were scattered lights burning in these massive houses—who knew why? It was gratifying somehow to take note of scattered lights in the windows of apartment buildings and two-storey woodframe rented houses on Langdon, Gorham, Henry streets as the early-morning shifted toward 6:00 A.M.; still darkness, for this was late autumn in a northerly climate, with a wan promise of dawn in the eastern sky. The nighthawk takes comfort in recognizing others, kindred souls, or anyway souls, at a distance: warm-lighted city buses wheezing on Gorham and University bearing a few passengers, and most of them dark-skinned women and men; headlights of vehicles, and (receding red) taillights; occasional pedestrians, alone, swiftly walking and bent against the wind. Among these there had to be some who were morning-insomniacs like me, relieved and grateful for the new day, the new chance, but most were of course workers, custodians, cafeteria staff, attendants at the university hospital, for whom there was no romance to the hour, nor probably any particular significance; beneath their coats they wore the uniforms of routine.

On Gorham Street sometimes I saw a man walking his dog; a man of indeterminate age, perhaps in his late thirties; I would see him leaving one of the sturdy old Victorian houses partitioned into rentals for graduate students, crossing the wide porch and descending, his dog held to a tight leash; the dog was a springer spaniel, buff-colored, thick-bodied but still youthful; my heart leapt at the sight of the spaniel, which reminded me of a dog out of my past, and behaved in a friendly way toward me even as his frowning master tugged him in another direction. On Gorham often I recognized certain lighted windows; I'd noticed glimpses of a couple behind a ground-floor window with a carelessly drawn blind; from less than ten feet away I could gaze into their kitchen, though not very clearly; I felt a stab of envy for to be awake at such an hour does not seem pathetic if there is another with you—if you are talking and laughing together, preparing breakfast. I wondered who this couple was, were they both students at the university, what were they studying, were they in love, were they married—of course they must be in love, and probably they must be married.

On Henry Street lived the man I would marry, by what concatenation of chance and fate I would never comprehend, in January 1961. Raymond lived on the ground floor of an attractively shabby wood-frame house, in a single-room "flat" with its own private entrance; the room was crowded with books, journals, papers—for Ray was completing his Ph.D. requirements in eighteenth-century English literature, writing a dissertation on Jonathan Swift under the direction of the eminent scholar Ricardo Quintana. In this flat, most evenings we prepared and ate supper together, and afterward worked, or read, side by side on a sofa. The little apartment was furnished, with an air of mismatched gaiety; though in retrospect it sounds cramped

and dreary, in fact it was a place of coziness, privacy, and contemplation. The man I would marry was not, and would never be, afflicted
by insomnia. *You would not wish to marry another like yourself: a night-*
hawk. My predominant feeling for Ray was a powerful wish to protect
him—which was strange, and groundless, for there was no reason to
feel this way, Ray was demonstrably capable of protecting himself.
He was eight years older than I was, a brilliant and bemused vet-
eran of the English graduate program at Madison; so kindly to me, a
naïve first-year student, that, on the first evening we met, while having an impromptu dinner in the Memorial Union overlooking Lake
Mendota, he led me patiently and painstakingly through the evolu-
tion of the "Great Vowel Shift" in the English language; Ray would
later indicate to me which titles were really important, and which
not so important, on the daunting list of titles on the department's
reading list for master's candidates. Begun in this way, our relationship was never one (it seemed to me) of "equals" precisely; in such
respects our marriage was a union of another era, about which I am
still hesitant to speak, for it is really not possible to speak of someone
whom you have loved, and who has loved you, for many years. I do
recall my initial shyness, even after we were engaged; even after we
saw each other each evening without fail; I would not have dared to
knock on the door of Ray's apartment, or tap lightly at the window
as I passed slowly by as if enchanted . . .

Instead, I walked on.

It was not really "early" any longer. Soon, it would be 7:00
A.M.—at which time normality begins.

At last I headed for the little diner on State Street, which was
open now. How warmly lighted it seemed, how welcoming, amid the
still-darkened storefronts of State Street at this hour. In this diner I'd
become a familiar customer, perhaps, like several others, though we
never acknowledged one another or spoke. We were individuals who

wanted to read at breakfast. We brought with us books, papers. We were solitary and silent and yet we were companions of a kind like the figures seated at the counter in Edward Hopper's *Nighthawks*, the most poignant and ceaselessly replicated romantic image of American loneliness. Like the red-haired woman in the painting I sat at the counter, since I would not have been allowed a booth unless I shared it with someone else. By this time after so much walking, and suffused with the optimism of the new day, I was ravenous with hunger. For no one is so happy, or so famished, as an insomniac who has survived the night.

And I was in love, and loved. I would not torment myself with the riddle—*How can he love* me? *Is his love predicated upon not precisely knowing* me?

I have yet to solve that riddle.

MID-MORNING, BASCOM HALL. THERE was "Joyce Carol" among the forty or more graduate students seated in a lecture room in Bascom Hall, in a hallucinatory drowse trying to take notes as the Renaissance scholar Mark Eccles lectured on the Elizabethan-Jacobean (non-Shakespearean) drama, reading from copious notes in a subdued, uninflected voice like that of a hypnotist. Professor Eccles was one of the most renowned of the Harvard-educated English faculty; one of those for whom a literary work exists for the sake of its footnotes, that cover it like barnacles; the more footnotes affixed to a work, the more valuable the work in its providing labor for the earnest scholar, if not exactly illumination. (Yet it was in Eccles's class that I first read the great tragedies of Marlowe, Middleton, and Webster; years later I would recall this soft-spoken man, and others at Madison, with more sympathy reasoning that they, too, had been trained in a particular sort of pedagogy for whom the "literary work" contained little pleasure; they, too, had been captives of the canon.) And afterward walking back to our residence with Marianna who had seemed increasingly distracted lately, complaining of the cold, worrying about a paper she was writing for Eccles, talking compulsively, very different from the young woman I'd met on my first day in Madison, back in September.

Though I would have been shocked to know it, this would be the last time I spoke with Marianna Churchland. Within a day or two she would have moved out of Barnard Hall and departed Madison, returning to North Carolina without a word of farewell to her friends.

Inside the residence Marianna went immediately to the row of mailboxes to look anxiously for mail though it was too early for mail, as she would have known. She was telling me that she had not heard from her fiancé since she'd been back home to visit at Thanksgiving—"We were talking about our wedding. I told him we need to set a date, next summer. I told him—'I love you so much! I want to have children with you. I want to live long enough to bury you.' I told him—"

(But at this point I was too distracted to listen for Marianna's words seemed uncanny to me, bizarre—*I want to live long enough to bury you*. Marianna's manner, her voice, her gaze were too intense. The remainder of our exchange was lost to me as I found myself in a hurry to get away from my friend.)

Not I but another. The wings of madness beating near.

ON JANUARY 23, 1961, at the Catholic chapel at Madison, Raymond Smith and I were married, and I vacated my room on the third floor of Barnard Hall to move my spare possessions of mostly winter clothes and books into a surprisingly spacious and airy five-room apartment on the second floor of a sturdy old Victorian house a mile away on University Avenue.

Though we were married by a Catholic priest, we were not married at the altar but in the sacristy, a sort of storage room at the front of the church; this was a compromise of sorts since Ray was no longer a practicing Catholic, and I had not wanted to upset my parents by being married "outside" the church.

It is true, I had not dared to marry "outside" the church—I had not dared to defy and disappoint my parents who were at this time, however nominally, members of the parish of the Pendleton Good Shepherd Church.

Hypocrisy is the compliment vice pays to virtue—as the eloquent La Rochefoucauld once observed.

One sunny morning in May, near the end of the spring term, I was examined for my master's degree in English, in venerable Bascom Hall. It would be my last visit to Bascom Hall. My examiners were, not surprisingly, all men; two were older professors with whom I'd taken seminars, and who had seemed to approve of my work; the third was a younger professor of American literature, perhaps an assistant professor. My heart sank—(yes, it is a cliché: but how appropriately visceral)—when I saw this stern individual staring at me doubtfully as if thinking—*Joyce Carol Smith?*—who'd been *Joyce Carol Oates?* A married woman? A serious scholar? It did seem suspicious, I could not blame him. In the young man's unsmiling eyes I saw my fate.

Yet, two-thirds of the exam seemed to go well. I had followed my husband's advice and memorized sonnets by Shakespeare, Sidney, and Donne which I could analyze and discuss, as he had done three years before in this very room; I could speak knowledgeably of "sources"—"influences." With feeling, but without an excess of feeling, I could recite the opening of *Paradise Lost* and key passages in *Lycidas, The Rape of the Lock,* and *The Prelude*; I could discuss the close reasoning of Milton's *Areopagitica*; but the American specialist was unimpressed, biding his time. When it was his turn to interrogate me, he didn't ask about primary works at all. I might have spoken knowledgeably about the poetry of Emily Dickinson and Walt Whitman, but I wasn't given an opportunity; as in a courtroom nightmare, I was asked only questions I couldn't answer with confidence about dates of poems, dates of drafts of poems, publications, editions; for instance, how did the 1867 *Leaves of Grass* differ from the 1855 edition, and what were the circumstances of the 1871 edition? Some of this I knew, in fact—but I did not know with certainty. (If I were teaching the material, I would simply have looked it up in a reference book.) Through a haze of headache and shame I heard myself murmur apologetically, "I don't know"—"I'm afraid I don't know." The experience brought back my having been interviewed for a Woodrow Wilson fellowship as an undergraduate at Syracuse, at the insistence of my professors; there, I had been virtually tongue-tied with shyness, feeling intrusively brash at having wished to be considered for a fellowship in which, it was mandated, only one in four recipients could be a woman.

Years later I would encounter my relentless interrogator in New York City at occasional literary luncheons and receptions; by this time he'd become a man deep into middle age, no longer a professor in the English Department at Madison but in manner and self-possession scarcely changed. Like torturer and torture victim meeting in a new, neutral environment, in new lives, this individual and I would never acknowledge the circumstances of our first meeting; never would we allude even elliptically to the fact, ironic in retrospect, that this man of no particular talent, distinction, or achievement had once hoped to defeat a young woman at the start of what he would have supposed to be my career as a university teacher. How vulnerable I'd been, that morning in May 1961! How negligible in his eyes, how expendable, a young woman, and married: not a likely candidate for the holy orders of the Ph.D., in which young men were always preferred. And it was so: though my love for literature was undiminished, I had become profoundly disillusioned with graduate study and could not have imagined continuing in Madison for another year, let alone several years; my subterranean despair would have choked me, and undermined the happiness of my marriage; it might have destroyed my marriage. The drudgery of scholarly research and the mind-numbing routines of academic literary study, above all the anxiety about pleasing and impressing one's elders, never displeasing, never upsetting or challenging one's sensitive elders, were not for me. My major effort of the year had been a one-hundred-page seminar paper on Herman Melville tailored to fit the expectations of a quirky, very senior professor named Harry Hayden Clark, who had a penchant for massive footnotes and "sources"; as I had learned my lesson in my early encounter with his colleague Merritt Hughes, I had not attempted an examination of Melville's prose as literature but only as a sort of historic document well rooted in nineteenth-century American whaling lore interlaced with the inescapable presence of Shakespeare. Amid the many footnotes of the paper were a considerable number citing Professor Clark, justifiably; though also expeditiously; the paper was well-received by Professor Clark but so depressed me that I tossed away my only copy soon afterward.

My normally even-mannered husband was astonished at such a gesture. How could I have done such a thing, after having worked so hard? *What if my grade hadn't been entered, and Clark wanted to see the paper again?*

I could not even contemplate this possibility. I had no idea why I hadn't made a carbon copy, either.

The master's oral exam ended. I was invited to leave the room, and to wait outside while the committee deliberated. My husband Ray was lurking somewhere in the English Department but I had asked him not to wait with me; not to be seen with me; afterward, I would seek him out, and that would be soon enough.

After a brief consultation during which time I waited in the hallway in a state of apprehension, knowing beforehand that the verdict would not be cause for euphoria, yet not wanting to think the worst, the senior member of the committee called me inside to inform me that "Joyce Carol Smith" would be granted a master's degree in English and American literature from the University of Wisconsin at Madison; but "Joyce Carol Smith" was not recommended to continue Ph.D. studies at Madison. The verdict was *You are not to be one of us.*

It is true that I felt relief, but disappointment as well. It is always painful to be rejected even by those by whom we would not really wish to be accepted.

When I went to seek out my husband, trying to smile, and trying also not to cry, Ray said with more vehemence than I could feel for myself: "You didn't want a Ph.D. anyway. Now you can write."

A QUARTER CENTURY LATER—(this is the great power of prose, that one can simply type *A quarter century later* and as in Alice's Wonderland we are catapulted there)—I was invited to return to the University of Wisconsin at Madison to be given an "honorary doctorate of humane letters" at an elaborate commencement ceremony. On this return to Madison in the spring of 1985 I went alone, without my husband; the experience was surreal, though not nightmare-surreal. Throughout my stay I was haunted by the irony of the situation, and the perversity, hearing the name "Joyce Carol Oates" intoned amid those of other "distinguished alumni" of the university: not that

I was an imposter exactly, for I did indeed have a master's degree in English and American literature from Madison, but rather that, if I had not been rejected as a Ph.D. candidate in 1961, if, instead, my examiners had urged me to continue with graduate work, I might have succumbed to the temptation; if I'd been a young man for instance, of equal talent; I might have refashioned myself into another person, a professional academic, and I certainly would not have written the books I'd written, and wouldn't as a consequence have been invited back to Wisconsin to be honored. The paradox was not one that might be elevated to a principle for others: to be accepted by my elders in one decade, I'd been required to be repudiated by my elders in an earlier decade.

Still later, in September 1999, I would compose an outline of this memoirist piece in a room at the Edgewater Inn in Madison, overlooking a rain-lashed Lake Mendota; I would be forced to recall the bittersweet irony of my situation once again. For here I was, the "nighthawk" of a bygone era, still alive, as in a picaresque novel! Another time I'd been invited back to Madison to give a public reading, this time in the beautiful Elvehjem Museum of Art (since renamed the Chazen Museum of Art) and to be honored at an elaborate dinner with the university chancellor, his wife, and a gathering of the university community. Honored at the age of sixty-one as a (circuitous, serendipitous) consequence of having failed at the age of twenty-two! I love it that our lives are not so crudely determined as some might wish them to be, but that we appear, and reappear, and again reappear, as unpredictably to ourselves as to those who would wish to oppress us.

I think we are all cats with nine lives, or even more. We must rejoice in our elusive *catness*.

Staring at the waves of Lake Mendota, where Ray and I had sometimes taken out a rowboat, I see that there is again a mist over the choppy water. I want to contemplate this moment, and not relinquish it too soon: that we are not absolutely determined by even crucial events in our lives; an initial failure may release us to a new, more appropriate, and even more challenging course of action. We have the power to redefine ourselves, to heal our wounds, to "be secret and take defeat" (W. B. Yeats) and re-emerge; like Henry James who had failed so ignominiously, and publicly, as a playwright in London, literally booed off the stage, yet bravely vowing in his journal, "I take up my *own* old pen again—the pen of all my old unforgettable efforts and sacred struggles. To myself—today—I need say no more. Large and full and high the future still opens. It is now indeed that I may do the work of my life. And I will."

In Madison, I have been made to feel at last that I do belong. I have arrived at an age when, if someone welcomes you, you don't question the motives. You don't question your own motives. Rejoice, and give thanks.

Of our wounds we fashion monuments of survival. If we survive.

A FRAGMENTARY MEMOIR OF *a lost time. A time of apprehension, a time of (near)-dissolution; hearing the nighthawk's beating wings, and not succumbing. For I'd become a kind of nighthawk myself, and I had persevered.*

Our lost selves are not really accessible. Our memories are fabrications, however well-intentioned. And so the effort turns upon itself like a Möbius strip, shrinking from its primary subject. I have been paralyzed by the taboo of violating the privacy of persons close to me and by the taboo, which seems a lesser one, of violating my own self; exposing my very heart, vulnerable and pulsing with life. There are intimacies, secrets, epiphanies and revelations and matters of historic fact of which I will never speak, much less write.

Yes, I did hear from my lost friend Marianna, a few years later, after I'd begun to publish my first books. After her abrupt departure from Madison, Marianna was living with her mother in their small hometown in North Carolina. She had not married her fiancé, evidently. She had not completed her courses at Madison, she had not earned a master's degree there but at a North Carolina college where she was now teaching. She had met "Ray Smith" (as she recalled him) a few times, and she knew that we were married. She asked after Ray, and after me. She asked me to please write back, and so I did—and never heard from her again.

And now I am thinking of that Sunday afternoon, October 23, 1960. I had come alone to a Graduate Students' Association reception in the Memorial Union overlooking this same lake, these waves, not far from where I am sitting, composing these words. I had come to that reception as a break from the obsessiveness of my reading. As a desperate plunge, to discover something outside my head. As a solace, for being unable to write. I knew no one, or nearly. I was one of several thousand graduate students at the university, and perhaps fifty had turned out for this reception; I was seated at a large, round, wooden table with a half-dozen others, their faces now forgotten, their names never known, and in the corner of my eye I saw, or believed that I saw, a figure approaching me. Or, approaching the table. I have no memory of myself that day except that I was likely to be dreamy-eyed, after insomniac nights in succession; I was listening to the conversation at the table without joining in, for I was too shy to join in; I would wait for someone to turn to me, to speak to me; I would not glance around with a bright hopeful smile at this person who was coming near, looming now above me. In one of my own works of fiction such a figure in the periphery of a young woman's vision, undefined, unbidden, mysterious, might turn out to be Death—but this was not fiction, this was my life.

Still, I didn't glance around. Until, when a man asked if he might join me, and pulled out a chair to sit beside me, I did, and lifted my eyes to his face.

DETROIT: LOST CITY 1962–1968

WE WERE SO HAPPY there, why did we ever leave?

THOSE STREETS, ROADS, EXPRESSWAYS. Those years.

Livernois. Gratiot. Grand River. Outer Drive. Telegraph. Michigan. Cass. 2nd. 3rd. 12th. Woodward. Jefferson. Vernor. Fort. Jos. Campau. Dequindre. Warren. Hancock. Beaubien. Brush. Freud. Randolph. Eight Mile. Six Mile. Shelby. Rouge. Faust. John R.

Motor City USA. Murder City USA.

Inside the city limits at Eight Mile and Woodward, the heartbeat quickens. Ceaseless motion, accelerated motion, the pulse of the city. The beat. The beat. The city of romance, wonder. The city of apprehension. The city not-knowing how its future is already receding like lights in a rearview mirror.

HAZY SKYLINES. CHEMICAL-RED SUNSETS. A yeasty gritty taste to the air—how easy to become addicted! And elsewhere, whatever comes to constitute elsewhere, will never quite satisfy. For here is Brownian motion—ceaseless, mesmerizing—a cityscape of grids interrupted by expressways snaking through neighborhoods, cutting streets and lives in two—and no looking back.

For it is a city to be traversed by automobile. It is a city that has sprung to life out of the automobile. Mass production! Overpasses, ramps, railroad tracks, razed buildings and vacant lots where weeds grow to the size of small trees, billboards, houses—blocks, acres, square miles of houses—stretching out forever. Shut my eyes and suddenly I am trembling with excitement, gripping the wheel of an automobile. Again driving south along Livernois in the rain, hoping to enter the John Lodge Expressway just above Fenkell. Or I am driving on Six Mile Road east to Woodward. Or making the turn off Eight Mile Road and Litchfield, grateful to be home. (But which home? It must be the first house my husband and I owned when we were new to Detroit, young instructors at Wayne State University and the University of Detroit respectively—a "Colonial" house of two storeys, four bedrooms, with white aluminum siding, blue shutters, and what seemed to us a large corner lot at the corner of Woodstock Drive and Litchfield. The price, in 1973?—$17,900.)

Shut my eyes, and there is Detroit. As if it has never gone out of my life.

WHEN YOU ARE YOUNG, *newly married, with new jobs and in a new city the future is open wide as an interstate highway crossing the Great Plains. All's ahead, massive open sky, horizon barely visible and the landscape behind so flat you can't see it.*

WE ARRIVED IN THE early summer of 1962 and we left in the early summer of 1968. A brief six years but a lifetime, in fact, a sentimental education never to be repeated for me.

For never underestimate the power—benevolent, malevolent, profound and irresistible—of *place*.

The first year, we lived on the second floor of a two-storey apartment building on Manderson Road, just south of prestigious Palmer Park with its beautiful old mansions, graceful curving drives and tall elms, and north of Six Mile/McNichols Road. A benevolent fate had brought me to teach English at the (Jesuit) University of Detroit (four courses of which two were expository writing—and I loved it) and my husband was an instructor at Wayne State University (though soon to be invited to join the faculty at the University of Windsor across the Detroit River in Canada). Our second residence, on Woodstock, was acquired perhaps a year later, or sometime in 1964 (I remember typing the final draft of *Expensive People* there—a novel not to be published until 1968 when I, too, was teaching at the University of Windsor). Our third and largest residence was a brick and wood Colonial on Sherbourne Road just above Seven Mile, on the corner of Berkeley and two or three blocks from Livernois. What a leafy, lovely neighborhood this was, an area known as Sherwood Forest—a less prestigious variant of Palmer Park, and very Jewish. During the 1967 "riot"—the most profound as it would be the most tragic and consequential of historical incidents in Detroit—there was looting, burning, and vandalism on then-stylish Livernois for a day and a night as we cowered in our house hoping only to be spared the wrath of fellow citizens who were strangers to us as we were strangers to them.

THE QUINTESSENTIAL AMERICAN CITY. That fast-beating stubborn heart.

May you live in interesting times is said to be an ancient Chinese curse but the fact is that for the writer/artist to live in "interesting"—

(i.e., turbulent, unsettled, dangerous)—times and places is likely to be the turning point in one's life.

IN DETROIT, THE LANDSCAPE of western New York State that had so long sustained me, like a riddle or a mystery eluding comprehension, began to fade, to a degree; my subjects for fiction were less likely to be rural, or rather mythic-rural; my obsessional nature began to fix itself upon the extraordinary, indeed unfathomable urban reality in which I was now living, and almost by accident the routes which I was obliged to drive, and which my husband Ray was obliged to drive, took us into parts of Detroit we might otherwise not have known. (As inhabitants of the affluent "white" suburbs of Detroit—Grosse Pointe, Birmingham, Bloomfield Hills predominantly—rarely drove into certain parts of the city but only—rapidly!—through them, on the John Lodge Expressway to the tip of "City Center" at the Detroit River.) Teaching night-school courses to adults in Detroit as well as more traditional students during the day was profoundly consequential: I have only to shut my eyes to see that first, to me intimidating, classroom at the University of Detroit, rows of students (of whom many were older than I was, at twenty-three) to the very back of the room (forty enrolled)—designated to be *mine*.

In such a place, the writer/artist vanishes as her surroundings come to life. The writer/artist becomes quiet as the individuals who surround her speak.

Always I will recall, following our first class, the tall middle-aged soft-spoken and very well-dressed African-American minister who shook my hand and told me *Thank you Mrs. Smith for giving us hope*.

SO MUCH OF MY writing from approximately 1963 to 1976 centers upon or has been emotionally inspired by Detroit and its suburbs that it is hardly possible for me, years later, to extract the historical and autobiographical from the fictional. Life is dazzlingly fecund but art must be selective.

Of course, I would have been a writer—I would have continued to be a writer (I'd already written my first two books before moving to Detroit)—whether I had come to live in Detroit or not. But Detroit so entered my soul, my subjects became almost immediately urban, and my settings were as "real" as the view from a moving automobile; my imagination shifted from a fascination with a quasi-surreal rural landscape to a hyper-realist cityscape. My younger and less experienced self might have recoiled from the sheer bombardment of stimulation in a place like Detroit of the 1960s when the "Motor Capital of the World" was not an ironic designation, and the city fairly simmered with pent-up excitement—Motown, culture, politics, civil rights issues.

After the "riot" of July 1967, there was a seismic shift in the soul of Detroit. You could try to ignore it—you could try, as an individual, to combat it—but you could not control its effect upon you, and you could not predict the ways in which you would be altered by it.

Recalling how our house was burglarized and we'd entered without realizing what danger we might have been in, though guessing that something was wrong—a sliding door at the rear, unlocked and open as we had not left it; the chagrin we'd felt, more than alarm or agitation at being burglarized, when Detroit police officers reprimanded us for having stepped inside a house in which a crime might have been "in progress."

That's how you get yourself killed, see? Next time stay outside.

Recalling how, though we'd always been on cordial, neighborly terms with the African-American family who lived next to us on Sherbourne Road, our neighbors' two young sons began to berate us, even to overturn our trash at the curb, in the months following the riot; once to our astonishment shouting at us as we approached our car in the driveway—*You think we're animals! You think we're animals!*

How furious they were, these boys! They were perhaps ten, twelve years old. They seemed to us much too young for such fury, and such hatred—surely they were repeating words their parents had said in their hearing, about us, their neighbors *the Smiths.*

We were too stunned to protest. Perhaps, in our white skins, we were too confounded by regret, and by guilt. And by fear, that something violent would happen very quickly, as such violent acts happened quickly in Detroit, altering the best-intentioned lives forever.

How we live what seems random, which we experience as fate.

A writer's work is a codified transcript of the writer's life. The (public) work is a record of the (private) life. As years pass, however, and the private/secret life is forgotten except in outline, even the key to the code is but haphazardly recalled, for past secrets are never so tantalizingly secret as those of the present. But the work remains, books remain, as testimonies of a kind.

To the modest extent to which any book, any work of the imagination, can define itself as a unique entity in the world.

IN 1968, WE LEFT Detroit to live in Windsor, Ontario, in a small white-brick house overlooking the Detroit River, across from Belle Isle; it is a geographical, or perhaps a political oddity, that Windsor, Ontario, Canada, is in fact south of Detroit, Michigan, USA.

In 1978, we left Windsor to live in Princeton, New Jersey, where I would teach at the university for several decades—though, in the vividness and starkness of memory, it seems very recent that we'd moved to Windsor; that air of bittersweet yearning, so associated, to me, with driving the endless streets and expressways of Detroit, often in miserable weather, prevails through decades.

The last time I returned to Detroit it was in fact to Grosse Pointe, where I gave a reading at the War Memorial in the fall of 2005, and was driven into the profoundly altered, depopulated and diminished city that had once been so vibrant, and so hopeful; this was an emotionally evocative sentimental journey, that took me to certain of the settings, the very addresses, memorialized in my novels *them*, *Expensive People*, *Do with Me What You Will* and any number of short stories and poems. For here too is a lost urban landscape, irrevocably lost to history, as that part of my life is irrevocably lost. *Turning onto Eight Mile Road from Livernois. A mile or so east, then turning onto Litchfield from Eight Mile. And before Woodstock Drive turning into the driveway of our corner house, driving my little black Volkswagen into our garage beside my husband's car, also a Volkswagen; opening the door that leads into the kitchen, and calling to my husband somewhere inside—* "Hello? I'm home."

STORY INTO FILM: "WHERE ARE YOU GOING, WHERE HAVE YOU BEEN?" AND *SMOOTH TALK*

SOME YEARS AGO IN the American Southwest there surfaced a tabloid psychopath known as "the Pied Piper of Tucson" whose specialty was the seduction and occasional murder of teenaged girls. This individual may or may not have had actual accomplices, but his murders were known among a circle of teenagers in the Tucson area who, for some reason, maintained their loyalty to him, and did not inform parents or police. It was this fact, the fact of the teenagers' loyalty to the psychopath, that struck me at the time as highly disturbing and yet perhaps not so very surprising. For had I not been a teenaged girl myself, not so very many years before?

This was a pre-Manson time, early or mid-1960s. It is worthy of note that the term "serial killer" did not yet exist.

The "Pied Piper" mimicked teenagers in talk, dress, and behavior, but he was not a teenager—he was a man in his early thirties. Rather short, he stuffed rags and crumpled newspapers in his leather boots to give himself height. (And sometimes walked unsteadily: did no one among his adolescent admirers notice?) He charmed his victims as charismatic psychopaths have always charmed their victims, to the bewilderment of others, elders, who fancy themselves free of all lunatic attractions. The Pied Piper of Tucson: a trashy dream, a tabloid archetype, sheer artifice, comedy, cartoon—surrounded, however improbably, and finally tragically, by real people. You think that, if you look twice, he won't be there. But there he is.

I had noticed the article—"The Pied Piper of Tucson"—in a copy of *Life* in our faculty lounge at the University of Detroit, where I was a young instructor. I recall skimming the article, staring at the photographs, and then quickly closing the magazine and laying it down. I did not want to be distracted by too much detail. I was in dread of knowing too much, and my imagination blocked. (It would be decades before I even learned the name of the serial killer: Charles Schmid, Jr.; it would be forty years before I read about him in a detailed online biographical entry, while preparing this memoir.) It was not after all the mass murderer himself who intrigued me, but the disturbing fact that a number of teenagers—from "good" families—aided and abetted his crimes. (In fact, two of the murdered girls were from a prominent Tucson family.) This is the sort of horror authorities, responsible adults, and the media call "inexplicable" because they can't find explanations for it. They would not have fallen under the maniac's spell, after all.

IN OUR SHERBOURNE ROAD house in Detroit, just north of Seven Mile Road, my study was a sparely furnished rosy-pink-walled room overlooking a tree-lined residential street in a neighborhood called, without irony, Sherwood Forest. In this room I would write my novel *them*, subsequent to the July 1967 "riot" that would have the effect of forever altering Detroit's history, and consequently my own, as a writer; in this room, quite clearly the former bedroom of a young girl, and radiating still something of the innocence and emotional volatility of a young girl, I would write the short story "Where Are

You Going, Where Have You Been?" which I mailed off to *Epoch*, a small but distinguished literary magazine published at Cornell University, where it was published in fall 1966. (*Epoch*'s editor James McConkey had been warmly friendly to me, having accepted for publication one of my first short stories, written when I was still an undergraduate at Syracuse University.) An early draft of the story was titled "Death and the Maiden"—which came to seem to me too explicit. The story was cast in a mode of fiction to which I am still partial—indeed, every third or fourth story of mine is probably in this mode— "realistic allegory," it might be called. It is in the mode, so to speak, of Nathaniel Hawthorne's romances, or parables; but its surface is meant to be totally realistic.

Like the medieval German engraving from which the original title was taken, the story was minutely detailed yet clearly an allegory of the fatal attractions of death (or the devil). An innocent young girl is seduced by way of her own vanity; she mistakes death for erotic romance of a particularly American/trashy sort.

In subsequent drafts the story changed its tone, its focus, its language, its title. It became "Where Are You Going, Where Have You Been?" Written at a time when the author was intrigued by the music of Bob Dylan, particularly the hauntingly elegiac song "It's All Over Now, Baby Blue," it was (eventually: not at the time of the writing) dedicated to Bob Dylan. The charismatic mass murderer drops into the background and his innocent victim, a fifteen-year-old, moves into the foreground. Connie becomes the true protagonist of the tale, courting and being courted by her fate, a self-styled 1950s pop figure, a grotesque descendant, in cultural terms, of Marlon Brando's biker-hero of *The Wild One* (1953). "Arnold Friend" is alternately absurd and winning—charismatic and frightening. (It was not my intention, I have to confess, that, as numerous sharp-eyed observers have noted, "Arnold Friend" can be deconstructed as "An Old Fiend.")

There is no suggestion in the story that "Arnold Friend" has seduced and murdered other young girls, or even that he unmistakably intends to murder Connie. Is his interest "merely" sexual? (Nor is there anything about the complicity of other teenagers. I saved that yet more provocative note for a current story, "Testimony.") Connie is shallow, vain, silly, hopeful, doomed—but capable nonetheless of an unexpected gesture of heroism at the story's end. Her smooth-talking seducer, who cannot lie, promises her that her family will be unharmed if she gives herself to him; and so she does. The story ends abruptly at the point of her "crossing over." We don't know the nature of her sacrifice, only that she is generous enough to make it.

IN ADAPTING A NARRATIVE so spare and thematically foreshortened as "Where Are You Going, Where Have You Been?" into the beautifully composed, emotionally engaging feature film *Smooth Talk*, director Joyce Chopra and screenwriter Tom Cole were required to do a good deal of imagining, inventing, expanding. Film is a visual medium, not a verbal medium: the camera is the narrator, not a prose voice-over. Connie's story becomes lavishly, and lovingly, textured from the perspective of a director who knows teenaged girls intimately; Connie is not an allegorical figure but rather a "typical" teenaged girl (if Laura Dern, highly attractive without being distractingly beautiful, can be so defined). Joyce Chopra, who had done documentary films on contemporary teenage culture and, yet more authoritatively, had an adolescent daughter of her own at the time of the film, creates in *Smooth Talk* a vivid and absolutely believable world for Connie to inhabit. Or worlds: as in the original story there is Connie-at-home, and there is Connie-with-her-friends. Two fifteen-year-old girls, two finely honed styles, two voices, sometimes (but not often) overlapping. It is one of the marvelous visual features of the film that we see Connie and her friends transform themselves, once they are safely free of parental observation. The girls claim their true identities as young, sexual beings with no idea of what "sex" actually is, as they walk together in the neighborhood shopping mall. What freedom, what joy! And what a risk.

WHERE THE STORY IS purely Connie's, narrated from her limited perspective, the film is as much Connie's mother's story as it is Connie's. Its center of gravity, its emotional nexus, is frequently with the mother—warmly and convincingly played by Mary Kay Place. (In the story, the mother is not so very nice. The film does not wish to explore the mother's sexual jealousy and resentment of her attractive daughter.) Connie's ambiguous relationship with her affable, somewhat mysterious father (Levon Helm) is an excellent touch: I had thought, subsequent to the story's publication, that I should have focused somewhat more on Connie's father, suggesting, as subtly as I could, an attraction there paralleling the attraction Connie feels for her seducer Arnold Friend. And Arnold Friend himself—"A. Friend" as he says—is played with appropriately overdone sexual swagger by Treat Williams, who is perfect for the part, and just the right age. We see that Arnold Friend isn't a teenager even as Connie, mesmerized by his superficial charm, does not seem to "see" him at all—she sees only his projected image. What is so difficult to accomplish in prose—directing the reader to look over the protagonist's shoulder, so to speak—is accomplished with enviable ease in film.

Treat Williams as Arnold Friend is supreme in his very awfulness, as, surely, the original Pied Piper of Tucson must have been. (Though no one involved in the film knew about the original source, evidently; they had not heard of Charles Schmid, Jr.) Williams brilliantly impersonates Arnold Friend as Arnold Friend awkwardly impersonates Marlon Brando—or is it James Dean? Brando, Dean, impersonating themselves in mirrors? That poor Connie's fate is so trashy is in fact her fate.

WHAT IS OUTSTANDING IN Joyce Chopra's *Smooth Talk* is its visual freshness, its sense of motion and life; the attentive intelligence the director has brought to the semi-secret world of the American adolescent—shopping mall flirtations, drive-in restaurant romances, highway hitchhiking, the fascination of rock music played very, very loud. (James Taylor's music for the film is wonderfully appropriate. We hear it as Connie hears it; it is the seductive music of her spiritual being.) Laura Dern is so dazzlingly right as "my" Connie that I may come to think I modeled the fictitious girl on her, in the way that writers frequently delude themselves about motions of causality.

MY DIFFICULTIES WITH THIS much-acclaimed adaptation of my short story have primarily to do with my hesitation at seeing/hearing work of mine abstracted from its contexture of language. All writers know that Language is our subject; quirky word choices, patterns of rhythm, enigmatic pauses, punctuation marks. Where the quick scanner sees "quick" writing, the writer conceals nine-tenths of the iceberg. Of course we all have subjects, and we feel great passion and commitment to these, but beneath the tale it is the tale-telling that grips us so very fiercely. The writer works in a single dimension, the director works in three. It is always my assumption that the film people who have adapted my work are professionals; authorities in their medium as I am an authority (if I am) in mine. I would fiercely defend the placement of a semicolon in one of my novels but I would probably have deferred in the end to Joyce Chopra's decision to reverse the story's conclusion, turn it upside down, in a sense, so that the film ends not with the death of vanity, not with a sleepwalker-maiden crossing over to Death, but with a scene of reconciliation, rejuvenation. Connie and her older sister reclaim music for themselves—celebrate themselves. Is this realistic? Is this probable? It is a satisfying ending.

A GIRL'S LOSS OF virginity, bittersweet but not necessarily tragic. Not today. A girl's coming-of-age that involves her succumbing to, but then rejecting, the "trashy dreams" of her pop teenage culture. "Where Are You Going, Where Have You Been?" defines itself as allegorical in its conclusion: Death and Death's chariot (a funky souped-up convertible) have come for the Maiden. Awakening is, in the story's final lines, moving out into the sunlight where Arnold Friend waits:

> My sweet little blue-eyed girl," he said in a half-sung sigh that had nothing to do with [Connie's] brown eyes but was taken up just the same by the vast sunlit reaches of the land behind him and on all sides of him—so much land that Connie had never seen before and did not recognize except to know that she was going to it.

—a vision perhaps impossible to transfigure into film.

PHOTO SHOOT: WEST ELEVENTH STREET, NYC, MARCH 6, 1970

Joyce Carol Oates, New York City, March 6, 1970.
(Jack Robinson for Vogue*)*

"ALMOST PATHETICALLY SERIOUS"—so *Vogue* wrote of the thirty-two-year-old novelist whose photograph appeared in the August 15, 1970, issue of the magazine. The writer went on to note that the novelist, whose fourth novel, *them*, had received the National Book Award for 1970, was "tentative, hush-voiced, with the fixed brown eyes of a sleepwalker" and that "daydreaming" had given to her writing a "peculiar floating quality" somewhat at odds with the violence of her subject. An excerpt from the novelist's National Book Award acceptance speech was quoted: "What an artist has to resist and turn to his advantage is violence." The photo-replica of the novelist's face of 1970, strangely without expression, masklike and dreamy and "serene," ironically gave no indication of the maelstrom of emotions she was feeling at the time of the photo-shoot: excitement, wonderment, stress, a kind of chronic ontological anxiety.

Photographed for *Vogue*! The most elegant, as it was the most daunting and mysterious, of the several glossy magazines my grandmother Blanche Morgenstern, herself a somewhat mysterious woman, brought to our house in Millersport, New York, when I was growing up in the 1950s. Other magazines were the more practical-minded *Redbook*, *McCall's*, *Cosmopolitan* (in an earlier, earnest and even "literary" incarnation), *Ladies' Home Journal* and *Good Housekeeping*; the career-girl *Mademoiselle* (where in 1959 my first published story, "In the Old World," appeared); and the *New Yorker*, most prized in our household for its cartoons, and inhabited by fey, epicene individuals we assumed were New York City sophisticates. My grandmother Blanche was an accomplished seamstress, sewing for me, and sometimes for my mother, not only skirts, blouses, jumpers but also suits and coats; my grandmother chose her designs from Butterick, Simplicity, McCall's, but also—at times—Vogue, which were the most difficult (and chic) patterns; it was for the sake of the fashion features in *Vogue* that my grandmother bought the expensive magazine, thick as a phone book with astonishing photographs. Of all the magazines that came into the house it was *Vogue* that evoked the most fascination to a girl living on a small not-very-prosperous farm in upstate New York, as it was *Vogue* that aroused in my father the most sardonic of remarks relating to women's fashions. (Many of Daddy's remarks, expressing bemused indignation, began with a scowl and a muttered "Jaysus—!") Both Daddy and I would have been stunned speechless if we could have known that, one day, the name *Oates* would appear in *Vogue*, as both byline and subject.

For here was a trove of the mystical, magically empowered feminine, distinct from the (merely) utilitarian female (on a farm, females have their specific uses, none of which is romantic in the slightest): *Vogue* was, among other things, a shrine honoring sheer nonutilitarian beauty, most of which happened to be, not *female*, but *feminine*. It would be decades before I encountered Sigmund Freud's remark in his late, melancholy *Civilization and Its Discontents*: "Beauty has no obvious use; nor is there any clear cultural necessity for it. Yet civilization could not do without it."

Already in early adolescence I had become an astute observer of worlds so foreign to my own, I might have been contemplating the photographs of women and men from another species, captured, for *Vogue*, by the lenses of such legendary photographers as Richard Avedon and Irving Penn. No more than I might have fantasized looking like any of these socialites and models wearing extraordinary clothes, jewels, and footwear could I have imagined seeing myself one day in *Vogue*.

On March 4, 1970, I had received the National Book Award for my novel *them* at a gala celebration in New York City; this portrait was taken in the late morning of March 6, in a studio in a town house on West Eleventh Street. Amid a flurry of interviews and photography sessions during my brief, vertiginous visit to New York City for the National Book Award event, this image is the only one that is dramatically imprinted in my memory. What is evoked in the portrait for me is a perverse sort of nostalgia: the recollection of that era of peril, beginning with the tragic and dispiriting assassination of John F. Kennedy in 1963, and continuing through a dazed, near-anarchic decade of assassinations and "race riots" in American cities (as infamously in Detroit in July 1967 when my husband Ray Smith and I were living in that beleaguered city) through the end of the bloody, protracted, and exhausting Vietnam War in 1973. It is an era difficult to evoke to those who didn't live through it: when paranoia flourished, and with justification; drug use became as commonplace as cigarettes; and isolated acts of terrorism, bombs on college campuses, for instance, or detonated at the Pentagon, were purely "American-revolutionary-radical" and not foreign. For on the morning of the photo shoot on West Eleventh Street, after a night of fitful sleep in a spacious, elegantly shabby Central Park West apartment listening to the nighttime noises of the great city (if sirens were neon-red traceries in the sky, how like a cat's cradle the sky above New York City would look!), as I sat stiff and self-conscious trying not to blink in the glaring lights, trying, as the photographer gently urged me, to "relax—smile," there came suddenly, from somewhere alarmingly close by, a deafening explosion. Windows in the photographer's studio rattled; the floors, walls, ceiling of the studio shook; for a terrible moment, it seemed that the very brownstone would shatter and collapse around us.

Abruptly, the photo shoot for *Vogue* ceased.

Perhaps it was at this instant that the image was "captured" on film: the instant when the private and inward is waylaid, appropriated, and redefined by an act of violence.

In such an instant you feel sick, animal fear. You become totally physical, visceral. Panic floods your veins, your heartbeat runs wild. Your confused thoughts are of the most primitive sort—*Am I injured? Am I alive? Am I in danger? Am I—all right?*

For it is not uncommon, that individuals who are terribly, even fatally injured will imagine, initially, that they are *all right*. If they can breathe, or move an arm—desperately the brain signals *Yes. I am alive—I am all right.*

I was reminded of the more protracted panic we'd felt, trapped in our house on Sherbourne Road, Detroit, several years before. From sometime in the early morning of July 23, 1967—(when Detroit police raided an unlicensed "drinking club" on Twelfth Street in an African-American neighborhood)—for forty-eight hours or more we'd remained in our house hoping it would not be set on fire, or that police or snipers wouldn't shoot into our windows; less than three blocks from our house, on Livernois Avenue, store windows were smashed, and stores were looted; there were arson fires, looting, gunfire, street violence, near-continuous sirens. It was as if— literally—the world had erupted into madness. At such times of peril you think, pleadingly—*This can't be happening to us!* And if you are very lucky, it isn't.

The photographer, the photographer's assistants, and I staggered out of the brownstone on West Eleventh Street, and onto the sidewalk, where the air was befouled—smoky and gritty. We were dazed, panicked. What had happened? Were we in danger—would there be another explosion? With stunning abruptness the intimate moment of "art" had ended to be replaced by this brute and utterly perplexing reality, of which we could make little sense. Around us were frightened pedestrians, stalled traffic, a cacophony of sirens and horns. No one had an idea what the explosion had been: a boiler? Gas line? Bomb?

A block away, in the direction of Fifth Avenue, it seemed that flames shot upward from what appeared to be a brownstone town house. It would turn out to have been an elegant nineteenth-century house with a Greek Revival facade, the boyhood home of the poet James Merrill.

Later, it would be revealed that the explosion had been inadvertently caused by an amateur bomb maker who'd triggered a timer on a homemade "antipersonnel" bomb being assembled in the basement of a house at 18 West Eleventh Street by members of the radical group Weathermen; their murderous intention had been to set off the bomb at a dance at the Fort Dix, New Jersey, army base. The bomb detonated that morning killed three individuals, two men and a woman named Diana Oughton, former debutante and Bryn Mawr graduate, whose body was grotesquely dismembered in the blast and who would be identified only by fingerprints; fleeing from the burning house, on foot, were two female Weathermen, one of them Kathy Boudin, later to acquire notoriety of her own. That season of peril. The sour, sick dregs of 1960s counter-culture idealism. In such rocky soil the seeds of nostalgia yet grow.

My husband and I left New York City the next morning, to drive back to Windsor, Ontario, Canada, where we now lived. It had come to seem an ironic commemoration: my novel *them*, set in Detroit, Michigan, in the era of the riot, and yet something of a valentine for the Detroit of those years, had been honored only after I'd departed Detroit forever, to move across the Detroit River to a more hospitable, as it was a Canadian, city, where the buildings and grounds of the University of Windsor partly fronted the river. Living in Ontario during the ongoing, spiritually exhausting crisis of the Vietnam War, in a foreign country with the advantage of hardly seeming foreign, I would gaze out the windows of my study at the fast-flowing, choppy, often lead-colored river at the foot of our lawn and I would feel a pang of loss, that I had been expelled from the United States, seemingly—out of despair and frustration with American politics of the time, and out of a genuine wish to work with those young Americans known contemptuously as "draft-dodgers"—individuals who seemed courageous to me, in their refusal to fight what appeared even then to be a futile and unjust war—as well as with excellent Canadian students, for whom high school was four years in contrast to the three years of American high school, and who were consequently much better prepared for university than American students. *Ten years in exile, in Ontario*—a fruitful and altogether wonderful decade, that ended too soon.

And often I would remember, seeing the *Vogue* photo which my practical-minded publisher would use on my book jacket covers for years, the circumstances of that dramatic photo shoot; how curious and fleeting is the intimacy between photographer and "subject," how abruptly it can end; and the image that remains can be both timeless and time-bound, a memory of nightmare crystallized in art.

JUST NOW, ON A balmy late morning in May 2014, I have walked past the brick town house at 18 West Eleventh Street, an entirely new building of course, refashioned, more "modern" than the old, amid a block of handsome, highly respectful, and very expensive West Village properties. From somewhere close by, on Fifth Avenue, a siren is wailing—but soon fades.

FOOD MYSTERIES

TOOTSIE ROLL, MALLOW CUP, Milky Way, Junior Mints, Snickers, Hershey Bar, Mars Bar, Oh Henry!

Juicy Fruit, Dentyne chewing gum.

Bubble gum. "Jawbreaker."

Hostess CupCake: chocolate with "cream" filling.

Pies in crinkly waxed paper that fit into the palm of the hand, to be devoured rapturously on the sidewalk outside the store in which they were purchased.

Magical syllables—"*Tastee-Freez.*" Transit Road, Lockport.

Orange, chocolate, cherry Popsicles slow-melting at first, then rapidly melting. Fingers sticky.

Fudgsicles, Creamsicles. Front of shirt stained, bare toes sticky.

At *The Royale* on Main Street, Lockport: hot fudge banana split with maraschino cherries, whipped cream, crown of sugar wafers.

At *Castle's Dairy* on Main Street, Lockport: vanilla malt so thick you could barely drink it through a straw; strawberry milk shakes, double-dip ice-cream cones, chocolate ice-cream sandwiches.

At *Rexall's* counter, chocolate Coke.

Freddie's Doughnuts: glazed, chocolate, frosted, cinnamon, sweet doughy filled to bursting with whipped cream/jelly and covered in confectioners' sugar that leave a guilty ghost-smile on your face.

MAYONNAISE SANDWICH

Mustard sandwich

Peanut butter sandwich

Baloney sandwich

Kraft American cheese sandwich

Grilled cheese sandwiches

Hamburgers/cheeseburgers/hot dogs

Ketchup, mustard-and-relish

French fries. Coleslaw. Salty, sugary.

Salty "buttery" popcorn sold at Palace Theater, Rialto Theatre hungrily devoured despite perennial rumors of rat droppings, cockroaches in popcorn boxes.

North Park Junior High cafeteria: (scorched) macaroni-and-cheese casserole, Chef Boyardee spaghetti and tomato sauce, grease-encrusted French fries.

Beef doves. Shepherd's pie. Texas hash.

(Canned) fruit cup.

Rice pudding, bread pudding. Chocolate pudding.

Shiny quivery red Jell-O in fluted mold.

Pizza: cheese, tomato, green pepper and coin-sized slices of pepperoni sausage glimmering with miniature pools of grease.

Tiny (canned) shrimp, macaroni with Kraft's mayonnaise on lettuce leaves.

Steaming-hot gluey oatmeal with milk, brown sugar.

Cheerios, Rice Krispies. Wheaties.

Gingerbread, fudge.

Triple-layer devil's food with fudge frosting.

Excitement of baking cookies: carefully placing Mom's cookie dough on baking tin. Chocolate chip, oatmeal, ginger, sugar.

Frosting Christmas cookies in the kitchen. Star-shaped, Christmas-tree-shaped sugar cookies with tiny sparkles like mica.

Excitement of coloring Easter eggs: carefully lowering egg into dye, on teaspoon.

PEPSI, COCA-COLA, DR PEPPER, Sunkist. Royal Crown Root Beer.

Sip of Daddy's dark ale—so bitter! hurtful on the tongue!

Foods fried in lard. Thickly coated in bread crumbs.

Southern-fried chicken, glazed ham baked with (canned) pineapple slices.

Campbell's soups: tomato, chicken noodle, cream of mushroom.

Heinz's Pork-and-Beans.

Breaded fish sticks dipped in Heinz's ketchup.

Breaded cutlets, breaded chicken parts.

Mashed potatoes with gravy-pools.

Mashed potatoes with slow-melting wedges of butter cold from the refrigerator.

Roast turkey. Bread stuffing. Cranberry sauce, pumpkin pie, Grandma's gravy boat brimming with fatty gravy.

Shame of Planters Peanuts eaten greedily out of the can in the car en route home from shopping at Loblaw's, Lockport.

Salt/grease acute. Interior of mouth smarting.

Cheese omelets the size of automobile hubcaps, preferred rubbery to "moist."

Iceberg lettuce wilting beneath spoonfuls of neon-pink "Russian" dressing.

From the dank earthen-floored cobweb-festooned cellar with its myriad odors, jars of canned applesauce, homemade—from the "fruit closet."

Canned pears, sweet cherries, peaches swimming in syrup— from the "fruit closet."

Blueberry pancakes. Waffles.

Vermont maple syrup in the sticky plastic pitcher.

Homemade spaghetti sauce, meatballs. Daddy's favorite meal simmering on the stove.

Wonderful lost foods of childhood, adolescence—where gone?

HOW COULD WE HAVE eaten such heavy, unhealthful food?
   Happily, mostly.

MY HUNGARIAN GRANDMOTHER LENA Bush made thick goulashes with sour cream and paprika. She made her own noodles rolling stiff chalky-white dough into layers on a breadboard, sprinkled with flour; stacking the layers together to be cut, precisely, with a long sharp knife. On her stove was a continuous simmering beef- or chicken-broth.

My grandmother's most intricate specialties were Hungarian pastries that required such patience, skill, and single-minded purpose that my mother rarely tried to make them after my grandmother's death. One of these consisted of thin pancakes prepared in a large iron skillet, filled with fruit (pears, cherries, peaches) and sour cream; another, yet more complicated, was rolled to airy thinness on the breadboard, filled similarly with fruit and sour cream, then rolled up tight, baked, cut, and served in small dishes. (Years later I would learn that these were variations of the traditional Hungarian Almás palacsinta, Egri félgömbpalacsinta, and rétesek.)

I never learned to prepare any Hungarian dish. I never learned a word of Hungarian except by osmosis, curse words of my grandfather's which I would never have dared repeat.

MEATLESS FRIDAYS. IT WAS a mystery to me, how, when our family "converted" to Catholicism after my grandfather's death, we could no longer eat meat on Friday.

There were *venial sins, mortal sins*. Eating meat on Friday was blatantly disobeying a decree of the Church (since rescinded), thus a *mortal sin* punishable by Hell.

I did not strongly question these decrees. I was not a confrontational or rebellious daughter, except inwardly, in secret; whatever I was expected to believe, a small still voice in my head assured me *You will do what you want to do. Nobody can make you do anything you don't want to do.*

Eating meat, not-eating meat—this issue meant little to me. But the idea behind it, the *Why?*—this was not so easily swept aside.

How strange and unsettling it seemed to me that my father, so skeptical by nature, had become mysteriously quiet, even passive, on this matter; as if to resist the strictures of Catholicism was in some way to betray the memory of John Bush, and to further upset Lena Bush and (for a while, at least) my mother Carolina.

And so on Fridays I would help my mother prepare "fish dishes" for us—salmon patties fried in a skillet, creamed tuna fish with peas on toast.

Except for the bread these ingredients were canned, of course. Packed in water and salt. Indeed, it would be years before I fully grasped the concept that "salmon" and "tuna" are in fact (large, beautiful) fish of the kind that swim in the ocean.

Does God care what we eat? Why?—in the Pendleton church in a haze of boredom I would ponder such questions, to which no adult had any answer except *This is what the Church teaches.*

Any young person will smartly counter *But somebody is making up these things, not the "Church"!*

Yet it is true in some way, that there is holiness bound up with the food we eat, when it is prepared for us with care and intention. And where there is holiness, there is the possibility of its reverse—the forbidden, the taboo.

By the standards of a world beyond Millersport these were crude meals—salmon patties, canned-tuna-on-toast. Also macaroni and cheese, "fish sticks." And yet, how we loved them! The memory of such meals, and my family at the small kitchen table upstairs in the old farmhouse in Millersport, now leaves me faint with hunger.

FACTS, VISIONS, MYSTERIES:
MY FATHER FREDERIC OATES,
NOVEMBER 1988

NOVEMBER 1988. IN MY study in our home in Princeton, New Jersey, I am listening, as dusk comes swiftly on, to my father playing piano in another part of the house. Unhesitatingly my father moves through the *presto agitato* of Schubert's "Erl-King," striking the urgent sequence of notes rapidly but firmly. There's a shimmering quality to the sound, and I am thinking of how the mystery of music is a paradigm of the mystery of personality: most of us "know" family members exclusive of statistical information, sometimes in defiance of it, in the way that we seem to know familiar pieces of music without having any idea of their thematic or structural composition. After a few notes we recognize them—that is all.

Neuroscientists can explain how such recognitions are instantaneously possible, or should be in a normally functioning human brain, but we who experience them have no idea of the astonishing circuits the brain has closed for us in a fraction of a second, a kind of learned knowledge that seems virtually instinctual. The powerful appeal of music is not easily explicable, forever mysterious, like the subterranean urgings of the soul; and so too, the appeal of certain individuals in our lives. We are rarely aware of the gravitational forces we embody for others (if we embody any at all) but we are keenly aware of the gravitational forces these certain others embody for us. To say *My father, my mother* is to name but not easily to approach one of the central mysteries of my life.

How did the difficult, malnourished, frequently violent circumstances of my parents' early lives allow them to grow, to blossom, finally to thrive into the people they've become?—is there no inevitable relationship between personal history and personality?—is character somehow bred in the bone, absolute fate? destiny? But what do we mean by "character"? What roles do "environment"—"family"—play?

I am determined to memorialize my father, my mother. But—how to begin?

In families, facts often come belatedly to us. Rarely are we told the most crucial facts of our parents' lives when we are most intimate with them, as young children; such knowledge comes, if it comes at all, when we are older. And what exactly are *facts*, that we should imagine they have the power to explain the world to us? On the contrary, it is facts that must be explained.

HERE ARE FACTS:

My father's father Joseph Carlton Oates left his young wife Blanche when their son, Frederic James, an only child, was two or three years old, in 1916. Abandoned them, to be specific, in Lockport, New York. There was no question of child support or alimony: this was the early 1900s, and such laws did not exist; even if they had, it isn't likely that Joseph Oates, allegedly a "heavy drinker," would have been willing or able to help support his family. My grandmother Blanche had to find work where she could (shopgirl? mill worker?

chambermaid?) in this small city on the Erie Barge Canal north of Buffalo; when Frederic was thirteen, he began to work part-time; at seventeen, he quit school to work full-time. Twenty-eight years after he'd left his family, one night in 1944, Joseph Carlton Oates reappeared in a country tavern in Swormville to seek out his son Frederic, now living a few miles away in the crossroads community of Millersport, not to ask forgiveness for his selfishness as a father, nor even to explain his abandonment of his family: he'd come, Joseph Carlton announced, to "fight" his son.

For it seemed that Joseph Carlton had been hearing rumors that his son Frederic had long held a grudge against him and wanted to fight him, so Joseph Carlton sought the younger man out to challenge him. (Since leaving Lockport he'd been living in the Buffalo area, not really far from his former wife and their son, but in those years twenty-five miles could seem distant, what one hundred miles might seem like today.) But when the swaggering and belligerent Joseph Carlton confronted Frederic, the elder in his mid-fifties, the younger a married man and father of thirty, it turned out that Frederic had no special grudge against Joseph, and didn't want to fight him.

How like a ballad or a folk song this story is, in the melancholy simplicity of its telling! Yet the story has an unexpectedly upbeat ending, a reversal of (Oedipal) expectations—the son doesn't fight the father, though the interior of a crude country tavern would be an ideal setting for such an encounter.

Said my father Frederic, now in his seventies, shaking his head with a bemused smile, "Jesus! I couldn't bring myself to hit anyone that old."

THE IRISH WILL BREAK your heart.

When I traveled to Ireland (to attend a literary festival) and made inquiries, I was told that "Oates" was not a common name but that there were "Oateses" in the west of Ireland—somewhere.

The Irishwoman who told me this did not sound very certain. I recall that she frowned thoughtfully—as if there might be something about "Oates" that wasn't so very positive, which she did not wish to suggest.

Very likely, these Oateses suspected to dwell somewhere in the west of Ireland were relatives of Joseph Carlton Oates, distant relatives by the time of the late twentieth century. My father's father had been born in Ireland, I think; or, he'd been brought to the United States as a young boy, in the late 1880s. How, why Joseph Carlton Oates found his way to the small barge canal town of Lockport where he met and married Blanche Morgenstern, and became a young, presumably restless father with a weakness for alcohol and no great love for domesticity—there was no one to tell me, and so I do not know.

In my novel *The Gravedigger's Daughter*, written after my grandmother Blanche's death, I have tried to evoke the mysterious life of my grandmother in those long-ago years. But Carlton Oates is present only by analogy: the hard-drinking, abusive and treacherous man who, if you make the mistake of loving him, will break your heart; if you make the mistake of marrying him, he will abandon you and your child.

It was said in the family—(though never when my grandmother Blanche was within earshot)—that Joseph Carlton and Frederic resembled each other dramatically. Identical thick, cresting black hair with a widow's peak, heavy brows, strikingly handsome features. The identical air of the quick-tempered, easily insulted male of a shabbily glamorous era best embodied, in popular culture, in the menacing swagger of Robert Mitchum (one of the few Hollywood actors whom my father admired, perhaps because Mitchum was the antithesis of the Hollywood leading man). Though I resemble my father, and so too this long-deceased Irish grandfather, I never saw Joseph Carlton's face, not even in a photograph.

And so, the "lost" Irish grandfather is an enigma to me. Never have I dared to ask questions directly, for in our family that isn't done, but by degrees I have come to form an impression of him from my father's offhanded remarks. This (seemingly) cruel, selfish, difficult and yet attractive man of whom my grandmother Blanche, who never speaks ill of anyone, will say only, stiffly, that he was "no good."

Yet Blanche Morgenstern must have fallen in love with Joseph Oates, as a girl of eighteen or nineteen; if she revised her judgment of the man afterward, still the fact remains—they were married, and my father was their only child. And I am descended from him, the elusive Irish Oates.

In this way Joseph Carlton Oates has become one of those phantom family members, common in many families perhaps, whose very historical existence must be taken on faith.

A paradigm, perhaps, for the elusive Other—the very romance of prose fiction that is both the quest for this obscure object of desire and the apprehension that the object's existence may be highly "fictitious."

THIS IS NOT FACT, but theory. *If Joseph Carlton Oates had not abandoned his young wife and son in 1916 but continued to live with them, isn't it likely that given his drinking and his predilection for settling matters with his fists he would have been abusive to both his wife and his son; would (probably) have beaten my father repeatedly, so infecting Frederic (if we can believe theories of the tragic etiology of domestic violence) with a similar predilection for violence. What then of my father's behavior as husband, father? In my life in Millersport I'd observed many times my father's quick temper, and his smoldering anger, but I had never observed him reacting violently, that is "physically," to anyone, nor even threatening to do so. And so it is possible that abandoning his young family to poverty in Lockport, in 1916, was an unintended gesture of kindness: perhaps the most magnanimous gesture my mysterious grandfather Joseph Carlton Oates could have made.*

But I won't suggest this to my father, I think. No one should try to come between a man and his memory of his father however embittered or bemused.

IN A MEMOIR OF her early childhood the poet Alicia Ostriker describes her father, a pharmacist, as a "kindly" man; a man of the Jewish tradition of "kindly" husbands, fathers, community members. *Kindness* as a tradition! In the America of my family's past there was no tradition of "kindness" in men; indeed, "kindness" as a cultivated virtue would have seemed unnatural, unmanly. (In fact, unknown to him, Fred Oates's maternal grandparents were German Jews who had emigrated to the United States in the late 1890s, changed their name and so successfully remade themselves into no-religion, no-ethnicity, that no one knew their background. The time-honored American-frontier tradition of making yourself into *nothing*.) But for much of his life my father Frederic Oates belonged to another tradition, you might say, in which (male) violence, the American romance of (male) violence, was unquestioned.

In this tradition there were two kinds of men: those who were willing/eager to fight, and those who were not willing/eager to fight, thus "unmanly."

The tradition has nothing inherently to do with guns. It is an American-frontier value of another kind, that has to do with male self-respect and male protectiveness of family. Despite my father's intelligence, talent (for art, music), and common sense, Fred Oates was no exception to the ethic of his time, place, and social class.

Though never stated explicitly, a code of ethics prevailed:

A man does not strike a woman or a child.

A man must maintain his dignity at all costs.

Except in special circumstances, a man does not back down from a fight.

Thus/and: A man *must always be prepared to fight*.

For such men, boxing was the most profound sport, as boxing would not have seemed like a "sport" at all but rather something deeper and more primal, analogous to their own lives as sports involving play, teams, balls would not.

No man would not follow American boxing. No man would have to stop to think who the current heavyweight or middleweight champion of the world was.

One of my childhood memories is of my mother pleading with my father not to drive back to confront a hitchhiker who had (evidently) made an obscene gesture when my father had driven past him on Transit Road, my mother in the passenger's seat and my brother and me in the backseat. My father was furious, red-faced; it wasn't just that he had been insulted, but that my mother had seen the gesture too, and possibly, as Daddy thought, my brother and me. (Reading comic books in the back of the car, I hadn't noticed a thing.) Despite my mother begging him not to drive back, my father did— with what results, we never knew. (At least, my brother and I never knew.) Did my father challenge the hitchhiker to a fight? *Did* they fight? Very likely, the hitchhiker was astonished that my father had driven back to confront him, and probably, or possibly, he had apologized and there was no exchange of blows.

(As an adult now, I am most sympathetic with my mother. I am trying to imagine how she must have felt when my father drove back to confront a stranger who might have been mentally ill, might have had a concealed weapon, or might have been stronger than my father, or more desperate—these possibilities my mother must have anxiously contemplated.)

A man never backs down from a fight.

It wasn't surprising to learn that my grandfather Joseph Carlton was a man who used his fists but it was surprising to learn that he'd sought out his own son to fight. And it was consoling to learn that my father, hotheaded as he'd been at thirty, had not cared to oblige him.

"We had a few beers together. That was it. My old man drove back to Buffalo, and I never saw him again."

IT WAS A FEATURE of his early life, with his (single) mother, that my father moved frequently in Lockport, from one low-priced rental to another. He worked at numerous jobs—Palace Theater organist, sign painter; machine shop at Harrison's—and soon became self-supporting. Eventually, his mother remarried, a man named Bob Woodside, whom my father did not like, or of whom he did not approve—I don't think we ever knew why. (When my grandmother Blanche came by Greyhound bus to visit us each week, my step-grandfather never accompanied her. My memory is of an older man, gray-haired, not unattractive, perhaps a factory worker, or an employee of a small Lockport business, who avidly read pulp magazines—*True Detective*, science fiction—and who smoked cigars.) For a brief while when my parents were first married they lived in Lockport, in "Lowertown"—then moved out to Millersport to live in the upper half of the Bushes' farmhouse.

At this time, in November 1988, my parents live on the same property on Transit Road, but in a small ranch-style house (built 1961) with white aluminum siding, neat brown trim, and an enormous front lawn which is my father's responsibility to mow with a tractor-mower. Some of the pear trees remain, but the old farmhouse of my childhood has long vanished.

The old hay barn, that had badly needed repair when I'd been a girl, has long vanished. My grandfather's smithy. The mound of rubble that contained broken horseshoes, rusted spikes. The silo in which a child might have suffocated, the chicken coop and all of the chicken yard and the wire fence surrounding it.

All of that ghostly flock of Rhode Island Reds, vanished. Beloved Happy Chicken a fading memory.

Yet nearby, on the Tonawanda Creek Road in the direction of Pendleton, the ruins of the old Judd house remain on an untended lot as if in mockery.

(Where has Helen Judd gone? What has become of the Judd children? No one in Millersport will claim to know.)

The generation that preceded my parents has long vanished. First-generation Americans, many of them; or immigrants from Hungary, Ireland, Germany.

My grandmother Blanche died after a lengthy illness, a form of cancer, in 1970. So reluctant were family members to speak of my grandmother's illness, and so undisposed was my grandmother to speak of herself, I never knew that my grandmother was seriously ill until her cancer was advanced. Belatedly I learned that my grandmother had not wanted me to know about her illness—she had not wanted to upset *me*.

In the hospital she assured me, with her calm smile: "I don't mind."

Gently Grandma squeezed my hand, to comfort me. I was stunned, stricken to the heart. I could not even cry—yet.

I don't mind. These words are so deeply imprinted in my soul, I think that a kind of anesthesia has overcome me; where I should be feeling strongly, there is a block, a cutting-short like a gentle rebuke—*I don't mind.*

(And so, when people ask me the maddening, socially mandated *how are you? how are you feeling?*—I have no reply except a bone-chillingly cheery, "Fine! And you?")

Of course, my grandmother was medicated. I know that. It was not my grandmother Blanche but the medication that spoke, to assure others what might have been true about her final hours of consciousness, or might not have been true in quite that way—*I don't mind*.

Joyce's grandmother Blanche Morgenstern, Lockport, New York, 1917.

On a windowsill in my study, facing my desk, is an old, precious photograph of Blanche Morgenstern in her early twenties: a delicately beautiful young woman in a stylish winter coat with fur collar and cuffs, holding a small purse in her ungloved hands; she is wearing a chic wide-brimmed dark hat; her stockings appear to be black, or black-tinged, and her legs and ankles are slim. Beside her is the rough wall of a stone house, behind her the front wheel of a bicycle. Tree limbs are bare and skeletal, the mood of the landscape is winter. Because it is black-and-white, and has no color, this image seems to belong to a time before time—certainly, a time before my birth— before even my parents' birth. Often for long minutes I stare at the photograph in wonderment: who took this picture? With what sort of camera, so long ago? What is the beautiful young woman in the picture thinking? *Is* she thinking? Her expression is somber, though she is half-smiling; a Mona Lisa—sort of smile; her beauty suggests a kind of antiquity. *This young woman—my grandmother-to-be!* How astonished she would have been, how disbelieving.

Everyone who sees this photograph, everyone to whom I have shown it, remarks how closely I resemble Blanche Morgenstern, despite the difference in our ages: the granddaughter now so much older than the grandmother in the photograph.

My Princeton friends also say, "But obviously, your grand-mother was Jewish."

If only my grandmother had acknowledged her Jewish back-ground, and allowed us to speak openly of these family "secrets"— perhaps she would have been less lonely. (*Was* my grandmother lonely? It is possible that I am imagining an isolation that my grand-mother didn't actually feel; it is just as likely that she felt, every hour of her life, a profound relief that her father had not murdered her, and that the gift of life was hers to accept without a backward glance.)

When Grandma died, her son Fred was deeply grieved, shaken. We had all been prepared for her death and yet—you are never pre-pared. My mother told me, "Dad is keeping what he feels to himself. He won't talk to me. You know how Dad is."

It is the way of some families, to keep emotion tight, tight, tight within—as if grasped by a fist. There is the fear that, if emotion is released, there will be no holding back, ever.

Especially for men like Fred Oates. The more "manly" the man, the more tightly restrained the emotion.

As the escalating notes of "The Erl-King" plunge forward.

FROM MY JOURNAL, 5/20/86:

> *Last week, my parents came to visit . . . They arrived on Wednesday, left on Saturday afternoon. Immediately the house is too large, empty, quiet, unused . . . My mother brought me a dress she'd sewed for me, blue print, long-sleeved, full-skirted. "Demure". . .*

> *(Another family secret revealed with a disarming casualness. Perhaps because of their ages my parents don't want to keep secrets? Not that they are old at seventy or seventy-one. My father told of how his grandfather Morgenstern tried to kill his grandmother in a fit of rage, then killed himself—gun barrel placed under his chin, trigger pulled, (his daughter) Blanche close by. My father was about fifteen at the time. They were all living in a single household . . . A sordid tale. Yet grimly comical: I asked what occupation my great-grandfather had, was told he was a gravedigger.)*

> *(Family secrets! So many! Or no—not so very many, I suppose, but unnerving. And I think of my sweet grandmother Blanche who nearly witnessed her own father's violent suicide . . . She had come home to find the door locked. Her father*

was beating her mother upstairs in their bedroom. Hearing her
at the door he came downstairs with his gun and for some
reason (frustration, drunkenness, madness) he killed himself
just inside the locked door. Several times I said to my father,
dazed, but you never told me any of this! and my father said
with his air of utter placidity, Didn't I?—I'm sure I did.
This is a counter-theme of sorts. The secret is at last revealed,
after decades; but it is revealed with the accompanying claim
that it had been revealed a long time ago and is not therefore
a secret.)

What is unexpected about this unhappy memory of a long-ago attempted murder and suicide is that my grandmother Blanche had already married Joseph Oates, and been divorced from him; if my father was fifteen, and born in 1914, this would date the suicide of his gravedigger-grandfather sometime in 1929. (In my re-imagining of the incident in *The Gravedigger's Daughter* the daughter of the suicidal gravedigger is not an adult but a girl, and her father contemplates killing her as well as her mother, before turning the gun on himself. What had not quite happened in actual life, but had been intended, was fulfilled in fiction—in this way, the desperate vengeance of my great-grandfather Morgenstern was fulfilled.)

ONLY BELATEDLY DID MY brother and I learn—my parents had had their fiftieth anniversary in 1987, and had not told us!

And, they had not celebrated the anniversary.

We protested: how could you do such a thing? Not celebrate your fiftieth anniversary? Not tell anyone?

My mother only smiled, and gestured toward my father. *He* was the one, of course, temperamentally disposed never to *make too much of things*.

(Was my mother's smile wistful? Would my mother have liked my father to have *made more of things* than he did, through their long marriage?)

When we were children my brother Robin and I had been astonished by our father's indifference to gifts. What meant so much to us, as children, meant literally nothing to him; Christmas and birthday presents for our father had to be opened by others (that is, by us) since Daddy thought so little of the ritual.

"Look, Daddy! This is for you"—my brother and I would plead with our father, who might be reading a newspaper, or involved in one or another household chore, and would barely glance at us.

We'd thought our father so strange, not to care—not to care about a *present*.

For children, even for teenagers, nothing seems quite so exciting as a *wrapped present*. For days beforehand my brother and I would speculate on the contents of packages beneath our Christmas tree, though our past experiences must surely have curbed our imaginations. But there was our father as indifferent to the excitement of gift-opening as he was to the gifts themselves (invariably shirts, neckties, socks).

Of all writers it is Henry David Thoreau who most speaks to my father's temperament—*Beware of all enterprises that require new clothes*.

And—*Simplify, simplify, simplify*.

From my father I have inherited my ambivalence about gift-giving. I understand that it is an ancient and revered social ritual and that, in human relations, it is, or should be, a genuine expression of love, affection, admiration, respect; yet, through my life I have rarely felt more anxiety than I feel at the prospect of being given a gift, and only slightly less anxiety at the prospect of giving a gift. For how grateful must one be, for a present which (probably) isn't at all needed, or wanted; how can one reciprocate a gift, without making a social or personal blunder? Will my gift be wildly inappropriate, too costly/ not costly enough? That gift-giving is so crucial to our society, the very wheel driving the capitalist-consumer economy, seems to me, as it seems to my father, unfortunate; the juggernaut of Christmas rolling around each year, overshadowing much else, invariably a season of apprehension and disappointment for many, seems particularly unfortunate. The very nicest "gifts" are those given spontaneously, without ritual or custom tied to a calendar, and these one can truly prize; the others, duly wrapped in expensive paper, part of a seasonal barrage of gifts, are likely to be dubious.

The gifts which I give to my parents now are more meaningful to Daddy than the perfunctory gifts of long ago—these are books, records, subscriptions to magazines (*Atlantic, Harper's, Hudson Review, Kenyon Review, Paris Review* in which from time to time work of mine might appear); of course, I've given my parents copies of each of my books, of which several have been dedicated to them. (Daddy has joked that he's had to build a special bookcase in their living room, to accommodate my books.) They have an ongoing subscription to *Ontario Review*.

It is natural that children mythologize their parents. Even adults mythologize their parents as a way of mythologizing themselves. Some of us make our parents into gods, some make them into demons. After all our parents are giants of the landscape into which we'd been born; we cast our eyes up to them, as we lay in our cribs, or tottered about at their feet.

The greatest of infantile mysteries must have been the sudden appearance of these giant beings: Mother, Father.

Equally great, though tinged with dread, their disappearance.

Yet it seems to me, though my parents are not gods, that they are extraordinary people *morally*; not in their accomplishments perhaps, but in themselves; in their souls, one might say. It has been a riddle of my own adulthood, as I contemplate my parents: how, given their difficult backgrounds, their impoverished and violence-ridden early lives, did they become the people they are? So many of my writer-friends speak wryly of their parents, or are critical of them, or angry at them; their adult lives are presented as triumphs over the limitations of parents, and rarely as a consequence of their parents. By contrast, I feel utterly sentimental about my parents *whose love and support have so informed my life, and who have become, in my adulthood, my friends.*

The writer is driven to commemorate what is past, or passing, if not what's to come; some of us are fascinated by tracking the generations that have preceded us, that seem to us stronger than our own, and stronger than the generations to follow, because more cruelly tested, more wounded, forced to grow up while still young, and to know of life's vicissitudes while making no claim, as subsequent generations of Americans have done, of "rights"—"privileges"—"entitlements."

Memory is a transcendental function. Its objects may be physical bodies, faces, facial expressions, but these are shot with luminosity like the light in a Caravaggio painting; an interior radiance that transfixes the imagination, signaling that Time has stopped and Eternity prevails. We are not able to perceive "soul" or "spirit" first-hand but this is the phenomenon we summon back by way of an exercise of memory.

And why the exercise of memory at certain times in our lives is almost too powerful to be endured.

THE PERFECT MAN OF *action is the suicide*. These words of William Carlos Williams have long fascinated me for I'd grown up in a world in which men were likely to be men *of action* rather than *of reflection*.

Growing up in the 1950s, I watched boxing matches on television with my father never less than once a week (Fridays), and sometimes twice a week (Wednesdays as well). The Gillette-sponsored fights were the only television programs my father watched including even news programs; my father preferred radio news, or the *Buffalo Evening News*.

Why this was, I have no idea. Why my father so disliked any sort of "fiction" on television or in the movies, while maintaining his respect for literature, seems paradoxical; it's possible that he had inherited his love for books from his mother, though when he was working forty hours a week, and distracted by part-time jobs, he had no time for reading anything but the newspaper.

Would I have watched boxing matches on television, as a girl, except for my father? Probably not. It's my theory that women who are emotionally attached to sports have been indoctrinated into such emotions by their fathers, or other men in their lives. Once you enter the particular culture of such a sport you acquire the vision, the sensibility, and the vocabulary for understanding it; you acquire a camaraderie with others who are similarly indoctrinated. You have little patience for those on the outside, who may be repelled by what engages you; you have little interest in "converting" them, and no interest at all in their opinion of *you*.

For men of my father's generation, and of my father's era generally, the boxing ring exuded a meaning it does not exude today. Boxing was the supreme sport, as it was the sport other sports aspired to be, in its very rawness and (relative) directness. For here was a contest in which men fought one another one-on-one—(that is, not team vs. team)—in a garishly lighted and pitilessly public exposure; here was the very paradigm of life's justice, or injustice: the elevated boxing ring, not the ballpark or the football field or any sort of tamed "court" or "game" space. *You can run but you can't hide*—to paraphrase Joe Louis's famous remark apropos his brash challenger, light-heavyweight Billy Conn, in 1946.

Indeed, my father was powerfully drawn to boxing: as a young man he'd sparred with a friend who'd been a semi-professional middleweight in Buffalo, and to this day he marvels at how fast his friend's hands were, how rapid his "footwork"; how astonished my father had been by being out-matched, so quickly—"In boxing, you either have the talent or you don't. You can be trained, but that's all. You have to be born with the talent to be trained."

One of the tragedies of my father's life was that this boxer-friend, as close to him at one time as a brother, had been carelessly mismatched by his manager with a more experienced boxer, who'd knocked him out and badly injured him; he'd retired from boxing in his late twenties, and a few years later, having failed at other prospects, he had killed himself with a rifle.

Boxing, the cruelest sport. The public sees only the great champions at the apex of their careers but the reality of boxing, the very culture of boxing, is permeated with failure—injuries, dementia, premature death. The boxer who simply prevails is a kind of hero, or would have seemed so in my father's era; the boxer is one who provides for men both like and unlike himself an emotional link with a (mythic) (masculine) past in which violence and grace, desperation and courage, raw talent and calculation are publicly entwined and communally celebrated. Boxing's dark fascination has always been as much with failure, and the moral strength to forbear failure, as it has been with success; boxing has always drawn its participants from the "lower depths"—hardly from the safety-concerned middle class. For the ring is a place of exposure as it is of celebration, and its failures and deceits are magnified many times larger than life.

For years, beginning when I was eleven, my father took me to Golden Gloves matches in Buffalo. No one would have questioned my being in such a hyper-masculine place, as Fred Oates's daughter; no one would have questioned my father's judgment in bringing me there to sit amid an audience comprised of virtually all men and boys. As I recall, I was more or less invisible—a slender, unobtrusive girl, and a silent girl, whose memory of the Buffalo arena is of a vast high-ceilinged space punctuated by shouts, screams, howls, catcalls and bells sharply rung as knife blades. Bluish cigarette and cigar smoke wafted everywhere.

Shouts and screams of triumph as a boxer is declared the winner of his match, and his hand in its big, balloon-like glove is raised aloft by the referee. Howls and catcalls of derision, as a young boxer is knocked to the floor, or tries to clinch with his more aggressive opponent, or scrambles on hands and knees to escape as one might naturally do, in instinctive panic.

Seeing such displays of aggression suggests a violation of taboo, thus the *frisson* of boxing, not so evident when seen on television as when it is seen "live" and there is no running verbal commentary to defuse and explain it; there is no TV screen to frame it, like a work of art or theater. In the arena, a boxing match is a raw and pitiless spectacle from which you can't hide your eyes—for whether you look or not, the spectacle is occurring before you.

My father subscribed to *The Ring*—"The Bible of Boxing"—a magazine absorbed in the history of its subject. (For boxing, far more obsessively than most sports, is not only about itself but about its history.) In those years—roughly, 1940s through the early 1960s—the names of boxers were household names, each evoking a distinct and colorful personality: *Rocky Marciano, Jersey Joe Walcott, Sugar Ray Robinson, Archie Moore, Carmen Basilio, Kid Gavilan, Rocky Graziano, Jake LaMotta, Bobo Olson, Tony DeMarco, Rocky Castellani,*

Roland LaStarza. Mention *Joey Maxim* and my father will react at once with contempt—for the mere name *Joey Maxim* summons up, for my father, memories of questionable decisions by referees and judges, rumors of fixed fights, the mob-controlled championship fights that became routine in the early 1950s (portrayed in Martin Scorsese's great boxing film *Raging Bull*).

Once, in fall 1952, I stayed home from a junior high school dance on a Friday night to watch, with my father, Rocky Marciano win the world heavyweight championship from Jersey Joe Walcott in a bout televised from Philadelphia. No dance could have been so thrilling—no occasion with classmates so profound as this with my father. I remember how respectful my father was of Walcott, and how impressed by Marciano—that exemplum of the triumph of sheer brute will in the face of an opponent's superior skill, intelligence, and experience.

Of this, I could not have spoken to my school friends. I could not have explained to anyone. Nor did my father speak so abstractly. That the Friday night fights illuminated dark, repressed, systematically denied aspects of our lives and by extension the communal life of America at that time might have been felt by us, but it could not have been articulated by either of us.

Who could have predicted, when Rocky Marciano won the heavyweight title in 1952, that he would be the last white (American) boxer to win this title; that, after Marciano's retirement in 1956, he would be most remembered for having been the single untied and undefeated champion in heavyweight history, and not for having been a great champion. By the time of Marciano's death, in the crash of a small, private plane in 1969, his era had long been over; the (predominantly white) boxing world that had so mesmerized my father and his friends had metamorphosed into something new and rich and strange and surely intimidating—the era of Muhammad Ali.

Since retiring from Harrison's my father has begun taking adult education courses at the University of Buffalo. He has begun taking piano lessons. In the evenings he reads, or practices piano. It is a new, rejuvenated life in which, as he says, he has no time for TV boxing.

FROM A LETTER OF my father's dated September 8, 1988.

> *Your postcard asking about my history came the day after I phoned. I don't quite know how to give you this information because I have no school records like you and Fred—all I can do is guess.*

> *Born in Lockport 3/30/14. Parents separated when I was 2 or 3. Started violin lessons in sixth grade (school instruction) then began private lessons with money earned peddling papers. My mother bought my violin for me otherwise I would have had to quit because the one I used belonged to the school. I played in the high school symphony orchestra as a freshman. My mechanical drawing teacher got me a job with Schine theaters in Lockport in the sign shop working after school. At summer vacation I worked full-time at the job and quit school in my second year. Worked at the theater until I was about 17 when the sign shop closed and I went into production advertising.*

> *Got a job in a commercial sign shop when I was 18 and bought a car. After about 4 years of this work got a job at Harrison Radiator in the punch press department and, thinking I had a steady job, learned to fly, got married, then found myself laid off for extended periods so I had to resume at the sign shop until the War began*

when I was able to get transferred into the engineering tool room
and learned the tool and die-making technique, later on was able,
after going to night school to learn trig and related subjects,
started tool and die design. At about 50 years of age I took piano
lessons for about four years at which time I was operated on to
remove herniated disc material and was out of commission for
about six months then worked about 10 more years and retired.
Took a course in stained glass, class in painting, four years ago
started classes in English & American literature as well as music
at SUNY (State University of New York, Buffalo) which I hope to
continue for a few more years.

Love
Dad

A FEW WEEKS AFTER I was born in June 1938 my twenty-four-year-old father reported to work at Harrison Radiator and was told that there was no work, the entire press room was laid off "indefinitely" . . . This was before the factory was unionized and my father became a member of the UAW (United Auto Workers) in the early 1940s.

And so, we ask Daddy, what did you do? How did you *feel*?

And Daddy looks at us with an expression of mild incredulity mingled with pity for our stupidity as if to say *Is that a serious question? How do you think a young husband and father would feel, having to come home early to his wife and tell her he has been laid off "indefinitely"?*— but he says only, "Yes. It was hard."

IT IS FASCINATING TO me, to be told that my grandmother, who'd had so little money as a young, single mother, had somehow purchased a violin for my father—the beautiful violin my father still owns, though he has not tried to play it in decades.

A piano is much easier, my father says. You don't have to create notes, the notes are there in the keyboard, to be played.

For as long as I could remember there was an upright piano in a corner of our living room in the farmhouse in Millersport, which my father played, or played at, virtually every night. Playing piano was a way of relaxing after hours of work, I suppose. Playing piano was a way of escaping into silence when a man did not wish to talk.

My piano lessons, paid for by my grandmother, began when I was ten and ended when I was sixteen. Like my father, but with more zeal and discipline than my father, since I was a "student," I sat at this piano rarely less than once a day, often two or three times a day, practicing scales, lessons. What sharp, visceral memories are contained in my fingertips, triggered by notes, sound, rhythm—it is a fraught exercise for me to approach any piano, and depress any chord no matter how innocuous.

For a musical instrument—piano, violin—inhabits a complex sort of space: it is both an ordinary three-dimensional object and an extraordinary object, a portal to another world; it exists as a physical entity solely so that the physical can be transcended. And so my father's old upright piano in the long-vanished living room in Millersport inhabits its own luminous space in my memory, as in this memoir.

For most of his life Fred Oates has played piano. He has loved to play piano. He plays classical music of a popular sort—"The Erl-King," "Für Elise," *Traümerei*, Beethoven's Fifth Symphony (transcribed for piano), *Moonlight Sonata*—and he plays American popular music—"Deep Purple," "St. James Infirmary," "As Time Goes By," "Night and Day," "Hong Kong Blues," "Frankie and Johnnie," "Blue Moon," "Melancholy Baby," "September Song," "Brother, Can You Spare a Dime?"; he plays Scott Joplin, jazz, "swing." He can sight-read music, to a certain degree of difficulty, and he can "play by ear" and improvise, impressively. Clearly I have inherited from my father a temperament that might be called "musical"—which isn't the same as having inherited talent.

Do you listen to music while you write?—this curious question is often asked of writers.

The more attentive you are to music, the more distracted you are by hearing music while you try to work. For music is an exquisite art, not white noise.

It must be a fairly modern custom, to ubiquitously "pipe in" music in public places. When did this custom begin, and how will it end? *Can* it end? There is something offensive in having to listen to music, particularly to "serious" music, as if it were but background noise, or a film score; for music exists in and of itself, and not as an accompaniment to anything else.

Music is the supreme solace, because it is so much more. It is the spiritual counterpoint to the world's cacophony, essential as a heartbeat.

When I am alone in any private place that is quiet I have only to shut my eyes and I can hear Daddy playing the old upright in our living room in Millersport. In the memory I am sitting beside Daddy on the piano bench as Daddy sings one of his favorite songs—"Melancholy Baby," "Blue Moon," "Brother, Can You Spare a Dime."

NOW IT IS NOVEMBER 1988. And I am listening to my father playing piano in a distant room in our house—now, Erik Satie's elegant *Gnossiennes*.

(This isn't a piano composition from the old days of Millersport, but a piano piece which I play myself, sometimes—Daddy has found the sheet music on the piano.)

When I think of my parents, I think of Colette's remark—*Happiness is a kind of genius*. How true this is! And yet, where genius is concerned, we become speechless, inadequate; we have nothing to say, for we are not able to understand what genius is.

In the case of Fred and Carolina Oates, no one would claim "genius" for them but only rather a kind of wisdom, as much acquired as instinctive. The quality of personality they embody, their magnanimity of spirit, the ways in which they enhance the lives of others around them—how oddly matched it is, with their origins and with the harsh and unsentimental world in which they were born.

I have taken it as a challenge, to evoke that world in its myriad complexities. And—how to write a memoir of Fred Oates? How even to begin?

A LETTER TO MY MOTHER
CAROLINA OATES ON HER
SEVENTY-EIGHTH BIRTHDAY,
NOVEMBER 8, 1994

Dear Mom,

    I have always meant to tell you.

    I have long rehearsed telling you.

    I have meant so many times to tell you.

    How the world divides, seemingly, into two: those who speak without hesitation saying I love you—*and possibly not mean it; and those too shy or constrained by family custom or temperament to utter the words* I love you—*though they mean it.*

HOW DIFFICULT IT HAS been to speak these simple words. To heave my heart into my throat—*I love you.*

WE CARRY OUR YOUNG parents inside us, so much more alive than any memory of ourselves as infants, children. We carry our young parents within us through our lives. No wonder is ever quite equal to that first, speechless wonder—gazing at the mysterious individuals leaning over us unable yet to say *Who are you? Why do you care for me? What does it mean, that you care for me? What does it mean, we are here together? Only feed me, only love me forever.*

"I GUESS WE WERE poor but it didn't seem that way. Somehow, we managed."

FROM MY PARENTS, A love of being busy, *at work*.

When we are not working, when we have nothing to do except entertain ourselves, we are restless and not so happy.

How many books dedicated *To my parents Carolina and Fred Oates with love.*

In memory of that landscape, now vanishing, that continues to nourish like an underground spring.

DAFFODILS, NARCISSI, TULIPS GROWING from bulbs you'd planted in the beds around the house. Scarlet peonies, pale pink peonies, bridal wreath, zinnias. Lilac bushes, azaleas.

Growing wild along the fence beyond the old hay barn, morning glories, sweet pea, and hollyhocks.

Wild and resilient as the tallest of weeds, sunflowers beyond the chicken yard.

Your favorite flower, roses. Your favorite rose, Double Delight.

Your favorite garden vegetable, tomatoes. Your favorite tomatoes, First Ladies.

AN INVENTORY OF OUR lives.

The lost world of (rural) laundry: clotheslines, clothespins, sheets, towels, trousers, dresses and underwear, socks flapping in the wind, a ceaseless wind it seemed, how crude by present standards, how primitive; yet there was pleasure in it, in the very repetition, familiarity. Each item of laundry lifted by hand, shook out, smoothed and affixed to the line by wooden pins. From my small narrow child's room on the second floor, at the rear of the house, I could look out at any time when the laundry was hanging on the line and see a reflection of our household, our family, like ghost-figures glimpsed in water.

Take me, take me with you! Don't let me go.

I am not a patient person but to the degree that I have been taught the virtues of patience, it is because of you. The consoling and comforting rituals of housekeeping. The very thought of *keeping house*: that there is a place, a *home*, that must be actively, ceaselessly *kept*. It cannot be neglected, or slighted.

For what is *housekeeping* but small simple finite tasks executed with attention, care, love. Pushing the carpet sweeper. "Vacuuming"—a thrilling task involving high-volume power. Clearing the kitchen table, helping you with the dishes—just the two of us in the kitchen after dinner.

You tried to teach me to knit, and to sew, without great success. For such (feminine) tasks I did not demonstrate much talent if, at the outset, energy and hope. You had more luck teaching me to cook, or at any rate to prepare meals. *This is how you prepare a baking pan. This is how you frost a cake with a knife. This is how you make bread stuffing. This is how you peel an orange without making a mess and getting the rind in your fingernails. This is how you stir the spaghetti sauce—with a wooden spoon.*

SO MANY BEAUTIFUL THINGS! Today here in Princeton I will lay them out on a bed, I will bring them out of closets to position in this room, and I will make an inventory.

- large knitted afghan of orange, brown, white wool
- large knitted afghan of white wool, with upraised floral designs
- smaller knitted quilt of many brightly colored wool squares, predominately red, yellow, green
- pale peach-colored coat sweater, belted
- crimson coat sweater, belted
- turquoise jacket and matching skirt (light fabric)
- dove-gray jacket and matching skirt (wool)
- dark red jacket and matching skirt (wool)
- fine-knit pale pink jacket-sweater with matching belt
- jacket of soft autumnal colors with a russet-red skirt (wool)
- camel's hair skirt
- lilac silk dress with lace trim, long sleeved
- dark blue velour dress, long
- crimson velour dress
- crimson evening skirt
- purple velvet skirt, long
- dark blue floral checked cocktail dress (silk)
- white long-sleeved blouse (raw silk)
- dark orange long-sleeved blouse (silk)
- dark pink blouse with fine-stitched collar (silk)
- dove-gray long-sleeved blouse (silk)
- dark gold long-sleeved blouse (silk)
- black vest (rayon, wool)
- beige vest (velour)
- pink flaring skirt with matching top (cotton)

All these, and more, you've made for me. How many hours of effort, concentration, skill in those things so delicately fashioned, exquisitely sewed or knitted. What infinite patience in such creation. What love.

An inventory of our lives.

THE OLD FARMHOUSE WAS demolished years ago (in 1960) and the very site of its foundation filled with earth, all trace of its existence obliterated. You'd lived there for virtually your entire life—how strange it must be to you, that it has vanished, to be replaced with a large patch of seeded grass grown thick as a shag rug.

Yet the house remains vivid in my mind's eye. And the small lilac tree that grew by the back door, a child-sized tree into which I climbed, in a crook of whose twisty limbs I sat, a dreamy child given to solitude in places near the house, near you.

Beneath this little tree chickens pecked in the dirt. Happy Chicken might be lifted onto a lower limb, to flutter his/her wings in sudden bird-panic.

For so many years, it seemed that I was rarely out of the range of your voice.

Joyce! Joy-ce!

In memory it is a misty-hazy summer day. That peculiar translucence to the light that means the air is heavy with moisture though the sky appears to be cloudless, a pure remote blue, and the sun dazzling overhead. In this place south of Lake Ontario and west of Lake Erie the sky is ever changing—this is the "lake effect"—so that a clear sky can be riddled with clouds within minutes; this too is deeply embedded in memory, a sudden crack of thunder, a dispirited darkening of the sky, pelting rain like bullets. *Joyce! Where are you, come inside!*

The houses of our earliest childhoods are houses of recurring dreams that are yet subtly altered, as if approximations of memory, or interpretations of memory, and not memory itself. In such dreams, the childhood houses are likely to be larger than the reality had been, with more rooms, mysterious doorways leading—where? Always there is the promise, alarming, yet tantalizing, of rooms not yet discovered, through a rear wall, in the attic perhaps, or in the earthen-floored cellar, places yet to be explored, beckoning. Your presence permeates the house, you are the house, its mysterious infinite rooms. You are the hazy light, the rich smell of damp earth, sunshine and grass, pears that are no sooner ripe than they are overripe, lightly bruised.

You are the humming buzzing not-quite-audible sounds of the orchard, and of the fields beyond the orchard. You are the uplifted cries of early-morning birds. I see you pushing me on the swing that Daddy built for me out of a six-foot pipe positioned between tall trees in the backyard, I see your hair reddish-brown, so wonderfully curly; you are wearing a shirt and pale blue "pedal pushers" and sandals. I am a lanky child of eight or nine gripping the rope swing with both hands tight, my legs stretch upward straining higher, higher, squealing with childish excitement, flying into the sky. It is like my airplane trips with Daddy: except this is Mommy pushing me, and we are safe on the ground. So often wanting to tell you how in patches of sudden sunshine hundreds of miles and thousands of days from home I am pulled back into that world as into the most nourishing of dreams, I am filled with a sense of wonder, and awe, and fear, sadness for all that has already passed from us and for what must be surrendered, in time.

What we imagine as life but cannot explain, cannot "put into words" for all our vocabulary; cannot utter aloud, dare not utter aloud, this succession of small perfect moments like the movement of the red second hand on the sunburst General Electric clock in the kitchen, moments linked together as pearls are linked together to constitute a necklace, linked by touch, invisible string, the interior mystery. We were lucky, and we were happy, and I think we've always known.

"WHEN I WAS A LITTLE GIRL, AND MY MOTHER DIDN'T WANT ME"

My father was killed and I never knew why.
Then, I was given away. By my mother.
I was so little—not a year old.
There were too many of us, ten of us,
my mother had to give me away.
When I was old enough to know, I cried a lot.

My father was killed and I never knew why.
No one would tell me.
Now there is no one I can ask.
"Why? Why?"
It happened in a fight, in a tavern, he was only
forty-four years old.
Forty-four! Now, he could be my son.

I wasn't always an old woman—this age that I am . . .
I was a girl for so long.
I was the youngest for so long.
I was nine months old when my father died

and there were too many of us to feed, and my mother
gave me away.

There were ten children. I was the baby.
I was born too late, I was the baby
that our mother could not keep.
My sisters and brothers did not miss me—I think.
They would have looked at me and tried to think why
I was the one to be given away, and not them.
They could not feel sorry for me for maybe then
they too would be given away by our mother.

My mother gave me to her sister-in-law Lena who
didn't have children. This was in 1918.
It was a shameful thing then, not to have babies.
This was in the Black Rock section of Buffalo,
the waterfront on the Niagara River.
Germans, Poles, Hungarians—immigrants.
We were Hungarians. We were called "Hunkies."
I don't know why people hated us.

Uncle John and Aunt Lena were my "parents."
We moved to a farm far away in the country.
And my real mother and my brothers and sisters
moved to a farm a few miles away.

I would learn one day that it happened often,
in immigrant families in those days.
In poor immigrant families.

My father was killed and I never knew why.

They said he was a "heavy drinker," he liked to
get into fights.
The Hungarians are the worst, they said—
the drinking, and the fighting.

They said he was so handsome, my father.
My mother Elizabeth was so pretty.
Curly red-brown hair like mine.
They said he had a temper "like the devil."
In the tavern there was a fight, and he died.
A man took up a poker and beat my father to death.
I never knew why, I never knew who it had been.
Yet this was how my life was decided.

There is the moment of conception—you don't know.
There is the moment of birth—you don't know.
There is the moment your life is decided—you don't know.
Yet you say, "This is my life."
You say, "This is me."

When I was a little girl and my mother didn't want me
I hid away to cry.
I felt so bad and so ashamed!
When I was old enough I would walk to the other farm.
There was a bridge over the creek a few miles away.
They didn't really want me there I guess.
My name was Carolina, but they didn't call me that.
They called me she, *and* her. *They called me* you.
They weren't very nice to me I guess.
They didn't want to see me, I was a reminder of—
something.

Elizabeth my mother never learned English.
She spoke Hungarian all her life.
She never learned to read. She never learned to drive
a car.
My Aunt Lena never learned to speak English well.
She never learned to drive so the two women didn't see
much of each other
though they were from the same street in Budapest and
lived only a few miles apart.
That was how women were in those days.

But—I loved my mother Elizabeth!
She was a pretty, plump woman.
Curly red-brown hair like mine.
People would say, "Carolina you look just like your momma!"
Then they would be surprised, I would start to cry.
My mother was always busy, she scolded me in Hungarian—
"Go away, go home where you belong. You have a home.
Your home is not here."
I did not know Hungarian but I understood these words
which I hear all the time, even now.

I loved my big brothers and sisters.
There was Leslie, he was the oldest.
He took over when our father died.
There was Mary, I never knew well.
They were born in Budapest.
There was Steve who'd been kicked and trampled
by a horse. His brain was injured, he would
never leave home.
There was Elsie who was my "big sister."

There was Frank who was my "big brother."
There was Johnny. There was Edith.
There was George, who went away in the army.
There was Joseph, I wasn't too close with.

They are all gone now.
I loved them, but—
I am the only one remaining.
Sometimes I think: The soul is just a burning match!
It burns a while and then—
And then that's all.

It's a long time ago now but I remember hiding away to cry.
When I was a little girl and my mother didn't want me.

(Written with permission from my mother Carolina Oates.)

EXCERPT, TELEPHONE CONVERSATION WITH MY FATHER FREDERIC OATES, MAY 1999

"THESE NIGHTS, I CAN'T read prose very well. I guess I won't get through your new novel. It's wonderful and I love it but my eyes . . . I read poetry. In the college anthologies. Frost, Dickinson, Whitman I already know by heart. That's how I spend my nights, now."

THE LONG ROMANCE

WE ARE YOUNG FOR so long, it seems. Entire lifetimes.

And when we're young we can't comprehend how personalities shift inexorably over time, as slowly, or nearly, as the wearing-away of granite by water or wind. Yet the wearing-away, invisible to the eye, is ceaseless and irrevocable. We can't begin to comprehend how the body shifts, shrinking by degrees into its frame, becoming ever less certain, humble. As if the very shadows of the elderly begin to fade. There come to dwell in these diminished bodies, if the bodies live long enough, unanticipated personalities as distinct from their predecessors as our child-selves are distinct and distant from our mature selves.

And one day, even those strangers are gone.

The long romance is ended, and we are alone.

MY DEAR FATHER FRED Oates passed away in May 2000. Daddy had been ill for several years with a variety of age-related illnesses, and he had long been losing his eyesight to macular degeneration—Daddy, who so loved to read; Fred Oates, whose signs had once been so prevalent in the countryside south of Lockport. In later years he'd even begun to paint, and to make stained-glass lamps which we have in our house here in Princeton. A portrait of me, modeled upon a photograph, hangs on a wall upstairs in our bedroom.

The last words Daddy spoke to me, over the telephone, in late April 2000, were to dissuade my husband Ray and me from driving up to see him just then. He'd seemed almost vehement, saying: "You don't need to make a special trip to see me right now. Hell, I'm not bad." It was the manly gesture, I realized afterward. *Manly* to dismiss his own mortality, and to insist that we shouldn't fuss over him just yet.

Daddy had wanted to shield me from the truth. In this, he was like his mother Blanche: he'd wanted to shield *me*. He had been so persuasive, I had not visited him in time; two days after this phone conversation he died, in his eighty-seventh year, in a hospice in Getzville, New York, much sooner than his doctors had expected.

"Your father just closed his eyes. As soon as he knew that your mother was all right and would be taken care of, he closed his eyes and fell asleep. He was so tired. He never woke up."

MY MOTHER'S LAST WORDS to me were spoken in person, in July 2002 in her nursing home in Getzville: "How could I forget Joyce?"

In her eighty-sixth year, my mother was living in a facility several miles from my brother and sister-in-law in Clarence, New York. They visited her often and each visit was, they said, a "happy surprise" to her—her memory had grown so porous.

The old farm-property had been sold, the "new" ranch house had been appropriated by strangers, my parents Fred and Carolina had been living in attractive quarters in an assisted-living residence in Clarence, for several years until my father's health deteriorated in the late winter of 2000. Now my dear mother was a widow, who had so long been dependent upon my father; for this she compensated by seeming to believe, or perhaps even believing, that "Freddy" was living in another wing of the nursing home, where "everybody knew him."

My father had been so dominant a personality, Fred Oates had been so marked a "character" among the circle of people who knew him in Lockport and northern Erie County, it would seem quite likely that, though no longer living, he was yet an individual whom "everybody knew."

My brother Fred had brought me to visit my mother. My brother, living near my parents, had become their caretaker, their overseer, and their protector; to Fred, Jr., I owe an enormous debt of emotion, gratitude, reverence. What a kind person your brother is!—one of the nursing staff told me.

Perhaps there is no higher value, when we think of it, than kindness.

We'd taken Mom outside, to sit in a sunny courtyard. It was not so difficult to speak as one might imagine, but I have no idea now what we spoke of; mainly, we looked at one another. We smiled, we looked at one another searchingly. We may have been breathless, giddy, with the exquisite wonder of simply being where we were— together. We may have talked of a dog at the facility, for the elderly nursing patients enjoyed the company of an obese, friendly Labrador, and my mother had always been fond of animals. We may have talked, or tried to talk, of the many cats and chickens on the old farm, perhaps even Happy Chicken—so long ago, who could remember a lone Rhode Island Red that had "bowed" when a child petted her—or, rather, him . . .

Though Mom's short-term memory had generally deteriorated by this time, my mother was ever alert to social subtleties; instinctively she tried to protect my brother's and my feelings, by disguising the degree of forgetfulness with which she was afflicted. To be extra cautious my brother said to her, when we'd first sat down in the courtyard, "This is your daughter Joyce, Mom. You remember Joyce."

And our mother smiled and replied with these words that haunt me through the years—"How could I forget Joyce?"

NOT LONG AFTERWARD, MY mother would die in her sleep also, of a massive stroke. When the phone rang, and my brother told me the news, it seemed for a moment that all of us had been stricken by this single terrible blow.

In this way ended my long romance of over sixty years with my beloved parents Carolina and Fred Oates.

MY MOTHER'S QUILTS

MY FAVORITE IS ALWAYS on my bed. Even in warm weather.

It is not a large quilt but very beautiful, I think: comprised of numerous brightly colored knitted-wool squares of every imaginable color—red, yellow, green, blue, purple, magenta, brown, cream.

The pattern is neither simple nor complex. It isn't, like some quilts, a labyrinthine design.

From the start, I loved this quilt. Just to look at it is to feel comforted.

Several generations of cats have slept on this quilt. (Even as I write this, my little gray cat Cherie is probably sleeping on it, asprawl in a patch of sunshine.) How many years have passed since my mother gave the quilt to me and my husband Ray Smith, I can only estimate: thirty years? Thirty-five?

The beautiful little quilt in all the colors of the rainbow has followed me from one residence to another. The same bed, in different bedrooms in different houses in different phases of my life.

In this most recent phase, in which the bright-colored quilt is laid on a pale blue comforter on my bed in a house in Princeton, New Jersey, into which I moved in 2009, with my second husband Charlie Gross, my mother has been absent from my life for nearly twelve years.

Twelve years! That seems so long, yet my memory of Mom is so vivid, I can glance up and "see" her in the doorway of my study—I can "see" the expression on her face, and (almost) hear what she is saying.

Of course, there are numerous photographs of my mother and father in this room, on windowsills, bulletin boards, and walls. My dear friend Gloria Vanderbilt did a collage of my most precious family photographs several years ago, incorporating snapshots of my grandmother Blanche (as a young woman in an elegant fur-trimmed coat), my parents and my husband Ray and me.

In this room, which is my writing room, thus my sanctuary, all times are present-tense. The past is not vanished but *now*.

My mother never visited this house. She would love it, I think—especially the large curving flower beds, so like the flower beds she'd tended in our yard in Millersport, New York, years ago. When she'd visited Ray and me in my former Princeton home, less than five minutes from this house, Mom had always helped out in the garden, as in the house; we would garden together, and we would prepare meals together, while my father played piano in the living room.

Whenever my parents came to visit us in Princeton my mother would bring gifts for us: mostly items she had knitted, crocheted, or sewn. The lovely afghans, sweater-coats, pullover tops and blouses, skirts, suits which for years I wore for "author's photos . . ." All are enshrined in my closets—I look at them often, marveling at the fine stitching and hemming, the exquisite small touches, mother-of-pearl buttons, pleated bodices. Dresses, skirts, vests, shawls. Often I wear the shirts she'd sewn for me—white, pink, red, magenta; one of my favorite sweaters is a pink sweater-coat with a knitted belt.

If you know me, you have seen me in my mother's clothes. Indeed, there is nothing so *comforting* as wearing clothes your mother has made for you.

In his seventies, in a burst of creative energy and enthusiasm my father began making Tiffany-inspired stained-glass lamps in a crafts class at SUNY Buffalo. (One of these, in subtle blues and reds, is on my piano; the very piano Daddy so enjoyed playing.) From a photograph Daddy painted a remarkably lifelike portrait of me, quite unlike anything he had ever done.

And Daddy's violin, purchased long ago by my grandmother Blanche Morgenstern in the early 1920s in Lockport, New York, is safe in my study, displayed on a shelf, a beautiful richly burnished red-brown, that always looks smaller than I expect it to be. After it became clear that my father would not be able to keep the violin much longer, after he and my mother had moved into smaller quarters in an assisted-living residence, he gave the violin to me with the enigmatic words, "I can't use it, where I'm going."

How those words echo, years after Daddy's death! He had never been one to speak with drama or urgency, which would have seemed to him excessively self-conscious, self-aggrandizing.

I can't use it, where I'm going.

It is a relief to me, that my father's violin had not become lost. Yet it is a loss of a kind, that this violin has played no music for fifty years.

After my mother died in 2003, for a long time I would imagine Mom with me, in my study in particular; though "imagine" is perhaps a weak word to describe how keenly I felt Mom's presence. In writing the novel *Missing Mom* I tried to evoke Carolina Oates—well, I'm sure that I did evoke her, not fully or completely but in part. My mother is so much a part of myself, writing the novel was the antithesis of an exorcism, a portrait in words of a remarkable person whom everyone loved and who lives on in our memories.

In the novel, when the daughter discovers some disturbing facts about her mother's early life, she thinks—*It just made me love Mom more*.

In February 2008 when my husband Ray Smith was hospitalized with pneumonia, and after Ray died unexpectedly a week later, often I lay in bed too exhausted to move, beneath the rainbow-colored quilt. The bed became my haven, my refuge, my sanctuary, my "nest"—with my mother's quilt predominant, a sign of how love endures in the most elemental and comforting of ways. Warmth, beauty, something to *touch*.

On a high shelf in this room is one of my father's stained-glass lamp shades, pearly-white, minimally ornamental, not attached to a lamp but simply set on the shelf like a work of art. And this too has been a solace to me.

Grief is a kind of illness. Severe grief, severe illness. The wish to do harm to oneself as penance for having survived the loved one, or as a way of joining the loved one, is very strong, and because it is totally unreasonable, it is difficult to refute with reason. At such times I could summon my parents to me—though I would not have wanted them to know that Ray, whom they had loved as a son, had died, yet I needed their counsel. My mother's calming voice, my father's chiding voice—these were the voices that carried me along, in a dark spell that lasted approximately four months.

In extremis we care very little for the public life—the life of the "career"—even the life of "literature": it is emotional comfort for which we yearn, but such comfort can come to us from only a few, intimate sources. I know that I have been very fortunate, and I never cease giving thanks for my wonderful parents who bequeathed me their love and their hope for me, that did so much to make my life as a writer possible; for this quilt on my bed, as singular and beautiful now as it was in the late 1970s when my mother gave it to me.

AFTERWORD

The root of the word *memoir* is *memory*. When memory is cast back decades it is likely to be imprecise as a torn net haphazardly cast that may drag in what is irrelevant as well as miss what is crucial. Our lives are enormous waves breaking on the shore, retreating and leaving only a few scattered things behind for us to contemplate—before the astonishing fact of a single day in our lives we are rendered speechless, if we are honest. And yet, as we are human, and our species' greatest achievement is speech, we are never speechless for long.

No one, especially a child, lives a life that can be summarized in a few deft words—"happy"—"unhappy." The most immediate fallacy of the memoir is that, from a perspective later in time, it seeks to cast a coherent emotional aura over the minutiae of life; perhaps unwittingly, it makes of the memoirist a kind of "character" as in a story. But our lives are not stories, and to tell them as narratives is to distort them.

The most reliable memoirs are those comprised of journal or diary entries, or letters, that attest to the immediacy of experience before it becomes subject to the vicissitudes of memory. As soon as you shift from the tense *I am* to *I was*, still more to *I had been* you are entering the realm of what might be called "creative recollection." My first memoir *A Widow's Story* (2011) was composed primarily of journal entries recording approximately four months following the hospital admission and the death of my husband Raymond Smith in February 2008. The memoir was not intended to present my subsequent life but to focus upon the raw, unassimilated, blindly head-on plunge of experience *in medias res* after an unexpected death; this is the great, the truly extraordinary adventure most of us will have to undergo at some point in our lives, though it is very difficult to speak of it coherently afterward. Not the phenomenon of grief as it might be calmly assessed and analyzed, but an evocation of grief itself—that which is unspeakable.

The Lost Landscape: A Writer's Coming of Age is an entirely different project. Except in two chapters about my parents that are, in fact, based upon journal entries, all of the chapters are "recollected"—with what that entails of the incomplete and abbreviated, the rounded-off and the summarized. In the midst of writing about "Joyce Carol" at the age of four, I might find myself leaping forward five decades to another landscape entirely. Such knowledge, and the irony of such knowledge, isn't available to those living *in time*—only to those casting their thoughts backward. If this is an advantage of the recollected memoir, it is also a disadvantage. In life, we don't see the shadows of things-to-come. It is always high noon, and we are likely to be blinded by such brightness.

Gazing back at more than six decades is a vertiginous feat but it would be impossible if the memoirist tried to be assiduously faithful to the immediacy of past experience. There are no written records in my family, probably not more than a dozen letters; in this era before computer technology, Americans did not trail much information in their wakes; "anonymity" was a blessed possibility. Until the early 1970s I did not begin to keep a detailed journal and have virtually no access to my younger life except by way of family snapshots, school yearbooks, a few extant anecdotes, and my memory.

(The novelist must have a considerable, elastic memory to retain even the "memory" of a single novel as it is in progress. You might think of a vacuum cleaner bag—filled to bursting with the necessary and the unnecessary alike. After completing a novel, this bag is emptied—to a degree. In life, something of the same principle might prevail, though it will not apply to the earliest decades of the life, most deeply imprinted in the brain; these memories, as they are our first, will be the last to vanish.)

The first principle of the recollected memoir is "synecdoche." A symbolic part is selected to stand for the whole. The reader should not expect anything like a full disclosure of a life but should understand that memoirs, like works of fiction and poetry, must be highly selective. (Unless one sets out to write an autobiography in many volumes, as some have done. But a memoir is not an autobiography, and should not be heavily footnoted.) By its very nature selectivity is distorting because it oversimplifies the complexity of our lives. "Helen Judd" was not the only girl whom I knew who was abused and victimized by members of her own family in that long-ago world of rural western New York State, but I chose to write about this girl because I knew her best; "Cynthia Heike" was not my only close friend in high school, but writing at length about Cynthia more or less nullified writing at length about my other friends, who did not commit suicide. (Writing about another high school friend who'd been the victim of "date rape"—a term that did not exist in 1956— was made redundant by my novel *We Were the Mulvaneys* [1996].) Writing about *Alice's Adventures in Wonderland* and *Through the Looking-Glass* precluded writing about many other childhood books that were close to my heart. Writing about a pet chicken, I could not reasonably write about pet cats though I have had many, many more pet cats than I'd had pet chickens. To charges of distortion I can only say—*mea culpa*.

It should also be disclosed: while each chapter of this memoir focuses upon events, circumstances, and persons from the author's life, several chapters contain material that is too painfully personal, even after decades, to be set forth transparently. In these, you will find composite characters given fictitious names: "Helen Judd," "Jean Grady," "Reverend Bender," "Cynthia Heike," "Lee Ann Krauser," "Emmet Heike." Knowing how painful such material would have been to my parents, who wished always to think, and perhaps always did think, that my sister Lynn Ann might one day "improve," I have chosen not to include much detail about this phase of my parents' lives; nor did I linger on their illnesses, and the last weeks of their lives. Nothing is more offensive than an adult child exposing his or her elderly parents to the appalled fascination of strangers, even with the pretense of openness, honesty.

In *A Widow's Story*, fictitious names for some persons might have been a good idea for it has never been my intention to write anything that disturbs, offends, or betrays any other person's privacy. Not individuals but rather events and occasions—prevailing "themes"—are what engage me most as a writer, for nothing merely particular and private can be of more than passing interest. In setting out to write *The Lost Landscape* I understood that in several chapters I would be obliged to write about excruciatingly painful subjects—the sexual abuse of young girls, including father-daughter incest ("'They All Just Went Away'"); the suicide of a high school friend ("An Unsolved Mystery: The Lost Friend"). Yet I could not bring myself to write of these individuals except obliquely, changing as many specific details as seemed required to disguise the persons about whom I was writing, and I could not find a way to represent myself in their stories except as a quasi-fictitious character named "Joyce"—who is almost entirely an observer of the girls' lives, more emotionally detached (and more naïve) in the memoir than I had been in actual life.

These quasi-fictitious chapters gave me the most difficulty. Each contains verbatim remarks made by individuals decades ago— (Cynthia Heike's aggressively friendly bully-father Dr. Heike, for one)—but to record these remarks necessitated imagining the (likely) context in which they were made, and this required invention. Memory is a patchwork in which much, if not most, is blank. Emotion is a sort of flash photography—if you feel something deeply, you are likely to remember it for a long time. But where emotion is not heightened, as in most of the hours of what we call our "daily" lives, memories fade like Polaroid pictures. The memoirist is one who has impulsively picked up a handful of very hot stones—and has to drop some, in order to keep hold of others.

A problem inherent in writing about childhood abuse of any kind, not exclusively sexual, is that such a theme may stand out to readers in a way that distorts its actual significance in the subject's life. For not all "abused" persons register the abuse profoundly; to a degree, we are haunted by things we are conditioned to be haunted by, through the expectations and admonitions of others. That my parents knew relatively little about the extent of my misery at the one-room rural schoolhouse may have saved me from a protracted reliving of it. That there were no "therapists" in the rural world of my childhood and girlhood may have saved me from a similar reliving. It is possible to consider such childhood experiences as "educational"—in a way—as well as "traumatic." Certainly I would not want to relive these experiences but, paradoxically, I would not want to have not lived them, for I would feel that my life was less complete; most importantly, my life as a writer, for whom the most crucial quality of personality is sympathy.

Indeed, to revise Henry James: Three things in human life are important. The first is to have sympathy; the second is to have sympathy; and the third is to have sympathy.

MRI

OF THE
Extremities

MRI
OF THE
Extremities
An Anatomic Atlas

Second Edition

Heung Sik Kang, MD
Professor of Radiology
Seoul National University College of Medicine
Chief, Musculoskeletal Section
Department of Diagnostic Radiology
Seoul National University Hospital
Seoul, Korea

Joong Mo Ahn, MD
Assistant Professor
Department of Radiology
Sungkyunkwan University School of Medicine
Samsung Seoul Hospital
Seoul, Korea

Donald Resnick, MD
Chief, Musculoskeletal Imaging
Professor of Radiology
University of California, San Diego
Veterans Affairs San Diego Healthcare System
San Diego, California

With the technical
assistance of
DEBRA TRUDELL

W.B. SAUNDERS COMPANY
An Imprint of Elsevier Science
Philadelphia London New York St. Louis Sydney Toronto

W.B. SAUNDERS COMPANY
An Imprint of Elsevier Science

The Curtis Center
Independence Square West
Philadelphia, Pennsylvania 19106

Library of Congress Cataloging-in-Publication Data

Kang, Heung Sik.

MRI of the extremities: an anatomic atlas / Heung Sik Kang, Joong Mo Ahn, Donald Resnick.—2nd ed.

p.   cm.

ISBN 0–7216–9695–3

1. Extremities—Magnetic resonance imaging—Atlases. I. Ahn, Joong Mo.
   II. Resnick, Donald.   III. Title.

QM548.K36 2002
617.5′80754—dc21   2001049842

Acquisitions Editor: Lisette Bralow
Developmental Editor: Gwen Wright
Project Manager: Robin E. Davis

MRI OF THE EXTREMITIES: AN ANATOMIC ATLAS, Second Edition   ISBN 0–7216–9695–3

Printed in Hong Kong.

Last digit is the print number: 9 8 7 6 5 4 3 2 1

To those who open this atlas for interpretation or
learning of musculoskeletal MRI.

H.S.K.

To my teachers, Heung Sik Kang and Donald Resnick,
who taught me the true meaning of bone radiology.

J.M.A.

To my co-authors, whose dedication and hard work
are in clear evidence in this Second Edition.

D.R.

Preface to the Second Edition

Advances in knowledge and accumulation of clinical experience during the past decade have allowed magnetic resonance imaging (MRI) to become the primary diagnostic tool in the assessment of many disorders of the musculoskeletal system, and MRI also allows staging of disease and monitoring of the effects of therapy. Because of these factors, knowledge of normal anatomy as displayed by MRI is clearly important and required for accurate interpretation of the images.

The First Edition of this atlas focused on the detailed anatomy of joints of the peripheral skeleton and used close correlation of MRI and specimen photography. This new edition supplements that material by illustrating anatomic features of those structures of the extremities that are located mainly between the joints. In the previous edition, the authors directly correlated MRI and specimen photography by employing cadaveric limbs. A similar method was attempted in this edition; however, distortion of those structures located between joints in cadavers derived from elderly persons, particularly muscles, proved problematic. Thus, we decided that a technique using in vivo imaging of normal volunteers and schematic anatomic drawings is more appropriate and effective for the material that is new to this edition.

Four new chapters appear in this Second Edition. They relate to the anatomy of the upper arm (Chapter 2), forearm (Chapter 4), thigh (Chapter 8), and lower leg (Chapter 10). In these new chapters, coronal, transverse, and sagittal planes are illustrated. The illustrations in these new chapters are presented in the same fashion as those of the previous edition, and they use the terminology and designations that were employed in the First Edition (see pp ix–x). At each anatomic level, two illustrations appear, with MRI presented before the corresponding schematic anatomic drawing, and a line drawing is used to indicate the location and orientation of the section. The anatomic drawings have been derived directly from the corresponding MRI to ensure accuracy. Identical colors are used in the anatomic drawings to facilitate differentiation of structures.

We believe the additions in this Second Edition strengthen the usefulness of this atlas. Furthermore, we are confident that the very detailed labeling used throughout the book is one of its greatest strengths and will prove useful during interpretation of clinical MRI scans. If we are correct, this atlas will be used on a daily basis, not left on the shelf!

Heung Sik Kang, MD
Joong Mo Ahn, MD
Donald Resnick, MD

Preface to the First Edition

Magnetic resonance imaging has been applied with great success to the assessment of a variety of musculoskeletal disorders. The advantages of this technique include an ability to provide sectional images in any plane with excellent spatial and contrast resolution and the capability of revealing considerable physiologic and histologic data. Unlike routine radiography, computer tomography, and scintigraphy, magnetic resonance imaging can accomplish these things without the use of ionizing radiation or radiation-emitting pharmaceutical agents. The accurate interpretation of the images provided by magnetic resonance, however, is not accomplished without difficulty, requiring foremost that the examiner have considerable knowledge of pertinent osseous and soft tissue anatomy. Unless one knows where to look for abnormalities of signal and morphology, missed diagnosed or misdiagnosis will result.

With this atlas, the authors have attempted to demonstrate the anatomic information that is necessary for correct interpretation of magnetic resonance images of the extremities. Although other atlases exist, it was our belief that there was a need for a publication based not on in vivo imaging or normal volunteers but rather on cadaveric imaging alone and precise correlation of the anatomic features depicted with magnetic resonance and with specimen photography. An atlas of this type required meticulous preparation and imaging of the cadaveric parts (see Introduction), which proved to be the most challenging aspect of the endeavor.

This atlas is divided into seven chapters: shoulder; elbow; wrist and hand; finger; hip; knee; and ankle and foot. For each region of the body, transverse, coronal, and sagittal planes are illustrated. With regard to the shoulder, coronal oblique and sagittal oblique data, rather than strict coronal and sagittal data, are illustrated because these are the planes most often used in clinical imaging. At each level, two illustrations are provided, with the magnetic resonance image presented before the corresponding sectional photograph, and a line drawing is used to indicate the orientation and location of the section. With the exception of the wrist and hand, the images in the transverse plane are presented as if viewed from the caudal aspect; medial structures are to the reader's right and lateral structures are to the reader's left. The reverse is true for the wrist and hand, and in the elbow, medial and lateral orientations are reversed. In the coronal plane, the images are presented as if viewed from the anterior aspect with medial structures located to the reader's right and lateral structures to the reader's left; the orientation of the coronal images of the wrist and hand is reversed. The images in the sagittal plane are presented as if viewed from the midline; posterior structures are to the reader's right and anterior structures to the reader's left.

In selected instances, we employed a specifically prepared solution that was injected into the articulation prior to magnetic resonance imaging. As described in the Introduction, the solution was composed of ingredients that ensured accurate monitoring with fluoroscopy during the injection procedure, a bright signal with T_1-weighted sequences, and rapid solidification before sectioning of the specimen was accomplished.

With regard to labeling of the illustrations, we have defined as many structures as possible at each level, been consistent in labeling from one level to another, and used the specific terminology that currently is generally accepted. Where controversy or inconsistency exists in the literature, we have employed the designations that most often are used.

The following abbreviations are utilized throughout this atlas:

anterior = ant	posterior = post
medial = med	lateral = lat
superior = sup	inferior = inf
internal = int	external = ext
muscle = m	muscles = mm
nerve = n	nerves = nn
tendon = t	tendons = tt
ligament = lig	ligaments = ligs
artery = a	arteries = aa
vein = v	veins = vv
aponeurosis = apon	joint = j

In the transverse sections of the finger, the following abbreviations also are used:

MC = metacarpal
MP = middle phalanx
PP = proximal phalanx

In the transverse sections of the wrist and hand, the following abbreviations also are used:

P = palmar interosseous muscle
D = dorsal interosseous muscle
1, 2, 3, 4, 5 = metacarpals

In coronal sections of the foot and ankle, one additional abbreviation was used:

I = interosseous muscle

This atlas represents the final product of 12 months of cadaveric preparation, image acquisition, specimen processing, photography, and labeling of illustrations. Although there were moments of considerable fatigue and frustration, we maintained our energy and enthusiasm throughout because of our strong belief that knowledge of anatomy, above all else, is essential to correct analysis of magnetic resonance images. Indeed, we ourselves profited immensely from the information gained during hours of investigation and probing of the specimens as we traced structures from one level to another, attempting to differentiate among the many muscles (mm) and tendons (tt) we encountered, to distinguish arteries (aa) from veins (vv), and to identify important nerves (nn), ligaments (ligs), and other structures. We gained new respect for the intricacy of human anatomy and derived considerable satisfaction in our increasing ability to identify this anatomy as depicted in the magnetic resonance images. It is our hope that the reader who studies these illustrations also will profit from the experience and that he or she will understand, more than before, the considerable challenge and splendid opportunity provided by the remarkable technique utilizing magnetic resonance.

H.S.K.
D.R.

Acknowledgments

The authors would like to acknowledge the considerable efforts of a number of persons involved in this Second Edition of *MRI of the Extremities: An Anatomic Atlas*. Debra Trudell worked tirelessly in the preparation of the cadaveric material, and Hyukjin Kwon prepared the schematic drawings. We thank them both. Numerous professionals at W.B. Saunders provided significant assistance, including Lisette Bralow (Medical Editor), Sally Grande (Marketing Manager), and Robin E. Davis (Project Manager). Finally, we thank our associates, fellows, and residents whose constant quest for knowledge keeps us all thinking and learning.

Contents

1

Shoulder

Shoulder, Coronal

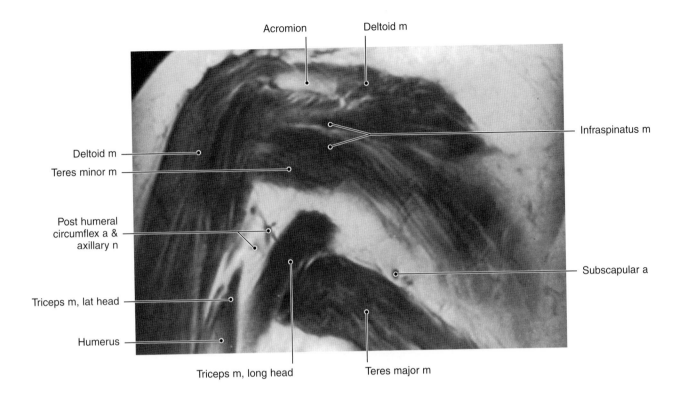

Acromion

Deltoid m

Infraspinatus m

Deltoid m

Teres minor m

Post humeral circumflex a & axillary n

Subscapular a

Triceps m, lat head

Humerus

Triceps m, long head

Teres major m

Acromion

Deltoid m

Infraspinatus m

Deltoid m

Teres minor m

Post humeral circumflex a & axillary n

Subscapular a

Triceps m, lat head

Triceps m, long head

Teres major m

Acromion

Deltoid m

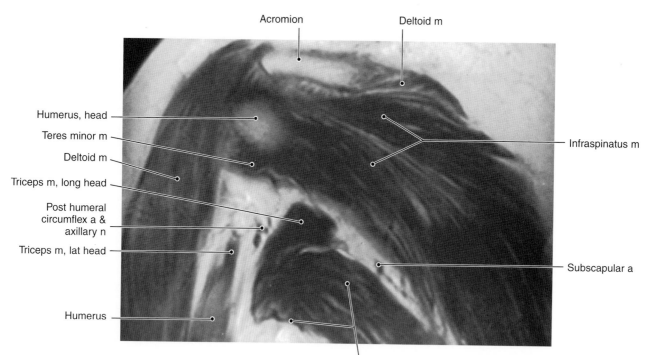

Humerus, head

Teres minor m

Deltoid m

Triceps m, long head

Post humeral
circumflex a &
axillary n

Triceps m, lat head

Humerus

Infraspinatus m

Subscapular a

Teres major & latissimus dorsi m & t

Acromion

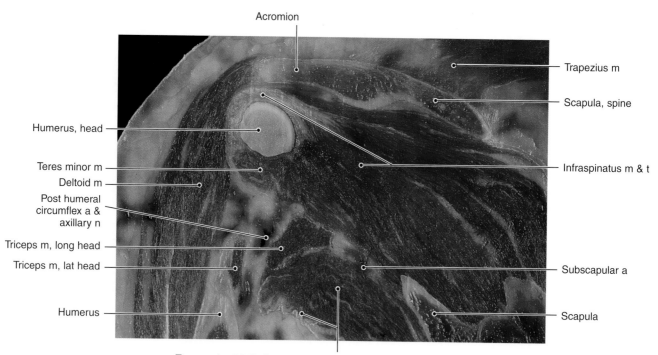

Trapezius m

Scapula, spine

Humerus, head

Teres minor m

Deltoid m

Post humeral
circumflex a &
axillary n

Triceps m, long head

Triceps m, lat head

Humerus

Infraspinatus m & t

Subscapular a

Scapula

Teres major & latissimus dorsi m & t

Shoulder, Coronal

Acromion Scapula, spine Trapezius m

Humerus, head

Deltoid m

Teres minor m & t

Triceps m, long head

Post humeral
circumflex a &
axillary n

Humerus

Infraspinatus m & t

Subscapular a

Teres major & latissimus dorsi m & t

Acromion Scapula, spine Trapezius m

Humerus, head

Teres minor m & t

Deltoid m

Triceps m, long head

Post humeral
circumflex a &
axillary n

Humerus

Infraspinatus m & t

Subscapularis m

Scapula

Teres major & latissimus dorsi m & t Subscapular a

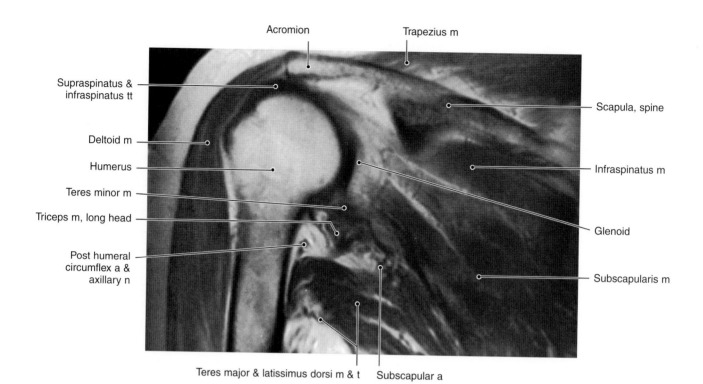

Acromion

Trapezius m

Supraspinatus & infraspinatus tt

Scapula, spine

Deltoid m

Humerus

Infraspinatus m

Teres minor m

Triceps m, long head

Glenoid

Post humeral circumflex a & axillary n

Subscapularis m

Teres major & latissimus dorsi m & t

Subscapular a

Acromion

Trapezius m

Infraspinatus t

Supraspinatus t

Supraspinatus m

Deltoid m

Scapula, spine

Humerus

Infraspinatus m

Glenoid

Teres minor m

Triceps m, long head

Scapula

Post humeral circumflex a & axillary n

Subscapularis m

Teres major & latissimus dorsi m & t

Subscapular a

Shoulder, Coronal

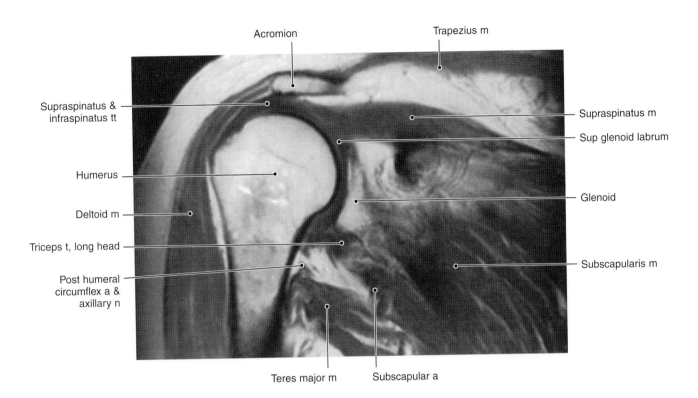

Acromion

Trapezius m

Supraspinatus & infraspinatus tt

Supraspinatus m

Sup glenoid labrum

Humerus

Glenoid

Deltoid m

Triceps t, long head

Post humeral circumflex a & axillary n

Subscapularis m

Teres major m

Subscapular a

Acromion

Trapezius m

Infraspinatus t

Supraspinatus m

Supraspinatus t

Sup glenoid labrum

Suprascapular a & n

Humerus

Glenoid

Deltoid m

Inf glenoid labrum

Articular capsule

Triceps t, long head

Post humeral circumflex a & axillary n

Subscapularis m

Teres major & latissimus dorsi m & t

Subscapular a

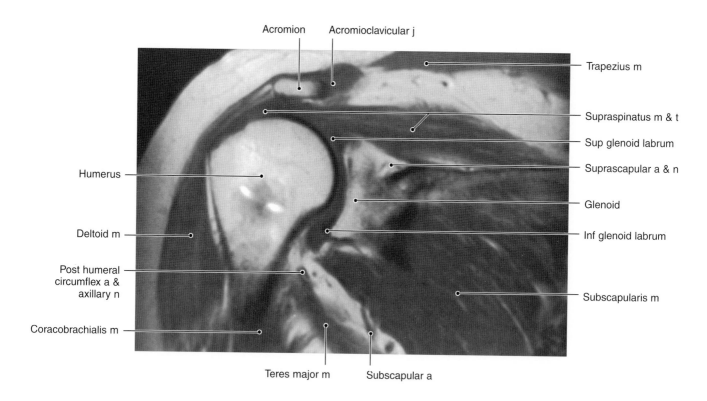

Acromion Acromioclavicular j

Trapezius m

Supraspinatus m & t

Sup glenoid labrum

Suprascapular a & n

Humerus

Glenoid

Inf glenoid labrum

Deltoid m

Post humeral circumflex a & axillary n

Subscapularis m

Coracobrachialis m

Teres major m Subscapular a

Acromion Acromioclavicular j

Trapezius m

Supraspinatus m & t

Sup glenoid labrum

Suprascapular a & n

Humerus

Glenoid

Subscapularis m

Articular capsule

Inf glenoid labrum

Post humeral circumflex a & axillary n

Deltoid m

Coracobrachialis m

Serratus ant m

Teres major & latissimus m & t Subscapular a

Shoulder, Coronal

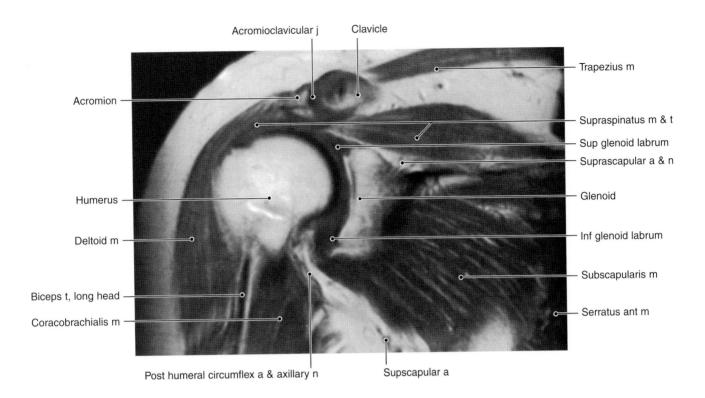

Acromioclavicular j
Clavicle
Acromion
Trapezius m
Supraspinatus m & t
Sup glenoid labrum
Suprascapular a & n
Humerus
Glenoid
Deltoid m
Inf glenoid labrum
Subscapularis m
Biceps t, long head
Coracobrachialis m
Serratus ant m
Post humeral circumflex a & axillary n
Supscapular a

Acromioclavicular j
Clavicle
Acromion
Trapezius m
Supraspinatus m & t
Sup glenoid labrum
Suprascapular a & n
Humerus
Glenoid
Deltoid m
Inf glenoid labrum
Articular capsule
Post humeral circumflex a & axillary n
Subscapularis m
Biceps t, long head
Coracobrachialis m
Serratus ant m
Latissimus dorsi t
Teres major t
Supscapular a

Acromioclavicular j   Clavicle

Acromion

Coracoacromial lig

Trapezius m

Humerus, head

Supraspinatus m

Suprascapular a & n

Coracoid process

Biceps t, long head

Glenoid

Deltoid m

Subscapularis m

Serratus ant m

Coracobrachialis m

Acromioclavicular j   Clavicle

Coracoacromial lig

Supraspinatus t

Biceps t, long head

Humerus, head

Trapezius m

Supraspinatus m

Suprascapular a & n

Coracoid process

Deltoid m

Glenoid

Biceps t, long head

Subscapularis m

Coracobrachialis m

Serratus ant m

Musculocutaneous n   Brachial a

Shoulder, Coronal

Coracoacromial lig

Clavicle

Trapezius m

Supraspinatus m

Coracoclavicular lig

Coracoid process

Coracohumeral lig

Biceps t, long head

Lesser tubercle

Subscapularis m & t

Deltoid m

Coracobrachialis m

Coracoacromial lig

Clavicle

Trapezius m

Coracoclavicular lig

Coracohumeral lig

Coracoid process

Biceps t, long head

Lesser tubercle

Subscapularis m & t

Deltoid m

Biceps m

Coracobrachialis m

Musculocutaneous n

Brachial a

Shoulder, Transverse

Acromioclavicular j

Trapezius m

Clavicle

Trapezius m

Acromioclavicular j

Trapezius m

Clavicle

Trapezius m

Deltoid m — Clavicle

Acromioclavicular j

Acromion

Deltoid m

Trapezius m

Omohyoid m

Serratus ant m

Scapula, sup angle

Supraspinatus m

Trapezius m

Deltoid m — Clavicle

Acromioclavicular j

Deltoid m

Acromion

Trapezius m

Omohyoid m

Serratus ant m

Scapula, sup angle

Supraspinatus m

Trapezius m

Shoulder, Transverse

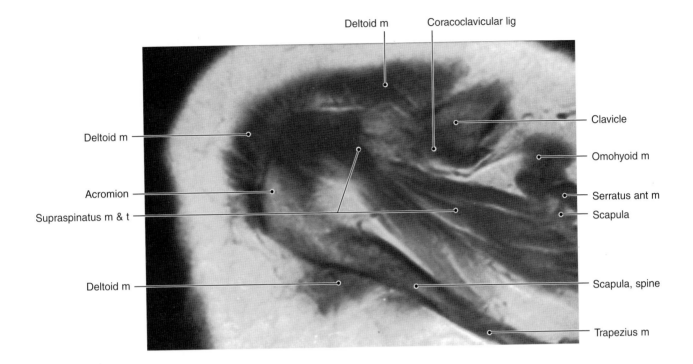

Deltoid m

Coracoclavicular lig

Deltoid m

Acromion

Supraspinatus m & t

Deltoid m

Clavicle

Omohyoid m

Serratus ant m

Scapula

Scapula, spine

Trapezius m

Deltoid m

Coracoclavicular lig

Coracoacromial lig

Deltoid m

Supraspinatus m & t

Acromion

Deltoid m

Clavicle

Omohyoid m

Serratus ant m

Scapula

Scapula, spine

Trapezius m

Deltoid m — Coracoacromial lig

Deltoid m

Humerus, head

Infraspinatus m & t

Deltoid m

Clavicle

Subclavius m

Coracoid process

Coracoclavicular lig

Serratus ant m

Supraspinatus m & t

Scapula, spine — Infraspinatus m

Deltoid m — Coracoacromial lig

Deltoid m

Humerus, head

Infraspinatus m & t

Deltoid m

Clavicle

Subclavius m

Coracoid process

Coracoclavicular lig

Sup transverse scapular lig

Serratus ant m

Scapula

Supraspinatus m & t

Infraspinatus m — Scapula, spine

Shoulder, Transverse

Glenoid labrum
Coracoid process
Deltoid m
Clavicle
Supraspinatus t
Calcification (supraspinatus t)
Subclavius m
Humerus, head
Coracoclavicular lig
Infraspinatus m & t
Glenoid
Serratus ant m
Subscapularis m
Deltoid m
Scapula, spine
Supraspinatus m

Coracohumeral lig
Deltoid m
Supraspinatus t
Clavicle
Coracoid process
Calcification (supraspinatus t)
Subclavius m
Glenoid labrum & long head of biceps t
Coracoclavicular lig
Humerus, head
Glenoid
Serratus ant m
Scapula
Infraspinatus m & t
Subscapularis m
Deltoid m
Supraspinatus m
Scapula, spine

Coracohumeral lig

Coracoid process

Deltoid m

Biceps t, long head

Calcification
(infraspinatus t)

Humerus, head

Infraspinatus m & t

Deltoid m

Clavicle

Pectoralis minor t

Subclavius m

Ant glenoid labrum

Subscapularis m

Serratus ant m

Scapula, spine

Glenoid

Suprascapular a & n

Coracohumeral lig

Coracoid process

Deltoid m

Biceps t, long head

Calcification
(infraspinatus t)

Humerus, head

Infraspinatus m & t

Deltoid m

Clavicle

Pectoralis minor t

Subclavius m

Ant glenoid labrum

Serratus ant m

Subscapularis m

Glenoid

Scapula, spine

Shoulder, Transverse

Ant glenoid labrum
Coracoid process
Deltoid m
Biceps t, long head
Greater tubercle
Lesser tubercle
Infraspinatus t
Humerus, head
Clavicle
Subclavius m
Pectoralis minor m & t
Subscapularis m & t
Glenoid
Serratus ant m
Deltoid m
Infraspinatus m
Post glenoid labrum
Suprascapular a & n

Ant glenoid labrum
Coracoid process
Deltoid m
Biceps t, long head
Greater tubercle
Lesser tubercle
Infraspinatus t
Humerus, head
Clavicle
Subclavius m
Pectoralis minor m & t
Subscapularis m & t
Glenoid
Serratus ant m
Deltoid m
Infraspinatus m
Post glenoid labrum
Suprascapular a & n

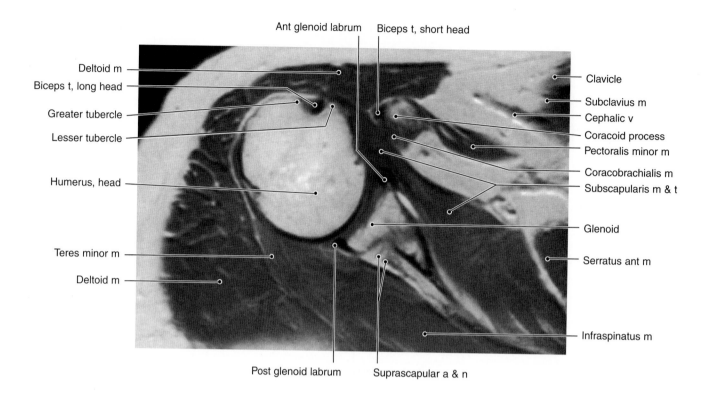

Ant glenoid labrum
Biceps t, short head
Deltoid m
Biceps t, long head
Greater tubercle
Lesser tubercle
Humerus, head
Teres minor m
Deltoid m
Clavicle
Subclavius m
Cephalic v
Coracoid process
Pectoralis minor m
Coracobrachialis m
Subscapularis m & t
Glenoid
Serratus ant m
Infraspinatus m
Post glenoid labrum
Suprascapular a & n

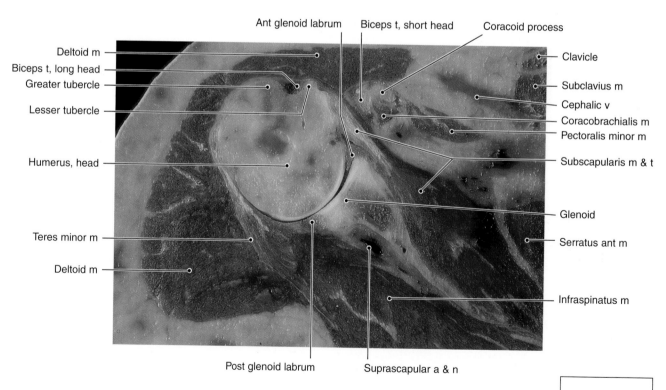

Ant glenoid labrum
Biceps t, short head
Coracoid process
Deltoid m
Biceps t, long head
Greater tubercle
Lesser tubercle
Humerus, head
Teres minor m
Deltoid m
Clavicle
Subclavius m
Cephalic v
Coracobrachialis m
Pectoralis minor m
Subscapularis m & t
Glenoid
Serratus ant m
Infraspinatus m
Post glenoid labrum
Suprascapular a & n

Shoulder, Transverse

Ant glenoid labrum   Biceps t, short head

Deltoid m
Biceps t, long head
Greater tubercle
Lesser tubercle
Teres minor t
Humerus, head
Teres minor m
Deltoid m

Cephalic v
Coracobrachialis m
Pectoralis minor m
Brachial plexus
Subscapularis m & t
Glenoid
Serratus ant m
Infraspinatus m

Post glenoid labrum   Suprascapular a & n

Ant glenoid labrum   Biceps t, short head   Coracobrachialis m

Deltoid m
Biceps t, long head
Greater tubercle
Lesser tubercle
Teres minor t
Humerus, head
Teres minor m
Deltoid m

Clavicle
Subclavius m
Cephalic v
Pectoralis minor m
Brachial plexus
Subscapularis m & t
Glenoid
Serratus ant m
Infraspinatus m

Post glenoid labrum   Suprascapular a & n

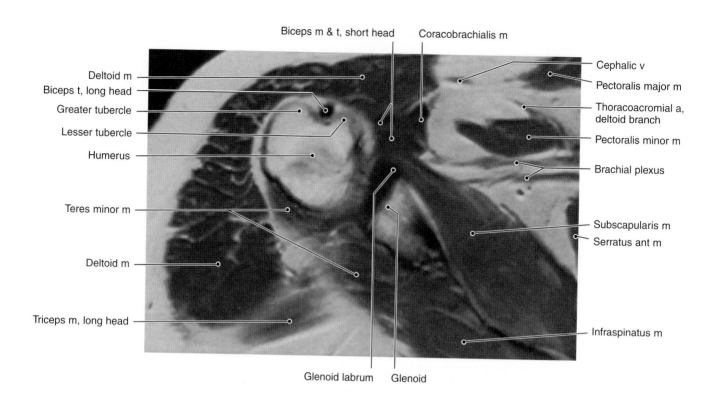

Biceps m & t, short head
Coracobrachialis m
Deltoid m
Biceps t, long head
Greater tubercle
Lesser tubercle
Humerus
Teres minor m
Deltoid m
Triceps m, long head
Cephalic v
Pectoralis major m
Thoracoacromial a, deltoid branch
Pectoralis minor m
Brachial plexus
Subscapularis m
Serratus ant m
Infraspinatus m
Glenoid labrum
Glenoid

Biceps m & t, short head
Coracobrachialis m
Deltoid m
Biceps t, long head
Greater tubercle
Lesser tubercle
Humerus
Teres minor m
Deltoid m
Triceps m, long head
Cephalic v
Pectoralis major m
Thoracoacromial a, deltoid branch
Pectoralis minor m
Brachial plexus
Ant glenoid labrum
Subscapularis m
Serratus ant m
Infraspinatus m
Post glenoid labrum
Glenoid

Shoulder, Transverse

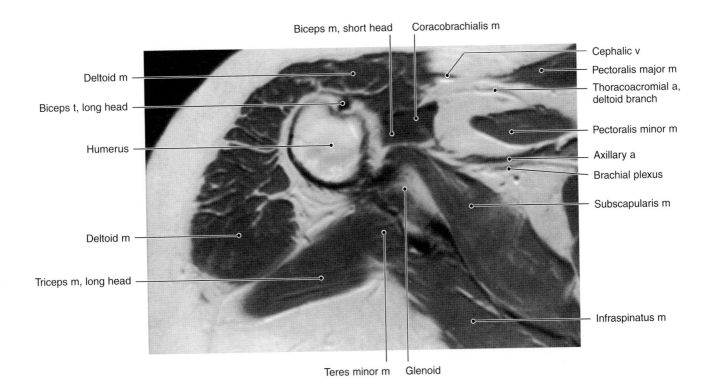

Biceps m, short head — Coracobrachialis m

Deltoid m

Biceps t, long head

Humerus

Deltoid m

Triceps m, long head

Cephalic v

Pectoralis major m

Thoracoacromial a, deltoid branch

Pectoralis minor m

Axillary a

Brachial plexus

Subscapularis m

Infraspinatus m

Teres minor m — Glenoid

Biceps m, short head — Coracobrachialis m

Deltoid m

Biceps t, long head

Humerus

Deltoid m

Triceps m, long head

Cephalic v

Pectoralis major m

Thoracoacromial a, deltoid branch

Pectoralis minor m

Axillary a

Brachial plexus

Subscapularis m

Infraspinatus m

Teres minor m — Glenoid

Biceps t, long head
Biceps m, short head
Deltoid m
Cephalic v
Pectoralis major m
Humerus
Pectoralis minor m
Coracobrachialis m
Triceps m, lat head
Axillary a &
brachial plexus
Post humeral
circumflex a &
axillary n
Deltoid m
Subscapularis m
Triceps m, long head
Scapula
Teres minor m
Infraspinatus m
Teres major m
Subscapular a

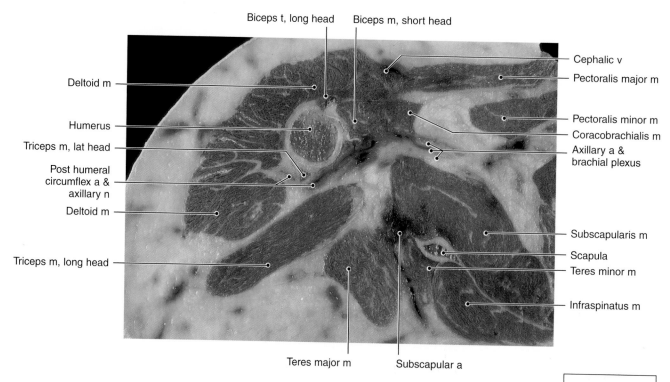

Biceps t, long head
Biceps m, short head
Deltoid m
Cephalic v
Pectoralis major m
Humerus
Pectoralis minor m
Triceps m, lat head
Coracobrachialis m
Axillary a &
brachial plexus
Post humeral
circumflex a &
axillary n
Deltoid m
Subscapularis m
Scapula
Triceps m, long head
Teres minor m
Infraspinatus m
Teres major m
Subscapular a

Shoulder, Transverse

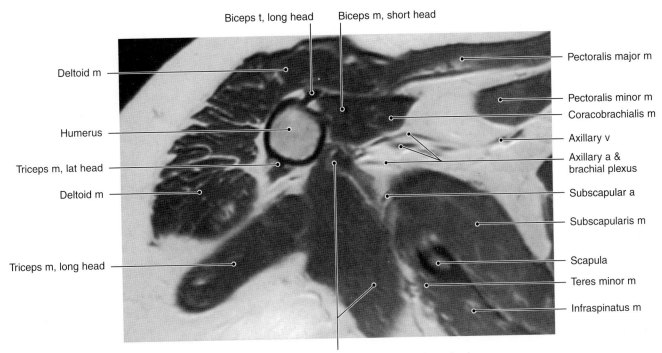

Biceps t, long head

Biceps m, short head

Deltoid m

Humerus

Triceps m, lat head

Deltoid m

Triceps m, long head

Pectoralis major m

Pectoralis minor m

Coracobrachialis m

Axillary v

Axillary a & brachial plexus

Subscapular a

Subscapularis m

Scapula

Teres minor m

Infraspinatus m

Teres major & latissimus dorsi mm

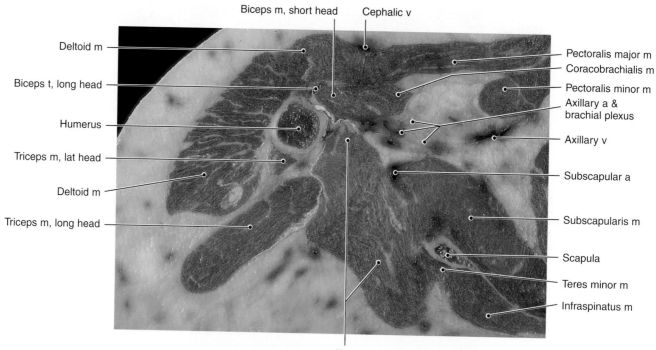

Biceps m, short head

Cephalic v

Deltoid m

Biceps t, long head

Humerus

Triceps m, lat head

Deltoid m

Triceps m, long head

Pectoralis major m

Coracobrachialis m

Pectoralis minor m

Axillary a & brachial plexus

Axillary v

Subscapular a

Subscapularis m

Scapula

Teres minor m

Infraspinatus m

Teres major & latissimus dorsi mm

Shoulder, Sagittal

Deltoid m

Coracoclavicular lig

Coracoid process

Thoracoacromial a,
pectoral branch

Pectoralis major m

Pectoralis minor m

Axillary a &
brachial plexus

Subscapularis m

Axillary v

Acromioclavicular j

Clavicle

Acromion

Supraspinatus m & t

Deltoid m

Infraspinatus m

Scapula, body

Teres minor m

Teres major m

Deltoid m

Coracoclavicular lig

Coracoid process

Thoracoacromial a,
pectoral branch

Pectoralis major m

Pectoralis minor m

Axillary a &
brachial plexus

Axillary v

Clavicle

Acromioclavicular j

Acromion

Supraspinatus m & t

Deltoid m

Scapula, body

Infraspinatus m

Subscapularis m & t

Teres minor m

Teres major m

Shoulder, Sagittal

Deltoid m — Acromioclavicular j

Clavicle — Acromion

Coracoclavicular lig

Coracoid process — Supraspinatus m & t

Thoracoacromial a,
pectoral branch — Glenoid

— Deltoid m

Pectoralis major m — Infraspinatus m
Pectoralis minor m

— Subscapularis m

Axillary a &
brachial plexus — Teres minor m

Axillary v

— Teres major m

Deltoid m

Clavicle

Coracoclavicular lig

Coracoid process

Thoracoacromial a,
pectoral branch

Pectoralis major m

Pectoralis minor m

Axillary a &
brachial plexus

Axillary v

Acromioclavicular j

Acromion

Supraspinatus m & t

Glenoid

Deltoid m

Infraspinatus m

Subscapularis m & t

Teres minor m

Teres major m

Shoulder, Sagittal

Deltoid m

Coracoacromial lig

Coracohumeral lig

Coracoid process

Thoracoacromial a,
pectoral branch

Pectoralis minor m

Coracobrachialis m

Pectoralis major m

Axillary a &
brachial plexus

Subscapular a

Acromioclavicular j

Acromion

Supraspinatus m & t

Glenoid

Deltoid m

Infraspinatus m

Subscapularis m & t

Teres minor m

Teres major m

Latissimus dorsi m

Deltoid m

Coracoacromial lig

Coracohumeral lig

Coracoid process

Thoracoacromial a,
pectoral branch

Pectoralis minor m

Corabrachialis m

Pectoralis major m

Axillary a &
brachial plexus

Axillary v

Subscapular a

Acromioclavicular j

Acromion

Supraspinatus m & t

Glenoid labrum

Gelnoid

Deltoid m

Infraspinatus m & t

Subscapularis m & t

Teres minor m

Teres major m

Latissimus dorsi m

Shoulder, Sagittal

Deltoid m

Coracoacromial lig

Coracohumeral lig

Coracoid process

Biceps t, long head

Corabrachialis m

Ant glenoid labrum

Subscapularis m & t

Pectoralis major m

Axillary a &
brachial plexus

Acromion

Supraspinatus m & t

Humerus, head

Infraspinatus m & t

Post glenoid labrum

Deltoid m

Glenoid

Teres minor m

Teres major m

Latissimus dorsi m

Deltoid m

Coracoacromial lig

Coracohumeral lig

Coracoid process

Sup glenohumeral lig

Middle glenohumeral lig

Coracobrachialis m

Subscapularis m & t

Axillary a &
brachial plexus

Axillary v

Pectoralis major m

Acromion

Supraspinatus m & t

Biceps t, long head

Humerus, head

Post glenoid labrum

Infraspinatus m & t

Glenoid

Deltoid m

Teres minor m

Teres major m

Latissimus dorsi m

Shoulder, Sagittal

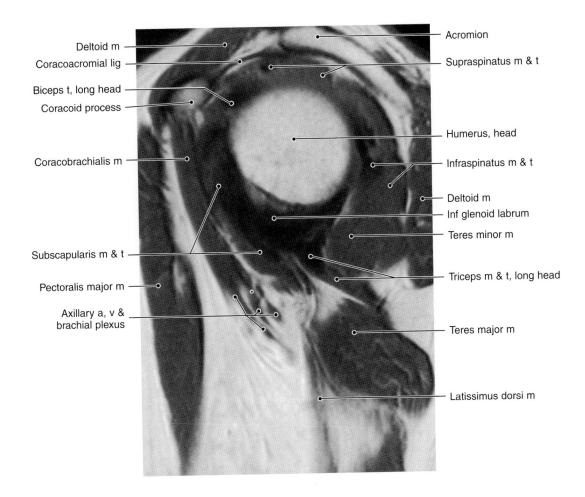

Deltoid m

Coracoacromial lig

Biceps t, long head

Coracoid process

Coracobrachialis m

Subscapularis m & t

Pectoralis major m

Axillary a, v &
brachial plexus

Acromion

Supraspinatus m & t

Humerus, head

Infraspinatus m & t

Deltoid m

Inf glenoid labrum

Teres minor m

Triceps m & t, long head

Teres major m

Latissimus dorsi m

Deltoid m

Coracoacromial lig

Biceps t, long head

Coracoid process

Coracobrachialis m

Pectoralis major m

Subscapularis m & t

Axillary a &
brachial plexus

Axillary v

Acromion

Supraspinatus m & t

Humerus, head

Infraspinatus m & t

Deltoid m

Inf glenoid labrum

Teres minor m

Triceps m & t, long head

Terest major m

Latissimus dorsi m

Shoulder, Sagittal

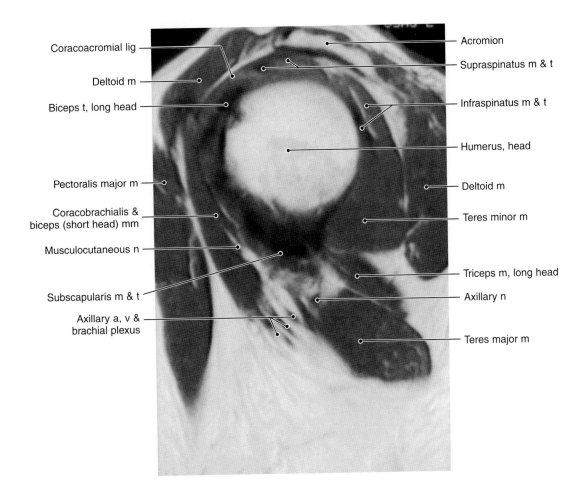

Coracoacromial lig

Deltoid m

Biceps t, long head

Pectoralis major m

Coracobrachialis &
biceps (short head) mm

Musculocutaneous n

Subscapularis m & t

Axillary a, v &
brachial plexus

Acromion

Supraspinatus m & t

Infraspinatus m & t

Humerus, head

Deltoid m

Teres minor m

Triceps m, long head

Axillary n

Teres major m

Coracoacromial lig

Supraspinatus m & t

Deltoid m

Transverse humeral lig

Biceps t, long head

Biceps t, short head

Subscapularis m & t

Musculocutaneous n

Coracobrachialis m

Pectoralis major m

Deltoid m

Acromion

Infraspinatus m & t

Humerus, head

Teres minor m

Articular capsule

Triceps m & t, long head

Axillary n

Teres major m

Latissimus dorsi t

Axillary a &
brachial plexus

Shoulder, Sagittal

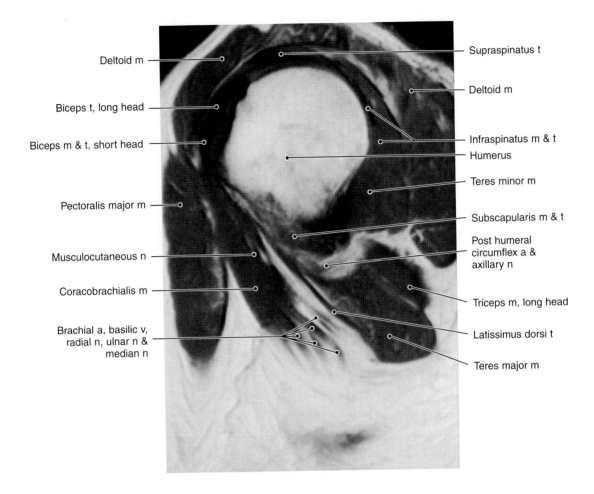

Deltoid m

Biceps t, long head

Biceps m & t, short head

Pectoralis major m

Musculocutaneous n

Coracobrachialis m

Brachial a, basilic v, radial n, ulnar n & median n

Supraspinatus t

Deltoid m

Infraspinatus m & t

Humerus

Teres minor m

Subscapularis m & t

Post humeral circumflex a & axillary n

Triceps m, long head

Latissimus dorsi t

Teres major m

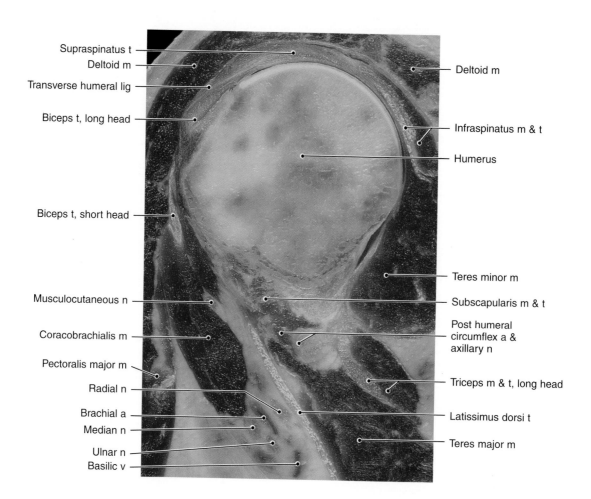

Supraspinatus t

Deltoid m

Transverse humeral lig

Biceps t, long head

Biceps t, short head

Musculocutaneous n

Coracobrachialis m

Pectoralis major m

Radial n

Brachial a

Median n

Ulnar n

Basilic v

Deltoid m

Infraspinatus m & t

Humerus

Teres minor m

Subscapularis m & t

Post humeral circumflex a & axillary n

Triceps m & t, long head

Latissimus dorsi t

Teres major m

Shoulder, Sagittal

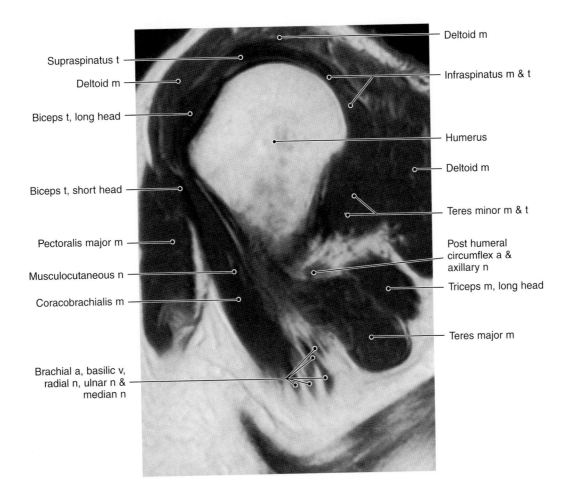

Supraspinatus t

Deltoid m

Biceps t, long head

Biceps t, short head

Pectoralis major m

Musculocutaneous n

Coracobrachialis m

Brachial a, basilic v, radial n, ulnar n & median n

Deltoid m

Infraspinatus m & t

Humerus

Deltoid m

Teres minor m & t

Post humeral circumflex a & axillary n

Triceps m, long head

Teres major m

Deltoid m

Supraspinatus t

Infraspinatus m & t

Biceps t, long head

Humerus

Deltoid m

Biceps t, short head

Teres minor m & t

Musculocutaneous n

Post humeral
circumflex a &
axillary n

Pectoralis major m

Coracobrachialis m

Triceps m & t, long head

Radial n

Latissimus dorsi t

Brachial a

Median n

Teres major m

Ulnar n

Basilic v

Shoulder, Sagittal

Deltoid m

Supraspinatus t

Infraspinatus m & t

Deltoid m

Humerus

Biceps t, long head

Deltoid m

Teres minor m & t

Pectoralis major m

Coracobrachialis &
biceps (short head) mm

Post humeral
circumflex a &
axillary n

Triceps m, long head

Teres major m

Brachial a, basilic v,
radial n, ulnar n &
median n

Supraspinatus t

Deltoid m

Biceps t, long head

Pectoralis major m

Biceps m, short head

Musculocutaneous n

Latissimus dorsi t

Coracobrachialis m

Radial n

Brachial a

Median n

Ulnar n

Deltoid m

Infraspinatus m & t

Humerus

Deltoid m

Teres minor m & t

Post humeral
circumflex a &
axillary n

Triceps m & t, long head

Teres major m & t

Basilic v

Shoulder, Sagittal

Deltoid m

Deltoid m

Humerus

Biceps t, long head

Pectoralis major m

Biceps m, short head

Coracobrachialis m

Brachial a, basilic v,
radial n, ulnar n &
median n

Infraspinatus m & t

Deltoid m

Teres minor m & t

Post humeral
circumflex a &
axillary n

Triceps m, long head

Teres major m

Deltoid m

Infraspinatus m & t

Deltoid m

Deltoid m

Humerus

Teres minor m & t

Biceps t, long head

Pectoralis major m

Post humeral
circumflex a &
axillary n

Latissimus dorsi t

Biceps m, short head

Musculocutaneous n

Triceps m & t, long head

Coracobrachialis m

Teres major m & t

Radial n

Brachial a

Basilic v

Median n

Ulnar n

Shoulder, Sagittal

Deltoid m

Infraspinatus t

Deltoid m

Deltoid m

Humerus

Teres minor m

Pectoralis major m

Post humeral circumflex a & axillary n

Biceps m

Triceps m, lat head

Coracobrachialis m

Triceps m, long head

Radial n

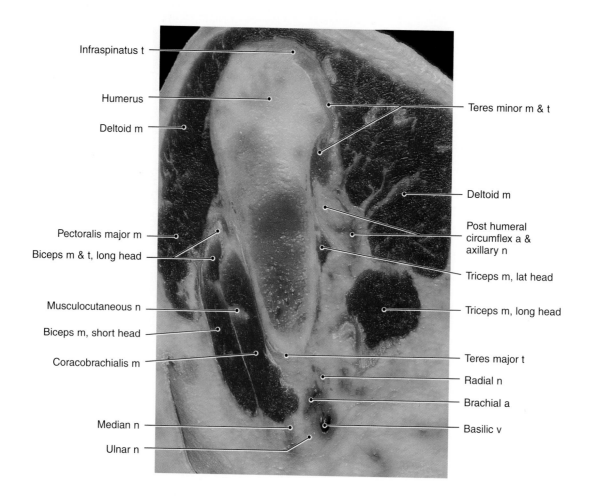

Infraspinatus t

Humerus

Deltoid m

Pectoralis major m

Biceps m & t, long head

Musculocutaneous n

Biceps m, short head

Coracobrachialis m

Median n

Ulnar n

Teres minor m & t

Deltoid m

Post humeral circumflex a & axillary n

Triceps m, lat head

Triceps m, long head

Teres major t

Radial n

Brachial a

Basilic v

Shoulder, Sagittal

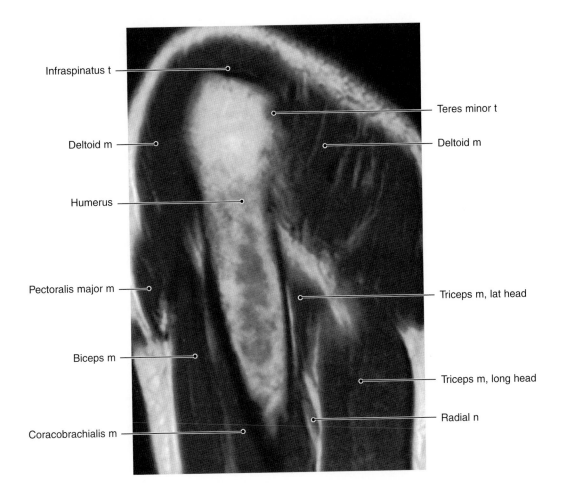

Infraspinatus t

Teres minor t

Deltoid m

Deltoid m

Humerus

Pectoralis major m

Triceps m, lat head

Biceps m

Triceps m, long head

Radial n

Coracobrachialis m

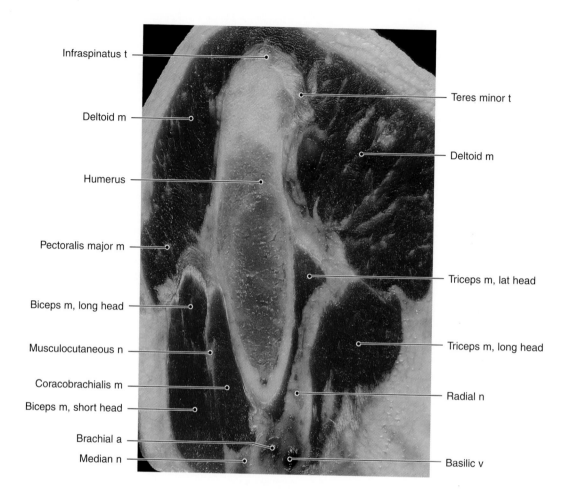

Infraspinatus t

Deltoid m

Humerus

Pectoralis major m

Biceps m, long head

Musculocutaneous n

Coracobrachialis m

Biceps m, short head

Brachial a

Median n

Teres minor t

Deltoid m

Triceps m, lat head

Triceps m, long head

Radial n

Basilic v

Shoulder, Sagittal

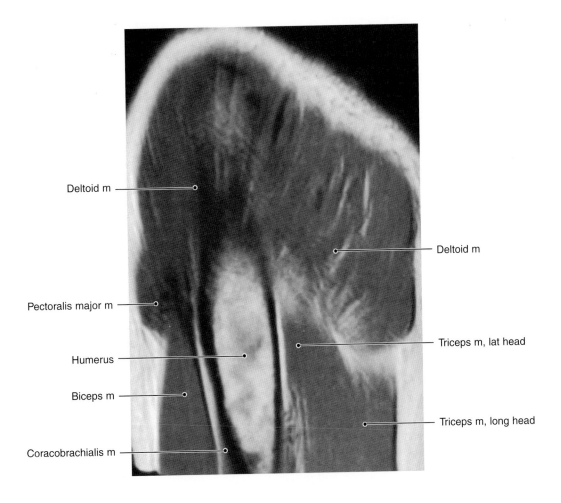

Deltoid m

Deltoid m

Pectoralis major m

Triceps m, lat head

Humerus

Biceps m

Triceps m, long head

Coracobrachialis m

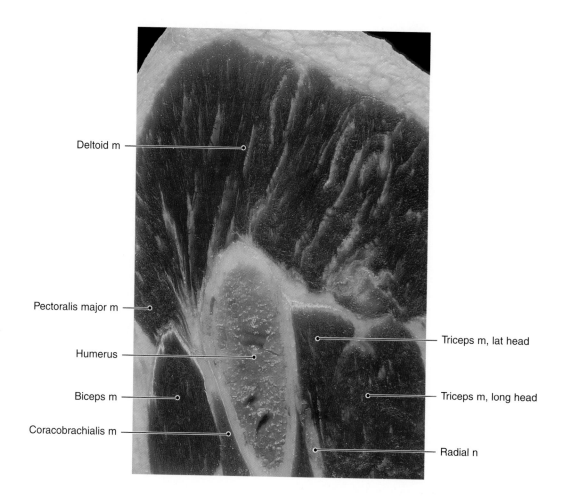

Deltoid m

Pectoralis major m

Humerus

Biceps m

Coracobrachialis m

Triceps m, lat head

Triceps m, long head

Radial n

2

Upper Arm

Upper Arm, Coronal

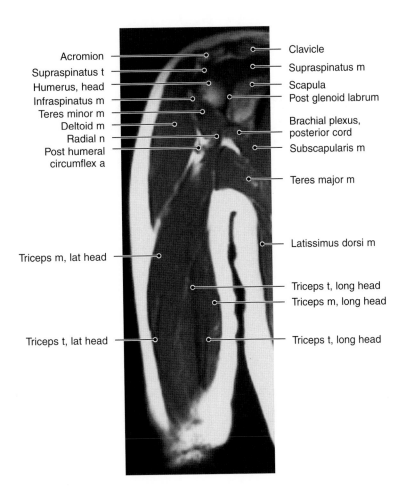

Acromion

Supraspinatus t

Humerus, head

Infraspinatus m

Teres minor m

Deltoid m

Radial n

Post humeral circumflex a

Triceps m, lat head

Triceps t, lat head

Clavicle

Supraspinatus m

Scapula

Post glenoid labrum

Brachial plexus, posterior cord

Subscapularis m

Teres major m

Latissimus dorsi m

Triceps t, long head

Triceps m, long head

Triceps t, long head

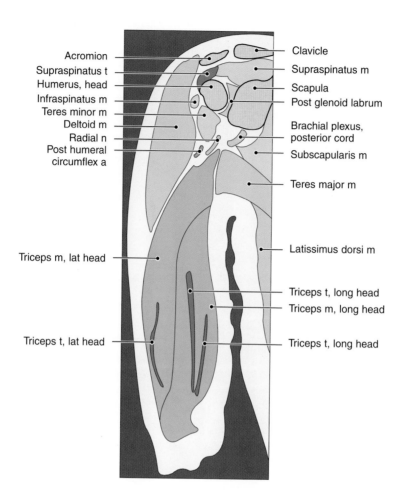

Acromion

Supraspinatus t

Humerus, head

Infraspinatus m

Teres minor m

Deltoid m

Radial n

Post humeral circumflex a

Clavicle

Supraspinatus m

Scapula

Post glenoid labrum

Brachial plexus, posterior cord

Subscapularis m

Teres major m

Latissimus dorsi m

Triceps m, lat head

Triceps t, long head

Triceps m, long head

Triceps t, lat head

Triceps t, long head

Upper Arm, Coronal

Acromion

Supraspinatus t

Humerus, head

Deltoid m

Triceps m, lat head

Post antebrachial cutaneous n

Radial n

Brachialis m

Extensor carpi radialis longus m

Lat epicondyle

Supinator m

Extensor digitorum m

Scapula

Subscapularis m

Subscapularis t

Subscapularis m

Brachial plexus

Teres major m

Ulnar n

Latissimus dorsi m

Humerus, shaft

Ulnar n

Triceps m, med head

Med epicondyle

Olecranon

Flexor digitorum superficialis m

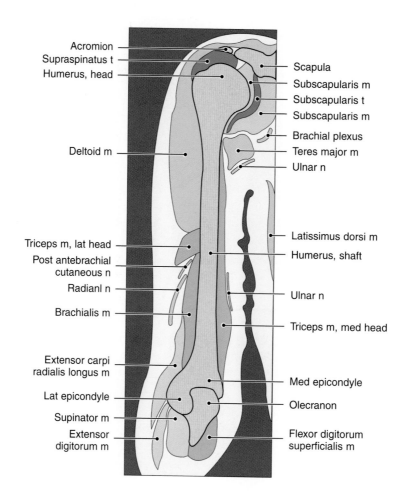

Acromion
Supraspinatus t
Humerus, head

Scapula
Subscapularis m
Subscapularis t
Subscapularis m
Brachial plexus
Teres major m
Ulnar n

Deltoid m

Triceps m, lat head
Post antebrachial
cutaneous n
Radianl n

Brachialis m

Latissimus dorsi m
Humerus, shaft

Ulnar n

Triceps m, med head

Extensor carpi
radialis longus m

Lat epicondyle

Supinator m

Extensor
digitorum m

Med epicondyle

Olecranon

Flexor digitorum
superficialis m

Upper Arm, Coronal

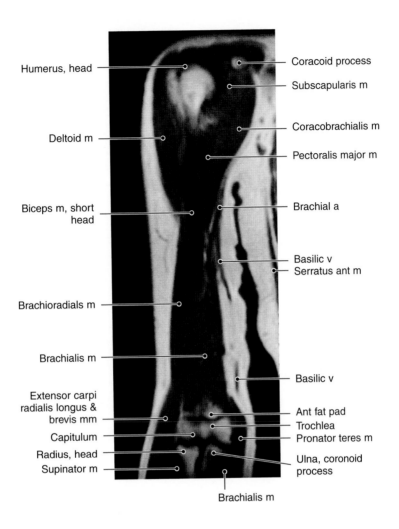

Humerus, head

Coracoid process

Subscapularis m

Deltoid m

Coracobrachialis m

Pectoralis major m

Biceps m, short head

Brachial a

Basilic v
Serratus ant m

Brachioradials m

Brachialis m

Basilic v

Extensor carpi radialis longus & brevis mm

Ant fat pad

Trochlea

Capitulum

Pronator teres m

Radius, head

Supinator m

Ulna, coronoid process

Brachialis m

Humerus, head

Coracoid process

Subscapularis m

Deltoid m

Coracobrachialis m

Pectoralis major m

Biceps m, short head

Brachial a

Basilic v

Serratus ant m

Brachioradials m

Brachialis m

Basilic v

Extensor carpi radialis longus & brevis mm

Ant fat pad

Trochlea

Capitulum

Pronator teres m

Radius, head

Ulna, coronoid process

Supinator m

Brachialis m

Upper Arm, Coronal

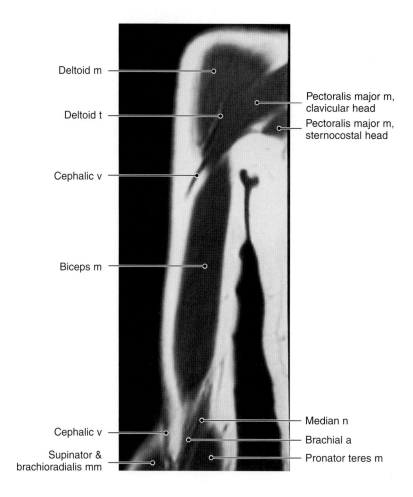

Deltoid m

Deltoid t

Cephalic v

Biceps m

Cephalic v

Supinator &
brachioradialis mm

Pectoralis major m,
clavicular head

Pectoralis major m,
sternocostal head

Median n

Brachial a

Pronator teres m

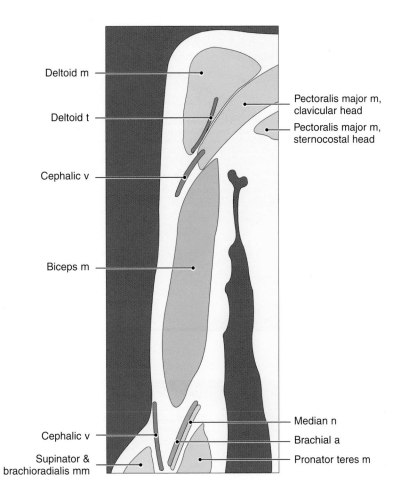

Deltoid m

Deltoid t

Cephalic v

Biceps m

Cephalic v

Supinator &
brachioradialis mm

Pectoralis major m,
clavicular head

Pectoralis major m,
sternocostal head

Median n

Brachial a

Pronator teres m

Upper Arm, Transverse

Superficial v — Cephalic v
Superficial v — Pectoralis major m
Deltoid tt — Biceps m, short head
— Biceps t, long head
— Coracobrachialis m
Deltoid tuberosity — Median n
Deltoid t — Brachial a
Biceps m, long head — Brachial vv
Humerus — Basilic v
Deltoid m — Ulnar n
Deltoid tt — Radial n
Triceps t, lat head — Med brachial cutaneous n
Triceps m, lat head — Teres major t
— Triceps m, med head
— Post humeral circumflex a
— Triceps m, long head
— Triceps t, long head

Superficial v — Cephalic v
Superficial v — Pectoralis major m
Deltoid tt — Biceps m, short head
— Biceps t, long head
— Coracobrachialis m
Deltoid tuberosity — Median n
Deltoid t — Brachial a
Biceps m, long head — Brachial vv
Humerus — Basilic v
Deltoid m — Ulnar n
Deltoid tt — Radial n
Triceps t, lat head — Med brachial cutaneous n
Triceps m, lat head — Teres major t
— Triceps m, med head
— Post humeral circumflex a
— Triceps m, long head
— Triceps t, long head

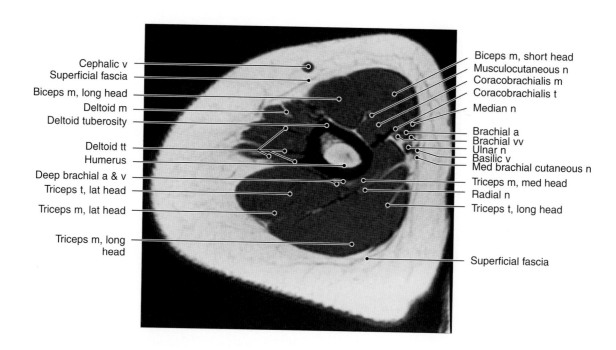

Cephalic v
Superficial fascia
Biceps m, long head
Deltoid m
Deltoid tuberosity
Deltoid tt
Humerus
Deep brachial a & v
Triceps t, lat head
Triceps m, lat head
Triceps m, long head

Biceps m, short head
Musculocutaneous n
Coracobrachialis m
Coracobrachialis t
Median n
Brachial a
Brachial vv
Ulnar n
Basilic v
Med brachial cutaneous n
Triceps m, med head
Radial n
Triceps t, long head
Superficial fascia

Cephalic v
Superficial fascia
Biceps m, long head
Deltoid m
Deltoid tuberosity
Deltoid tt
Humerus
Deep brachial a & v
Triceps t, lat head
Triceps m, lat head
Triceps m, long head

Biceps m, short head
Musculocutaneous n
Coracobrachialis m
Coracobrachialis t
Median n
Brachial a
Brachial vv
Ulnar n
Basilic v
Med brachial cutaneous n
Triceps m, med head
Radial n
Triceps t, long head
Superficial fascia

Upper Arm, Transverse

Cephalic v
Biceps m, long head
Superficial fascia
Musculocutaneous n
Brachialis m
Superficial fascia
Humerus
Lat intermuscular septum
Radial n
Triceps m, lat head
Triceps t, lat head

Biceps m, short head
Brachialis m
Musculocutaneous n
Median n
Brachial a
Brachial vv
Basilic v
Ulnar n
Med intermuscular septum
Med brachial cutaneous n
Brachial fascia
Triceps m, med head
Triceps m, long head

Cephalic v
Biceps m, long head
Superficial fascia
Musculocutaneous n
Brachialis m
Superficial fascia
Humerus
Lat intermuscular septum
Radial n
Triceps m, lat head
Triceps t, lat head

Biceps m, short head
Brachialis m
Musculocutaneous n
Median n
Brachial a
Brachial vv
Basilic v
Ulnar n
Med intermuscular septum
Med brachial cutaneous n
Brachial fascia
Triceps m, med head
Triceps m, long head

Cephalic v
Superficial fascia

Musculocutaneous n

Brachialis m

Humerus
Deep brachial a & v
Radial n
Lat intermuscular septum
Triceps m, lat head
Superficial fascia

Biceps m
Median n
Brachial a
Brachial vv
Brachial fascia
Basilic v
Brachial fascia
Ulnar n
Med brachial cutaneous n
Triceps m, long head

Triceps m, med head
Triceps t

Triceps m, long head

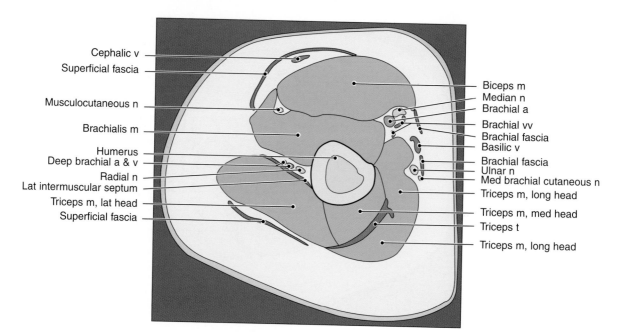

Cephalic v
Superficial fascia

Musculocutaneous n

Brachialis m

Humerus
Deep brachial a & v
Radial n
Lat intermuscular septum
Triceps m, lat head
Superficial fascia

Biceps m
Median n
Brachial a
Brachial vv
Brachial fascia
Basilic v
Brachial fascia
Ulnar n
Med brachial cutaneous n
Triceps m, long head

Triceps m, med head
Triceps t

Triceps m, long head

Upper Arm, Transverse

Cephalic v
Biceps m

Brachialis m
Brachial fascia
Deep brachial a & v
Post antebrachial cutaneous n
Radial n
Brachioradialis m
Lat intermuscular septum
Triceps m, lat head

Biceps t
Brachial fascia
Median n
Brachial a
Brachial v
Brachial v
Basilic v
Brachial fascia
Ulnar n
Med brachial cutaneous n
Humerus
Triceps m, long head
Triceps m, med head
Triceps t

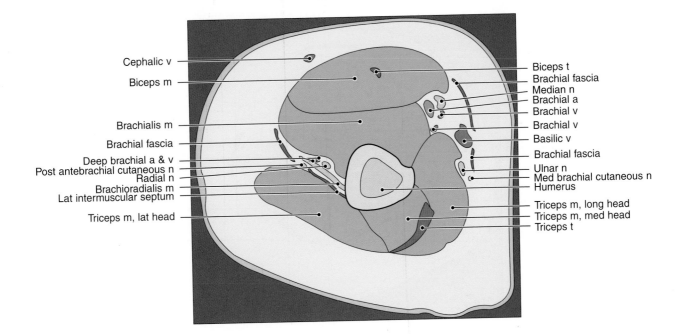

Cephalic v
Biceps m

Brachialis m
Brachial fascia
Deep brachial a & v
Post antebrachial cutaneous n
Radial n
Brachioradialis m
Lat intermuscular septum
Triceps m, lat head

Biceps t
Brachial fascia
Median n
Brachial a
Brachial v
Brachial v
Basilic v
Brachial fascia
Ulnar n
Med brachial cutaneous n
Humerus
Triceps m, long head
Triceps m, med head
Triceps t

Cephalic v
Biceps t
Biceps m

Brachialis m

Radial n
Brachial fascia
Post antebrachial cutaneous n
Brachioradialis m
Humerus

Triceps m, lat head

Biceps t
Brachial v
Median n
Brachial a
Brachial v
Basilic v

Brachial fascia

Ulnar n

Med brachial cutaneous n
Triceps m, long head
Triceps m, med head
Triceps t

Cephalic v
Biceps t
Biceps m

Brachialis m

Radial n
Brachial fascia
Post antebrachial cutaneous n
Brachioradialis m
Humerus

Triceps m, lat head

Biceps t
Brachial v
Median n
Brachial a
Brachial v
Basilic v

Brachial fascia

Ulnar n

Med brachial cutaneous n
Triceps m, long head
Triceps m, med head
Triceps t

Upper Arm, Sagittal

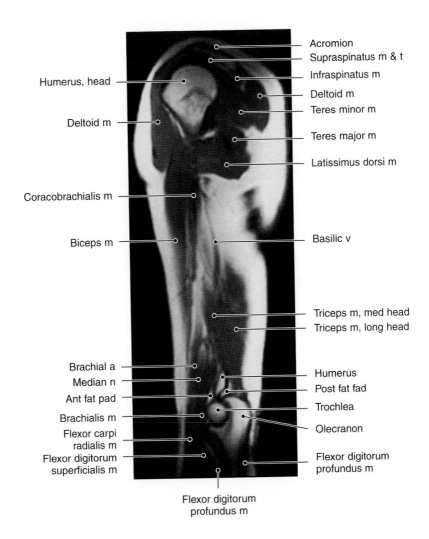

Humerus, head

Deltoid m

Coracobrachialis m

Biceps m

Brachial a
Median n
Ant fat pad
Brachialis m
Flexor carpi radialis m
Flexor digitorum superficialis m

Acromion
Supraspinatus m & t
Infraspinatus m
Deltoid m
Teres minor m
Teres major m
Latissimus dorsi m

Basilic v

Triceps m, med head
Triceps m, long head

Humerus
Post fat fad
Trochlea
Olecranon

Flexor digitorum profundus m

Flexor digitorum profundus m

Humerus, head

Deltoid m

Coracobrachialis m

Biceps m

Brachial a
Median n
Ant fat pad
Brachialis m
Flexor carpi
radialis m
Flexor digitorum
superficialis m

Acromion
Supraspinatus m & t
Infraspinatus m
Deltoid m
Teres minor m

Teres major m

Latissimus dorsi m

Basilic v

Triceps m, med head
Triceps m, long head

Humerus
Post fat fad
Trochlea
Olecranon

Flexor digitorum
profundus m

Flexor digitorum
profundus m

Upper Arm, Sagittal

Humerus, head

Deltoid m

Cephalic v

Humerus, shaft

Biceps m

Brachialis m

Ant fat pad

Capitulum

Radius, head

Median antebrachial v

Supinator m

Pronator teres m

Supraspinatus t

Deltoid m

Infraspinatus m

Teres minor m

Post humeral circumflex a

Teres major m

Latissimus dorsi m

Triceps m, long head

Triceps m, lat head

Post fat pad

Extensor carpi ulnaris m

Supinator m

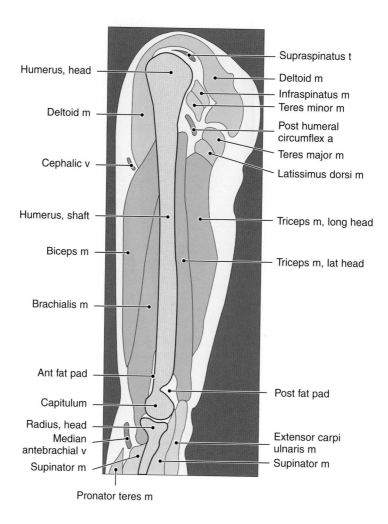

Humerus, head

Deltoid m

Cephalic v

Humerus, shaft

Biceps m

Brachialis m

Ant fat pad

Capitulum

Radius, head

Median
antebrachial v

Supinator m

Pronator teres m

Supraspinatus t

Deltoid m

Infraspinatus m

Teres minor m

Post humeral
circumflex a

Teres major m

Latissimus dorsi m

Triceps m, long head

Triceps m, lat head

Post fat pad

Extensor carpi
ulnaris m

Supinator m

Upper Arm, Sagittal

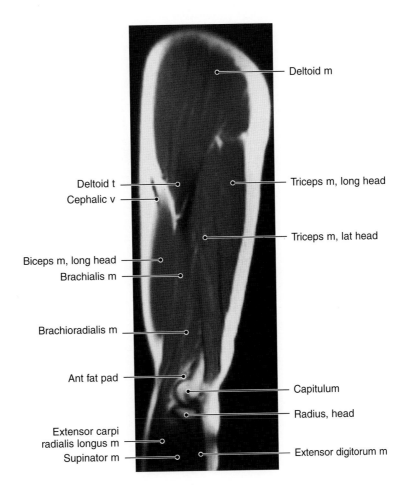

Deltoid m

Deltoid t

Cephalic v

Triceps m, long head

Triceps m, lat head

Biceps m, long head

Brachialis m

Brachioradialis m

Ant fat pad

Capitulum

Radius, head

Extensor carpi
radialis longus m

Supinator m

Extensor digitorum m

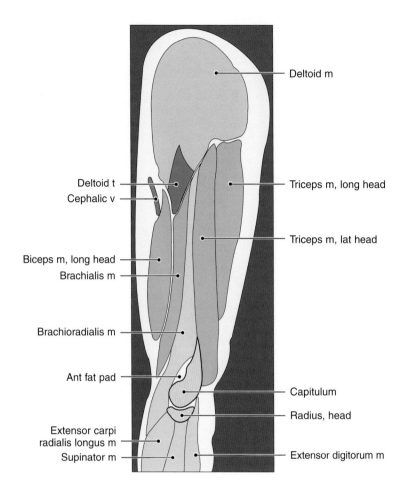

Deltoid m

Deltoid t

Cephalic v

Triceps m, long head

Triceps m, lat head

Biceps m, long head

Brachialis m

Brachioradialis m

Ant fat pad

Capitulum

Radius, head

Extensor carpi
radialis longus m

Supinator m

Extensor digitorum m

Upper Arm, Sagittal

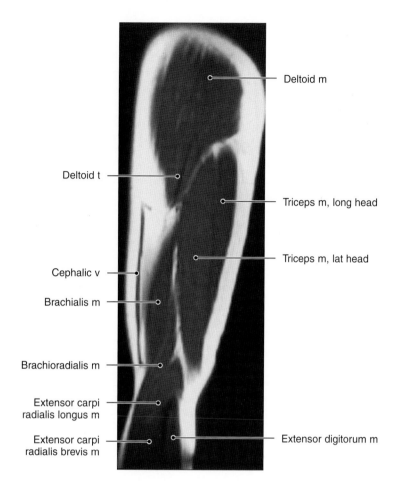

Deltoid m

Deltoid t

Triceps m, long head

Triceps m, lat head

Cephalic v

Brachialis m

Brachioradialis m

Extensor carpi
radialis longus m

Extensor carpi
radialis brevis m

Extensor digitorum m

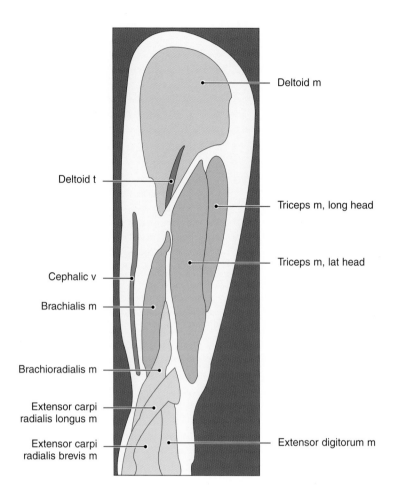

Deltoid m

Deltoid t

Cephalic v

Brachialis m

Brachioradialis m

Extensor carpi radialis longus m

Extensor carpi radialis brevis m

Triceps m, long head

Triceps m, lat head

Extensor digitorum m

3

Elbow

Elbow, Coronal

Triceps m & t

Olecranon

Anconeus m

Extensor carpi
ulnaris m

Ulnar n

Med collateral lig

Flexor carpi
ulnaris m

Ulnar n

Flexor digitorum
profundus m

Triceps m & t

Olecranon

Anconeus m

Ulnar n

Flexor carpi
ulnaris m

Extensor carpi
ulnaris m

Flexor digitorum
profundus m

Elbow, Coronal

Triceps m & t

Ulnar n

Olecranon

Med epicondyle

Common flexor t

Capitulum

Trochlea

Lat collateral &
annular ligs

Med collateral lig

Radius, head

Flexor digitorum
superficialis m

Brachialis t

Supinator &
anconeus mm

Flexor digitorum
profundus m

Extensor carpi
ulnaris m

Ulnar n

Extensor
digitorum m

Flexor carpi
ulnaris m

Triceps m & t

Olecranon

Capitulum

Anconeus m

Extensor carpi
ulnaris m

Supinator m

Extensor
digitorum m

Ulnar n

Med epicondyle

Ulnar n

Trochlea

Med collateral lig

Flexor digitorum
superficialis m

Ulnar n

Flexor digitorum
profundus m

Flexor carpi
ulnaris m

Elbow, Coronal

Triceps m & t

Ulnar n

Post fat pad

Extensor
radialis longus m

Med epicondyle

Olecranon

Common flexor t

Common extensor t

Med collateral lig

Radius, head

Coronoid

Extensor carpi
radialis longus &
brevis mm

Flexor digitorum
superficialis m

Lat collateral &
annular ligs

Brachialis t

Supinator m, deep
portion

Flexor digitorum
profundus m

Extensor
digitorum m

Ulnar n

Supinator m,
superficial portion

Flexor carpi
ulnaris m

Triceps m

Ulnar n

Extensor
radialis longus m

Post fat pad

Med epicondyle

Common flexor t

Olecranon

Lat collateral lig

Med collateral lig

Common extensor t

Coronoid

Annular lig

Radius, head

Flexor digitorum
superficialis m

Brachialis t

Supinator m, deep
portion

Flexor digitorum
profundus m

Extensor
digitorum m

Flexor carpi
ulnaris m

Supinator m,
superficial portion

Ulnar n

Elbow, Coronal

Triceps m

Brachialis m

Extensor carpi
radialis longus m

Olecranon

Common extensor t

Lateral collateral &
annular ligs

Radius, head

Extensor
digitorum m

Supinator m, deep
portion

Radial n, deep
branch

Supinator m,
superficial portion

Med epicondyle

Common flexor t

Med collateral lig

Coronoid

Palmaris longus m

Brachialis t

Pronator teres t,
ulnar head

Flexor digitorum
superficialis m

Flexor digitorum
profundus m

Brachioradialis m

Brachialis m

Olecranon fossa

Lat epicondyle

Extensor carpi
radialis longus m

Common extensor t

Lat collateral &
annular ligs

Radius, head

Supinator m, deep
portion

Extensor
digitorum m

Radial n, deep branch

Supinator m,
superficial portion

Triceps m

Med epicondyle

Common flexor t

Med collateral lig

Coronoid

Brachialis m & t

Palmaris longus m

Flexor digitorum
superficialis m

Flexor digitorum
profundus m

Flexor carpi ulnaris m

Ulnar n

Elbow, Coronal

Brachioradialis m

Brachialis m

Olecranon

Lat epicondyle

Common extensor t

Lat collateral &
annular ligs

Extensor carpi
radialis longus &
brevis mm

Radius, head

Supinator m, deep
portion

Radial n, deep
branch

Supinator m,
superficial portion

Extensor
digitorum m

Triceps m

Pronator m

Med epicondyle

Common flexor t

Med collateral lig

Coronoid

Pronator teres m

Brachialis m & t

Median n

Pronator teres t,
ulnar head

Ulnar a

Palmaris longus m

Flexor digitorum
superficialis m

Triceps m

Brachioradialis m

Brachialis m

Pronator teres m

Olecranon

Extensor carpi
radialis longus m

Med epicondyle

Lat epicondyle

Common flexor t

Common extensor t

Med collateral lig

Lat collateral &
annular ligs

Pronator teres m

Coronoid

Radius, head

Extensor carpi
radialis brevis m

Brachialis m & t

Supinator m, deep
portion

Pronator teres t,
ulnar head

Radial n, deep branch

Palmaris longus m

Supinator m,
superficial portion

Flexor carpi radialis m

Ulnar a

Extensor
digitorum m

Flexor digitorum
superficialis m

Elbow, Coronal

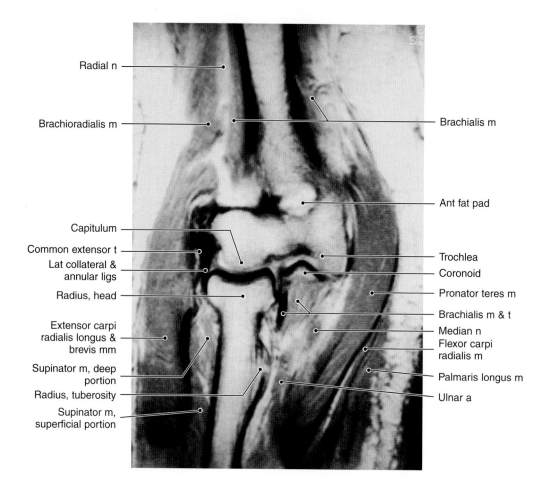

Radial n

Brachioradialis m

Brachialis m

Ant fat pad

Capitulum

Common extensor t

Lat collateral & annular ligs

Radius, head

Trochlea

Coronoid

Pronator teres m

Brachialis m & t

Median n

Extensor carpi radialis longus & brevis mm

Flexor carpi radialis m

Supinator m, deep portion

Radius, tuberosity

Palmaris longus m

Ulnar a

Supinator m, superficial portion

Brachioradialis m

Brachialis m

Olecranon fossa

Lat epicondyle

Extensor carpi
radialis longus m

Common extensor t

Lat collateral &
annular ligs

Radius, head

Supinator m, deep
portion

Extensor
digitorum m

Radial n, deep branch

Supinator m,
superficial portion

Triceps m

Med epicondyle

Common flexor t

Med collateral lig

Coronoid

Brachialis m & t

Palmaris longus m

Flexor digitorum
superficialis m

Flexor digitorum
profundus m

Flexor carpi ulnaris m

Ulnar n

Elbow, Coronal

Radial n

Brachioradialis m

Brachialis m

Ant fat pad

Capitulum

Common extensor t

Lat collateral & annular ligs

Radius, head

Trochlea

Coronoid

Pronator teres m

Brachialis m & t

Median n

Flexor carpi radialis m

Palmaris longus m

Ulnar a

Extensor carpi radialis longus & brevis mm

Supinator m, deep portion

Radius, tuberosity

Supinator m, superficial portion

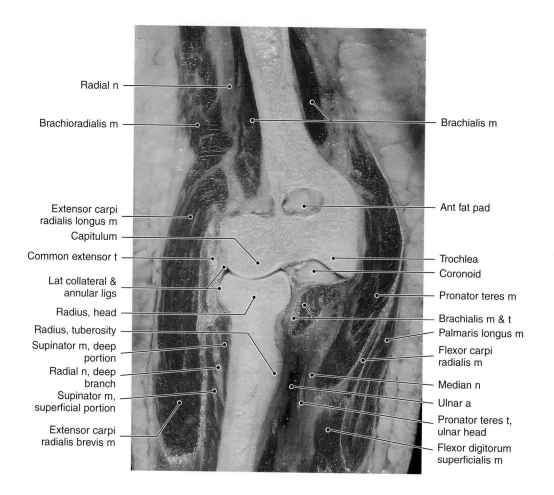

Radial n

Brachioradialis m

Brachialis m

Extensor carpi
radialis longus m

Ant fat pad

Capitulum

Common extensor t

Trochlea

Coronoid

Lat collateral &
annular ligs

Pronator teres m

Radius, head

Brachialis m & t

Radius, tuberosity

Palmaris longus m

Supinator m, deep
portion

Flexor carpi
radialis m

Radial n, deep
branch

Median n

Supinator m,
superficial portion

Ulnar a

Extensor carpi
radialis brevis m

Pronator teres t,
ulnar head

Flexor digitorum
superficialis m

Elbow, Coronal

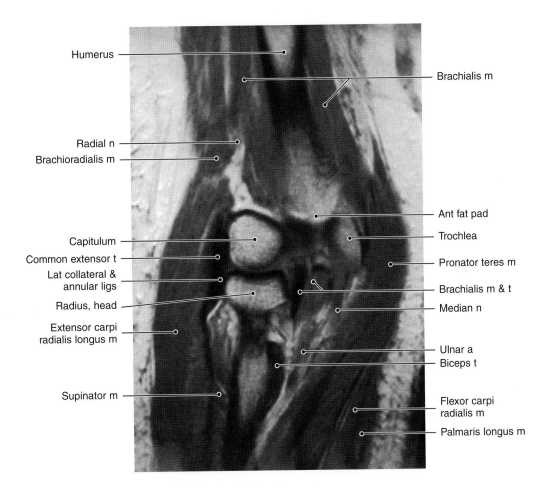

Humerus

Brachialis m

Radial n

Brachioradialis m

Ant fat pad

Capitulum

Trochlea

Common extensor t

Pronator teres m

Lat collateral &
annular ligs

Brachialis m & t

Radius, head

Median n

Extensor carpi
radialis longus m

Ulnar a

Biceps t

Supinator m

Flexor carpi
radialis m

Palmaris longus m

Humerus

Radial n

Brachioradialis m

Capitulum

Common extensor t

Lat collateral &
annular ligs

Radius, head

Extensor carpi
radialis longus m

Radial n, deep
branch

Radius, tuberosity

Supinator m

Brachialis m

Ant fat pad

Trochlea

Pronator teres m

Brachialis m & t

Median n

Ulnar a

Biceps t

Flexor carpi
radialis m

Palmaris longus m

Elbow, Coronal

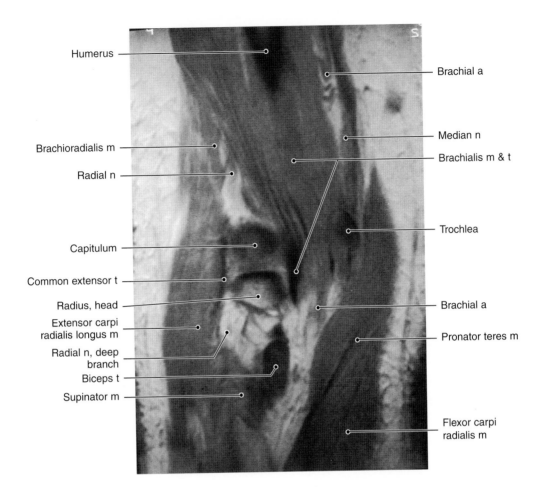

Humerus

Brachioradialis m

Radial n

Capitulum

Common extensor t

Radius, head

Extensor carpi radialis longus m

Radial n, deep branch

Biceps t

Supinator m

Brachial a

Median n

Brachialis m & t

Trochlea

Brachial a

Pronator teres m

Flexor carpi radialis m

Humerus

Radial n

Brachioradialis m

Capitulum

Radius, head

Extensor carpi
radialis longus m

Radial n, deep
branch

Biceps t

Supinator m

Brachial a

Median n

Brachialis m & t

Trochlea

Pronator teres m

Median n

Ulnar a

Flexor carpi
radialis m

Palmaris longus m

Elbow, Coronal

Brachioradialis m

Radial n

Brachialis m & t

Biceps m & t

Extensor carpi
radialis longus m

Median n

Brachial a

Pronator teres m

Brachioradialis m

Radial n

Biceps m & t

Extensor carpi
radialis longus m

Supinator m

Brachialis m

Median n

Pronator teres m

Brachial a

Flexor carpi
radialis m

Elbow, Transverse

Brachial a

Biceps m & t

Median n

Brachialis m

Brachioradialis m

Humerus

Ulnar n

Radial n

Triceps m & t

Extensor carpi radialis longus m

Brachial a

Biceps m & t

Median n

Brachialis m

Ant fat pad

Brachioradialis m

Ulnar n

Radial n

Humerus

Post fat pad

Extensor carpi radialis longus m

Triceps m & t

Brachial a
Brachialis m
Median n
Biceps m & t
Pronator teres m
Med epicondyle
Brachioradialis m
Ulnar n
Radial n
Ant fat pad
Olecranon
Extensor carpi radialis longus m
Post fat pad
Lat epicondyle
Triceps m & t

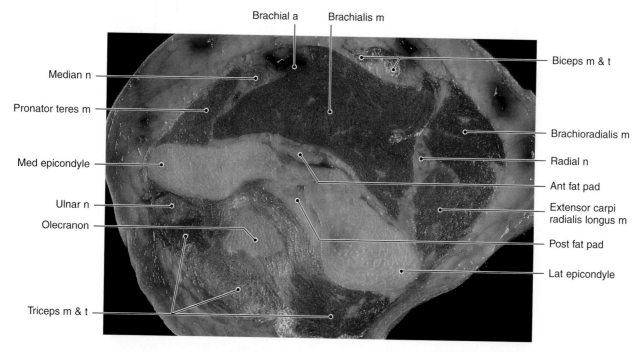

Brachial a
Brachialis m
Median n
Biceps m & t
Pronator teres m
Med epicondyle
Brachioradialis m
Ulnar n
Radial n
Olecranon
Ant fat pad
Extensor carpi radialis longus m
Post fat pad
Lat epicondyle
Triceps m & t

Elbow, Transverse

Brachial a — Brachialis m

Median n

Pronator teres m

Common flexor t

Med epicondyle

Ulnar n

Olecranon

Biceps t

Brachioradialis m

Radial n

Ant fat pad

Extensor carpi radialis longus m

Common extensor t

Lat epicondyle

Anconeus m

Triceps m & t

Brachial a — Brachialis m

Median n

Pronator teres m

Common flexor t

Med epicondyle

Ulnar n

Olecranon

Biceps t

Brachioradialis m

Radial n

Ant fat pad

Extensor carpi radialis longus m

Common extensor t

Lat epicondyle

Anconeus m

Triceps m & t

Brachial a   Brachialis m

Median n
Pronator teres m

Trochlea
Common flexor t

Med epicondyle

Ulnar n

Olecranon

Biceps t

Brachioradialis m
Radial n, superficial
& deep branches

Extensor carpi
radialis longus m
Capitulum

Common extensor t

Lat epicondyle

Anconeus m

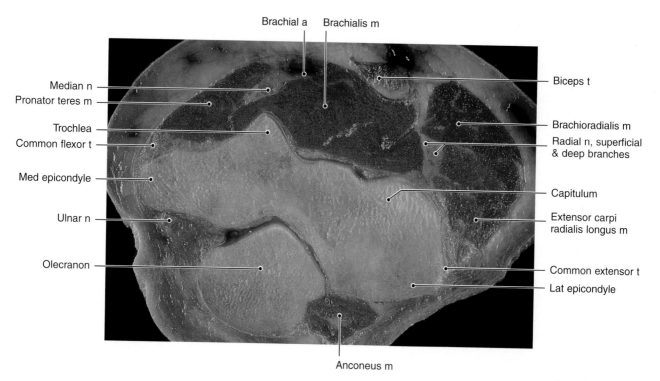

Brachial a   Brachialis m

Median n
Pronator teres m

Trochlea
Common flexor t

Med epicondyle

Ulnar n

Olecranon

Biceps t

Brachioradialis m
Radial n, superficial
& deep branches

Capitulum

Extensor carpi
radialis longus m

Common extensor t
Lat epicondyle

Anconeus m

Elbow, Transverse

Brachial a   Brachialis m

Median n

Pronator teres m

Trochlea

Common flexor t

Ulnar n

Med collateral lig

Flexor carpi ulnaris m

Olecranon

Biceps t

Brachioradialis m

Radial n, superficial & deep branches

Extensor carpi radialis longus m

Capitulum

Extensor digitorum m

Common extensor t

Anconeus m

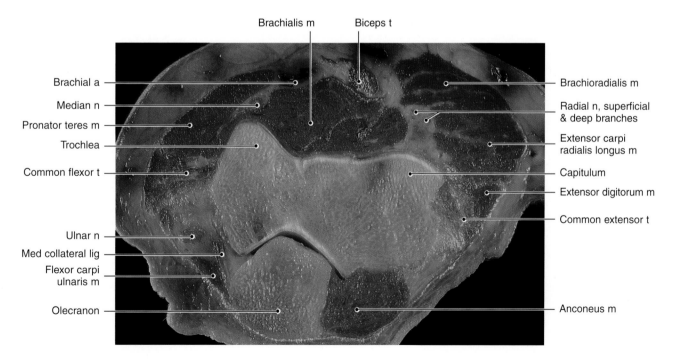

Brachialis m   Biceps t

Brachial a

Median n

Pronator teres m

Trochlea

Common flexor t

Ulnar n

Med collateral lig

Flexor carpi ulnaris m

Olecranon

Brachioradialis m

Radial n, superficial & deep branches

Extensor carpi radialis longus m

Capitulum

Extensor digitorum m

Common extensor t

Anconeus m

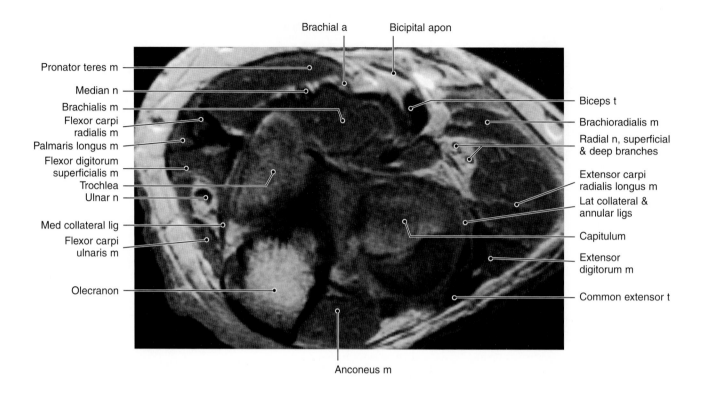

Brachial a — Bicipital apon

Pronator teres m
Median n
Brachialis m
Flexor carpi radialis m
Palmaris longus m
Flexor digitorum superficialis m
Trochlea
Ulnar n
Med collateral lig
Flexor carpi ulnaris m
Olecranon

Biceps t
Brachioradialis m
Radial n, superficial & deep branches
Extensor carpi radialis longus m
Lat collateral & annular ligs
Capitulum
Extensor digitorum m
Common extensor t

Anconeus m

Brachial a — Bicipital apon

Pronator teres m
Median n
Brachialis m
Coronoid
Flexor carpi radialis m
Palmaris longus m
Flexor digitorum superficialis m
Trochlea
Ulnar n
Med collateral lig
Flexor carpi ulnaris m
Flexor digitorum profundus m
Olecranon

Biceps t
Brachioradialis m
Radial n, superficial & deep branches
Extensor carpi radialis longus m
Lat collateral & annular ligs
Capitulum
Extensor digitorum m
Lat collateral lig
Common extensor t

Anconeus m

Elbow, Transverse

Brachialis m & t — Brachial a

Pronator teres m
Median n
Flexor carpi radialis m
Palmaris longus m
Coronoid
Flexor digitorum superficialis m
Trochlea
Ulnar n
Flexor carpi ulnaris m
Flexor digitorum profundus m

Bicipital apon
Biceps t
Brachioradialis m
Radial n, superficial & deep branches
Supinator m
Extensor carpi radialis longus m
Radius, head
Extensor digitorum m
Common extensor t
Annular lig

Olecranon   Anconeus m

Brachialis m & t   Brachial a   Bicipital apon

Pronator teres m
Median n
Ant ulnar recurrent a
Flexor carpi radialis m
Coronoid
Palmaris longus m
Trochlea
Flexor digitorum superficialis m
Ulnar n
Flexor carpi ulnaris m
Flexor digitorum profundus m

Brachioradialis m
Biceps t
Radial n, superficial & deep branches
Extensor carpi radialis longus m
Supinator m
Extensor digitorum m
Radius, head
Common extensor t
Annular lig

Olecranon   Anconeus m

Brachialis m & t — Bicipital apon — Brachial a

Pronator teres m
Median n
Ant ulnar recurrent a
Flexor carpi radialis m
Palmaris longus m
Coronoid
Flexor digitorum superficialis m
Ulnar n
Flexor carpi ulnaris m
Flexor digitorum profundus m
Olecranon

Brachioradialis m
Biceps t
Radial n, superficial branch
Radial n, deep branch
Supinator m
Extensor carpi radialis longus m
Radius, head
Extensor digitorum m
Common extensor t
Extensor carpi ulnaris m

Anconeus m

Brachialis m & t — Bicipital apon — Brachial a

Pronator teres m
Median n
Ant ulnar recurrent a
Flexor carpi radialis m
Palmaris longus m
Coronoid
Flexor digitorum superficialis m
Ulnar n
Flexor carpi ulnaris m
Flexor digitorum profundus m
Olecranon

Brachioradialis m
Biceps t
Radial n, superficial branch
Radial n, deep branch
Supinator m
Extensor carpi radialis longus m
Radius, head
Extensor digitorum m
Common extensor t
Extensor carpi ulnaris m

Anconeus m — Annular lig

Elbow, Transverse

Median n
Brachial a

Pronator teres m
Ant ulnar recurrent a
Flexor carpi radialis m
Palmaris longus m
Brachialis m & t
Flexor digitorum superficialis m
Ulnar n
Flexor carpi ulnaris m
Ulna
Flexor digitorum profundus m

Bicipital apon
Biceps t
Brachioradialis m
Radial n, superficial branch
Radial n, deep branch
Extensor carpi radialis longus m
Supinator m
Radius, head
Extensor digitorum m
Extensor carpi ulnaris m

Anconeus m
Annular lig

Median n
Brachial a

Pronator teres m
Flexor carpi radialis m
Palmaris longus m
Ant ulnar recurrent a
Flexor digitorum superficialis m
Brachialis m & t
Ulnar n
Flexor carpi ulnaris m
Flexor digitorum profundus m
Ulna
Anconeus m

Bicipital apon
Brachioradialis m
Biceps t
Radial n, superficial branch
Radial n, deep branch
Extensor carpi radialis longus m
Supinator m
Radius, head
Extensor digitorum m
Extensor carpi ulnaris m

Annular lig

Ulnar a

Pronator teres m

Flexor carpi
radialis m

Median n

Palmaris longus m

Ant ulnar
recurrent a

Flexor digitorum
superficialis m

Brachialis m & t

Ulnar n

Flexor carpi
ulnaris m

Flexor digitorum
profundus m

Ulna

Radial a

Brachioradialis m

Radial n, superficial
branch

Biceps t

Radial n, deep
branch

Extensor carpi
radialis longus m

Supinator m

Extensor
digitorum m

Extensor carpi
ulnaris m

Anconeus m

Radius

Pronator teres m, ulnar head

Ulnar a

Flexor carpi
radialis m

Palmaris longus m

Pronator teres m

Median n

Flexor digitorum
superficialis m

Ant ulnar
recurrent a

Ulnar n

Flexor carpi
ulnaris m

Brachialis m & t

Flexor digitorum
profundus m

Ulna

Anconeus m

Radial a

Brachioradialis m

Radial n, superficial
branch

Biceps t

Radial n, deep
branch

Extensor carpi
radialis longus m

Supinator m

Extensor
digitorum m

Extensor carpi
ulnaris m

Radius

Elbow, Transverse

Pronator teres m, ulnar head — Ulnar a — Radial a

Pronator teres m

Flexor carpi radialis m

Palmaris longus m — Brachioradialis m

Median n — Radial n, superficial branch

Ant ulnar recurrent a — Biceps t

Flexor digitorum superficialis m — Supinator m, superficial portion

Brachialis m & t — Extensor carpi radialis longus m

Ulnar n — Radial n, deep branch

Flexor carpi ulnaris m — Extensor carpi radialis brevis m

Flexor digitorum profundus m — Supinator m, deep portion

Ulna — Extensor digitorum m

Radius

Anconeus m — Extensor carpi ulnaris m

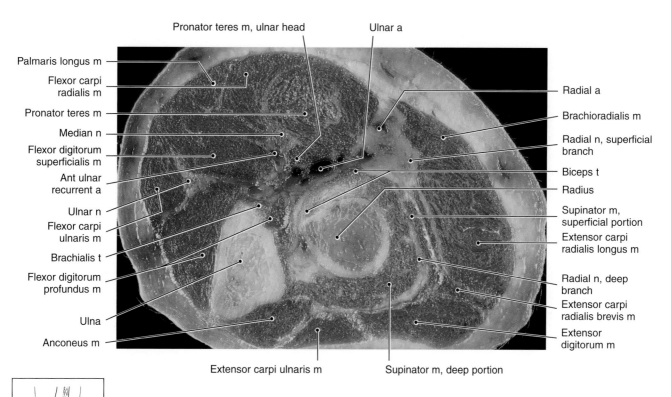

Pronator teres m, ulnar head — Ulnar a

Palmaris longus m — Radial a

Flexor carpi radialis m — Brachioradialis m

Pronator teres m — Radial n, superficial branch

Median n — Biceps t

Flexor digitorum superficialis m — Radius

Ant ulnar recurrent a — Supinator m, superficial portion

Ulnar n — Extensor carpi radialis longus m

Flexor carpi ulnaris m

Brachialis t — Radial n, deep branch

Flexor digitorum profundus m — Extensor carpi radialis brevis m

Ulna — Extensor digitorum m

Anconeus m

Extensor carpi ulnaris m — Supinator m, deep portion

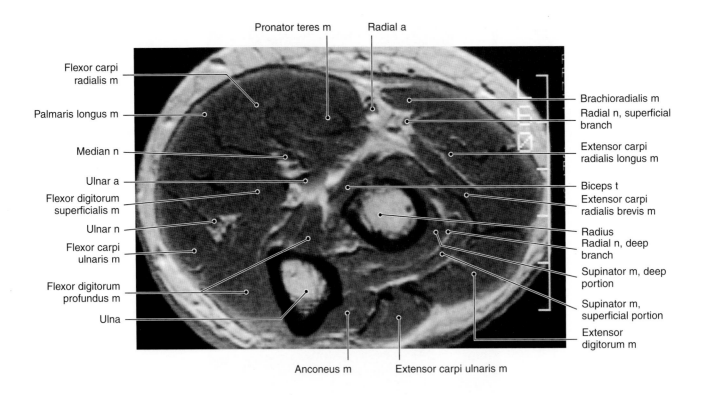

Pronator teres m Radial a

Flexor carpi radialis m

Palmaris longus m

Median n

Ulnar a

Flexor digitorum superficialis m

Ulnar n

Flexor carpi ulnaris m

Flexor digitorum profundus m

Ulna

Brachioradialis m

Radial n, superficial branch

Extensor carpi radialis longus m

Biceps t

Extensor carpi radialis brevis m

Radius

Radial n, deep branch

Supinator m, deep portion

Supinator m, superficial portion

Extensor digitorum m

Anconeus m Extensor carpi ulnaris m

Pronator teres m Radial a

Flexor carpi radialis m

Palmaris longus m

Median n

Ulnar a

Flexor digitorum superficialis m

Ulnar n

Flexor carpi ulnaris m

Flexor digitorum profundus m

Ulna

Brachioradialis m

Radial n, superficial branch

Extensor carpi radialis longus m

Biceps t

Extensor carpi radialis brevis m

Radius

Supinator m, deep portion

Radial n, deep branch

Supinator m, superficial portion

Extensor digitorum m

Anconeus m Extensor carpi ulnaris m

Elbow, Sagittal

Biceps m

Brachial a

Brachialis m

Median n

Bicipital apon

Pronator teres m

Triceps m

Med epicondyle

Ulnar n

Flexor carpi
ulnaris m

Flexor digitorum
superficialis m

Palmaris longus m

Biceps m

Brachialis m

Brachial a

Median n

Bicipital apon

Pronator teres m

Flexor carpi
radialis m

Triceps m

Med epicondyle

Ulnar n

Flexor carpi
ulnaris m

Flexor digitorum
superficialis m

Palmaris longus m

Elbow, Sagittal

Biceps m

Brachialis m

Bicipital apon

Brachial a

Median n

Pronator teres m

Brachioradialis m

Triceps m & t

Olecranon

Trochlea

Coronoid

Flexor digitorum profundus m

Flexor digitorum superficialis m

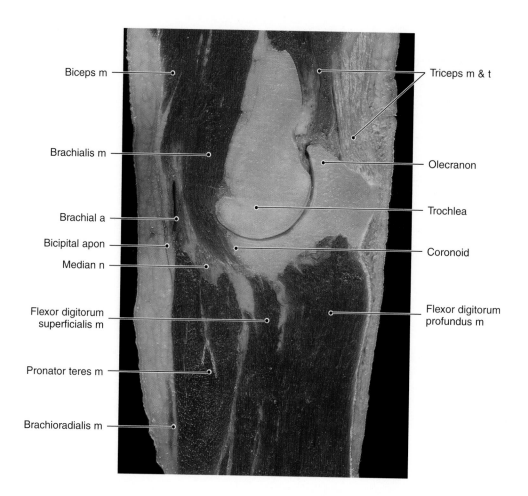

Biceps m

Brachialis m

Brachial a

Bicipital apon

Median n

Flexor digitorum superficialis m

Pronator teres m

Brachioradialis m

Triceps m & t

Olecranon

Trochlea

Coronoid

Flexor digitorum profundus m

Elbow, Sagittal

Biceps m

Ant fat pad

Brachialis m

Trochlea

Bicipital apon

Coronoid

Pronator teres m

Brachioradialis m

Triceps m & t

Post fat pad

Olecranon

Flexor digitorum profundus m

Median n

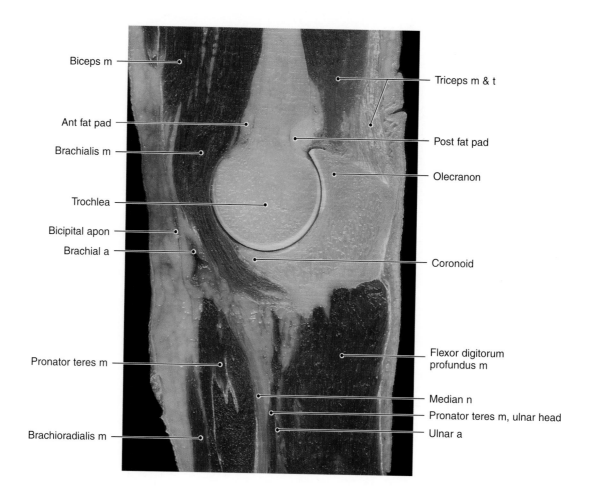

Biceps m

Ant fat pad

Brachialis m

Trochlea

Bicipital apon

Brachial a

Pronator teres m

Brachioradialis m

Triceps m & t

Post fat pad

Olecranon

Coronoid

Flexor digitorum profundus m

Median n

Pronator teres m, ulnar head

Ulnar a

Elbow, Sagittal

Biceps m & t

Ant fat pad

Trochlea

Brachialis m

Coronoid

Brachioradialis m

Pronator teres m

Post fat pad

Triceps m & t

Olecranon

Ulnar a

Flexor digitorum profundus m

Biceps m & t

Ant fat pad

Trochlea

Brachialis m

Coronoid

Brachial a

Brachioradialis m

Ulnar a

Pronator teres m

Post fat pad

Triceps m & t

Olecranon

Flexor digitorum
profundus m

Elbow, Sagittal

Biceps m

Brachialis m

Ant fat pad

Trochlea

Coronoid

Biceps t

Brachialis t

Brachioradialis m

Radial a

Ulnar a

Pronator teres m

Post fat pad

Triceps m & t

Olecranon

Flexor digitorum profundus m

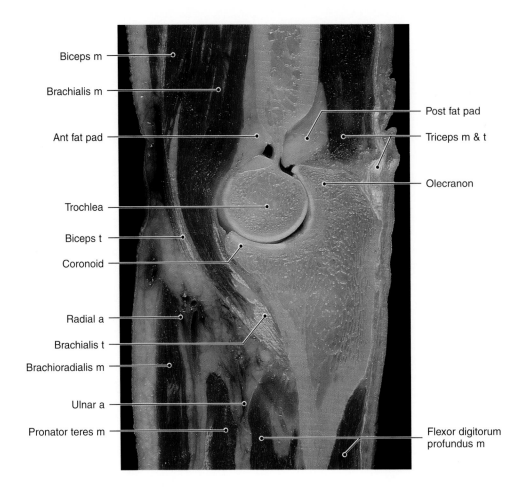

Biceps m

Brachialis m

Ant fat pad

Post fat pad

Triceps m & t

Olecranon

Trochlea

Biceps t

Coronoid

Radial a

Brachialis t

Brachioradialis m

Ulnar a

Pronator teres m

Flexor digitorum profundus m

Elbow, Sagittal

Biceps m

Ant fat pad

Brachialis m & t

Biceps t

Brachioradialis m

Supinator m

Radial a

Pronator teres m

Triceps m & t

Post fat pad

Olecranon

Trochlea

Coronoid

Anconeus m

Flexor digitorum
profundus m

Biceps m

Ant fat pad

Brachialis m & t

Biceps t

Brachioradialis m

Radial a

Pronator teres m

Triceps m & t

Post fat pad

Olecranon

Trochlea

Coronoid

Anconeus m

Flexor digitorum
profundus m

Elbow, Sagittal

Biceps m & t

Brachialis m & t

Trochlea

Brachioradialis m

Radial recurrent a

Supinator m

Triceps m & t

Post fat pad

Olecranon

Radial notch

Anconeus m

Biceps t

Radius, tuberosity

Ulna

Flexor digitorum profundus m

Biceps m & t

Brachialis m & t

Brachioradialis m

Radial recurrent a

Supinator m

Radius, tuberosity

Pronator teres m

Triceps m & t

Post fat pad

Trochlea

Radial notch

Anconeus m

Biceps t

Ulna

Flexor digitorum
profundus m

Elbow, Sagittal

Biceps m

Brachialis m

Brachioradialis m

Radial recurrent a

Supinator m

Radial n, superficial branch

Triceps m

Capitulum

Radius, head

Anconeus m

Biceps t

Radius, tuberosity

Supinator m

Ulna

Flexor digitorum profundus m

Biceps m

Brachialis m

Annular lig

Brachioradialis m

Radial recurrent a

Supinator m

Radial n, superficial branch

Triceps m

Capitulum

Radius, head

Anconeus m

Biceps t

Radius, tuberosity

Ulna

Supinator m

Flexor digitorum profundus m

Elbow, Sagittal

Biceps m

Radial n

Brachialis m

Brachioradialis m

Radial recurrent a

Supinator m

Extensor carpi radialis longus & brevis mm

Triceps m

Capitulum

Radius, head

Anconeus m

Radius, tuberosity

Supinator m

Biceps m

Radial n

Brachialis m

Brachioradialis m

Annular lig

Radial n &
radial recurrent a

Extensor carpi radialis
longus & brevis mm

Supinator m

Triceps m

Capitulum

Radius, head

Annular lig

Anconeus m

Radius, tuberosity

Supinator m

Extensor carpi
ulnaris m

Elbow, Sagittal

Extensor carpi radialis longus m

Brachioradialis m

Annular lig

Radius, head

Radial n, deep branch

Extensor carpi radialis longus & brevis mm

Supinator m, superficial portion

Brachioradialis m

Triceps m

Capitulum

Annular lig

Common extensor t

Supinator m, deep portion

Extensor carpi ulnaris m

Triceps m

Extensor carpi
radialis longus m

Brachioradialis m

Capitulum

Annular lig

Lat collateral lig

Radius, head

Common extensor t

Annular lig

Radial n, deep
branch

Supinator m,
deep portion

Supinator m,
superficial portion

Brachioradialis m

Extensor carpi
radialis longus &
brevis mm

Extensor carpi
ulnaris m

Elbow, Sagittal

Extensor carpi radialis longus m

Brachioradialis m

Lat epicondyle

Common extensor t

Annular lig

Radius, head

Radial n, deep branch

Supinator m, deep portion

Supinator m, superficial portion

Extensor digitorum m

Extensor carpi radialis longus & brevis mm

Extensor carpi ulnaris m

Extensor carpi radialis longus m

Brachioradialis m

Lat epicondyle

Radius, head

Radial n, deep branch

Supinator m, superficial portion

Extensor carpi radialis longus & brevis mm

Common extensor t

Lat collateral lig

Annular lig

Supinator m, deep portion

Extensor carpi ulnaris m

Extensor digitorum m

Elbow, Sagittal

Brachioradialis m

Extensor carpi
radialis longus &
brevis mm

Lat epicondyle
Common extensor t

Radius, head

Extensor
digitorum m

Extensor carpi
ulnaris m

Brachioradialis m

Common extensor t

Radius, head

Annular lig

Extensor carpi
radialis longus &
brevis mm

Extensor
digitorum m

Extensor carpi
ulnaris m

4

Forearm

Forearm, Coronal

Anconeus m

Superficial v

Ulna

Flexor digitorum profundus m

Superficial v

Extensor carpi ulnaris m

Flexor carpi ulnaris m

Extensor digiti minimi m

Flexor digitorum profundus t

Flexor carpi ulnaris t

Extensor digiti minimi t

Extensor carpi ulnaris t

Superficial v

Superficial v

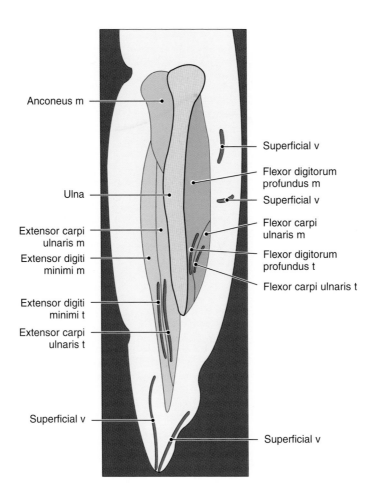

Anconeus m

Superficial v

Flexor digitorum
profundus m

Ulna

Superficial v

Extensor carpi
ulnaris m

Flexor carpi
ulnaris m

Extensor digiti
minimi m

Flexor digitorum
profundus t

Flexor carpi ulnaris t

Extensor digiti
minimi t

Extensor carpi
ulnaris t

Superficial v

Superficial v

Forearm, Coronal

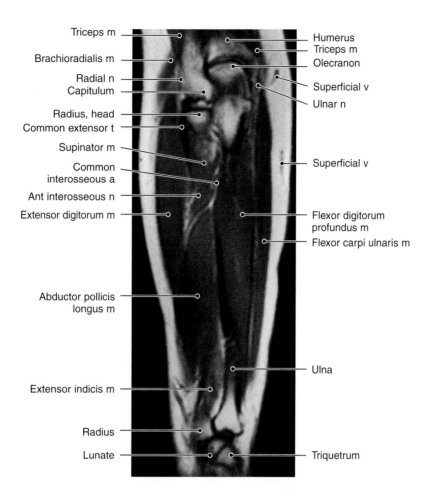

Triceps m

Brachioradialis m

Radial n

Capitulum

Radius, head

Common extensor t

Supinator m

Common interosseous a

Ant interosseous n

Extensor digitorum m

Abductor pollicis longus m

Extensor indicis m

Radius

Lunate

Humerus

Triceps m

Olecranon

Superficial v

Ulnar n

Superficial v

Flexor digitorum profundus m

Flexor carpi ulnaris m

Ulna

Triquetrum

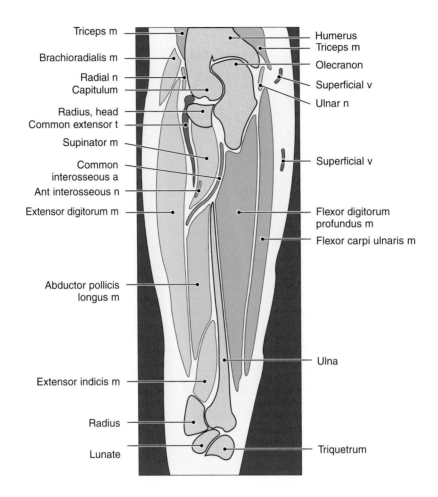

Triceps m

Brachioradialis m

Radial n

Capitulum

Radius, head

Common extensor t

Supinator m

Common
interosseous a

Ant interosseous n

Extensor digitorum m

Abductor pollicis
longus m

Extensor indicis m

Radius

Lunate

Humerus

Triceps m

Olecranon

Superficial v

Ulnar n

Superficial v

Flexor digitorum
profundus m

Flexor carpi ulnaris m

Ulna

Triquetrum

Forearm, Coronal

Basilic v

Capitulum

Extensor carpi
radialis longus m

Radius, head
Brachioradials m
Biceps t

Supinator m

Brachioradialis t

Extensor carpi
radialis brevis m

Extensor carpi
radialis brevis t

Abductor pollicis
longus t

Scaphoid
Extensor carpi
radialis longus t

Trapezoid

Common flexor t
Olecranon fossa
Trochlea
Basilic v
Ulna, coronoid process

Brachialis m

Flexor carpi
radialis m

Flexor pollicis
longus m

Flexor carpi
ulnaris m

Flexor digitorum
superficialis m

Flexor digitorum
superficialis t

Basilic v

Flexor carpi ulnaris t

Lunate
Triquetrum
Capitate
Pisiform

Basilic v

Capitulum

Extensor carpi
radialis longus m

Radius, head
Brachioradialis m
Biceps t

Supinator m

Brachioradialis t

Extensor carpi
radialis brevis m

Extensor carpi
radialis brevis t

Abductor pollicis
longus t

Scaphoid
Extensor carpi
radialis longus t

Trapezoid

Common flexor t
Olecranon fossa
Trochlea
Basilic v
Ulna, coronoid process

Brachialis m

Flexor carpi
radialis m

Flexor pollicis
longus m

Flexor carpi
ulnaris m

Flexor digitorum
superficialis m

Flexor digitorum
superficialis t

Basilic v

Flexor carpi ulnaris t

Lunate
Triquetrum
Capitate
Pisiform

Forearm, Coronal

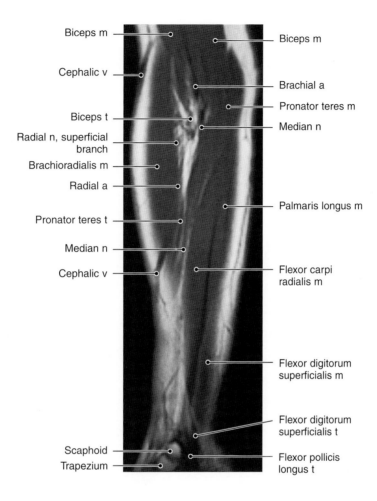

Biceps m

Cephalic v

Biceps t

Radial n, superficial branch

Brachioradialis m

Radial a

Pronator teres t

Median n

Cephalic v

Scaphoid

Trapezium

Biceps m

Brachial a

Pronator teres m

Median n

Palmaris longus m

Flexor carpi radialis m

Flexor digitorum superficialis m

Flexor digitorum superficialis t

Flexor pollicis longus t

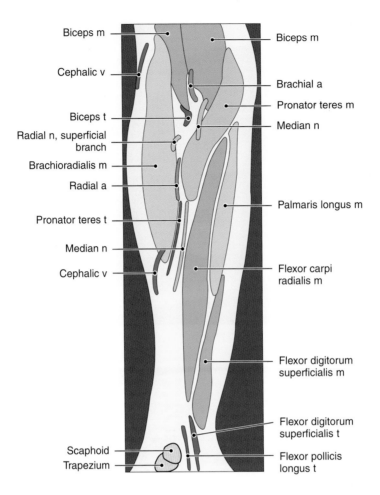

Biceps m

Cephalic v

Biceps t

Radial n, superficial branch

Brachioradialis m

Radial a

Pronator teres t

Median n

Cephalic v

Scaphoid
Trapezium

Biceps m

Brachial a

Pronator teres m

Median n

Palmaris longus m

Flexor carpi radialis m

Flexor digitorum superficialis m

Flexor digitorum superficialis t

Flexor pollicis longus t

Forearm, Transverse

Cephalic v
Brachioradialis m
Radial n, superficial branch
Extensor carpi radialis longus m
Supinator m
Extensor carpi radialis brevis m
Biceps t
Radius
Extensor digitorum m
Extensor carpi ulnaris m
Anconeus m
Ulna

Median cubital v
Radial a
Radial vv
Pronator teres m
Flexor carpi radialis m
Ulnar v
Ulnar a
Ulnar v
Median a
Median n
Palmaris longus m
Flexor digitorum superficialis m
Ulnar n
Flexor carpi ulnaris m
Flexor digitorum profundus m
Basilic v

Cephalic v
Brachioradialis m
Radial n, superficial branch
Extensor carpi radialis longus m
Supinator m
Extensor carpi radialis brevis m
Biceps t
Radius
Extensor digitorum m
Extensor carpi ulnaris m
Anconeus m
Ulna

Median cubital v
Radial a
Radial vv
Pronator teres m
Flexor carpi radialis m
Ulnar v
Ulnar a
Ulnar v
Median a
Median n
Palmaris longus m
Flexor digitorum superficialis m
Ulnar n
Flexor carpi ulnaris m
Flexor digitorum profundus m
Basilic v

Cephalic v
Brachioradialis m
Radial n, superficial branch
Extensor carpi radialis longus t
Extensor carpi radialis longus m
Supinator m
Extensor carpi radialis brevis m
Radius
Extensor digitorum t
Extensor digitorum m
Radial n, deep branch
Extensor pollicis longus t
Extensor digiti minimi m
Extensor carpi ulnaris t
Ulna
Extensor carpi ulnaris m

Median cubital v
Radial a & vv
Flexor carpi radialis t
Flexor carpi radialis m
Pronator teres m & t
Palmaris longus m
Palmaris longus t
Median n
Ulnar a & v
Ant interosseous a, v & n
Flexor digitorum superficialis m
Ulnar n
Flexor digitorum profundus t
Flexor carpi ulnaris t
Flexor digitorum profundus m
Flexor carpi ulnaris m
Basilic v

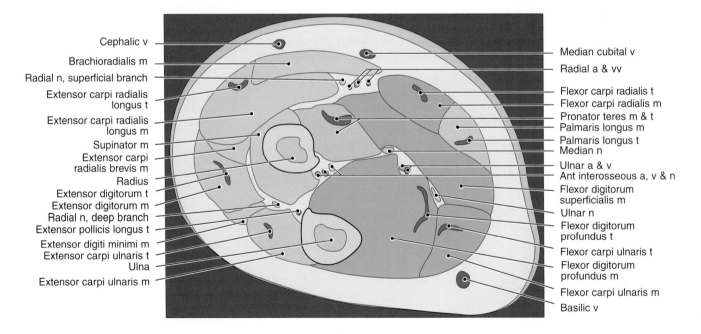

Cephalic v
Brachioradialis m
Radial n, superficial branch
Extensor carpi radialis longus t
Extensor carpi radialis longus m
Supinator m
Extensor carpi radialis brevis m
Radius
Extensor digitorum t
Extensor digitorum m
Radial n, deep branch
Extensor pollicis longus t
Extensor digiti minimi m
Extensor carpi ulnaris t
Ulna
Extensor carpi ulnaris m

Median cubital v
Radial a & vv
Flexor carpi radialis t
Flexor carpi radialis m
Pronator teres m & t
Palmaris longus m
Palmaris longus t
Median n
Ulnar a & v
Ant interosseous a, v & n
Flexor digitorum superficialis m
Ulnar n
Flexor digitorum profundus t
Flexor carpi ulnaris t
Flexor digitorum profundus m
Flexor carpi ulnaris m
Basilic v

Forearm, Transverse

Cephalic v
Brachioradialis m
Extensor carpi radialis longus t
Pronator teres m
Extensor carpi radialis longus m
Radius
Extensor carpi radialis brevis m
Interosseous membrane
Supinator m
Radial n, muscular branch of deep branch
Extensor digitorum t
Extensor digitorum m
Abductor pollicis longus m
Post interosseous a & n
Extensor digiti minimi m & t
Extensor pollicis longus m
Extensor carpi ulnaris t

Median cubital v
Radial a & vv
Radial n, superficial branch
Flexor carpi radialis t
Flexor carpi radialis m
Palmaris longus m
Palmaris longus t
Flexor digitorum superficialis t
Ant interosseous a & n
Flexor digitorum superficialis m
Flexor digitorum superficialis t
Ulnar a & v
Ulnar n
Median n
Flexor carpi ulnaris t
Flexor digitorum profundus m & tt
Ulna
Flexor carpi ulnaris m
Basilic v

Extensor carpi ulnaris m

Cephalic v
Brachioradialis m
Extensor carpi radialis longus t
Pronator teres m
Extensor carpi radialis longus m
Radius
Extensor carpi radialis brevis m
Interosseous membrane
Supinator m
Radial n, muscular branch of deep branch
Extensor digitorum t
Extensor digitorum m
Abductor pollicis longus m
Post interosseous a & n
Extensor digiti minimi m & t
Extensor pollicis longus m
Extensor carpi ulnaris t

Median cubital v
Radial a & vv
Radial n, superficial branch
Flexor carpi radialis t
Flexor carpi radialis m
Palmaris longus m
Palmaris longus t
Flexor digitorum superficialis t
Ant interosseous a & n
Flexor digitorum superficialis m
Flexor digitorum superficialis t
Ulnar a & v
Ulnar n
Median n
Flexor carpi ulnaris t
Flexor digitorum profundus m & tt
Flexor carpi ulnaris m
Ulna
Basilic v

Extensor carpi ulnaris m

Cephalic v
Brachioradialis t
Extensor carpi radialis longus t

Extensor carpi radialis longus m
Flexor pollicis longus m

Radius
Extensor carpi radialis brevis m
Abductor pollicis longus m & t

Interosseous membrane

Extensor digitorum m & t

Extensor pollicis longus m & t

Post interosseous n
Extensor digiti minimi m & t

Extensor carpi ulnaris m & t

Median cubital v
Median antebrachial v

Radial n, superficial branch
Radial a & vv

Flexor carpi radialis m & t

Superficial fascia
Palmaris longus m & t

Flexor digitorum superficialis m & tt

Median n
Ant interosseous a & n

Ulnar a & vv
Ulnar n
Flexor carpi ulnaris t

Flexor digitorum profundus m & tt

Flexor carpi ulnaris m

Ulna
Basilic v

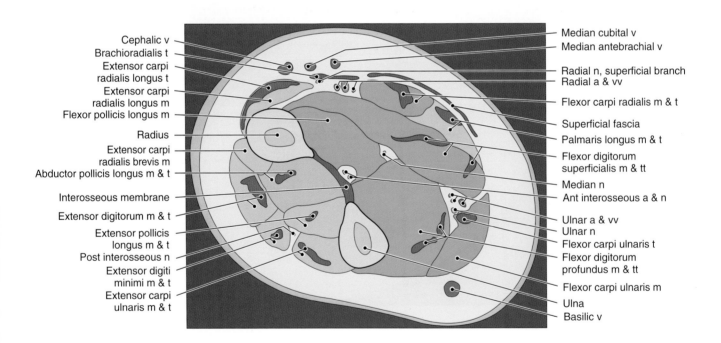

Cephalic v
Brachioradialis t
Extensor carpi radialis longus t

Extensor carpi radialis longus m
Flexor pollicis longus m

Radius
Extensor carpi radialis brevis m
Abductor pollicis longus m & t

Interosseous membrane

Extensor digitorum m & t

Extensor pollicis longus m & t

Post interosseous n
Extensor digiti minimi m & t

Extensor carpi ulnaris m & t

Median cubital v
Median antebrachial v

Radial n, superficial branch
Radial a & vv

Flexor carpi radialis m & t

Superficial fascia
Palmaris longus m & t

Flexor digitorum superficialis m & tt

Median n
Ant interosseous a & n

Ulnar a & vv
Ulnar n
Flexor carpi ulnaris t
Flexor digitorum profundus m & tt

Flexor carpi ulnaris m

Ulna
Basilic v

Forearm, Transverse

Radial n, superficial branch
Brachioradialis t
Abductor pollicis longus t
Cephalic v
Extensor carpi radialis longus t
Flexor pollicis longus m & t
Extensor carpi radialis brevis t
Radius

Abductor pollicis longus m
Interosseous membrane
Extensor digitorum t
Extensor pollicis longus m & t
Extensor indicis m & t
Extensor digiti minimi m & t
Extensor carpi ulnaris m & t

Median antebrachial v
Flexor carpi radialis t
Radial a & vv
Palmaris longus t
Flexor digitorum superficialis m & t
Median n
Flexor digitorum profundus t
Flexor digitorum profundus m & t
Ant interosseous a & n
Ulnar a
Ulnar n
Flexor carpi ulnaris t
Ulnar n, dorsal branch
Flexor carpi ulnaris m
Ulna
Basilic v

Radial n, superficial branch
Brachioradialis t
Abductor pollicis longus t
Cephalic v
Extensor carpi radialis longus t
Flexor pollicis longus m & t
Extensor carpi radialis brevis t
Radius

Abductor pollicis longus m
Interosseous membrane
Extensor digitorum t
Extensor pollicis longus m & t
Extensor indicis m & t
Extensor digiti minimi m & t
Extensor carpi ulnaris m & t

Median antebrachial v
Flexor carpi radialis t
Radial a & vv
Palmaris longus t
Flexor digitorum superficialis m & t
Median n
Flexor digitorum profundus t
Flexor digitorum profundus m & t
Ant interosseous a & n
Ulnar a
Ulnar n
Flexor carpi ulnaris t
Ulnar n, dorsal branch
Flexor carpi ulnaris m
Ulna
Basilic v

Median antebrachial v
Radial n, superficial branch
Abductor pollicis longus t
Brachioradialis t
Extensor pollicis longus t

Extensor carpi
radialis longus t
Radius
Extensor carpi
radialis brevis t

Cephalic v
Extensor pollicis
longus m & t
Extensor digitorum t
Extensor indicis m & t
Extensor digiti minimi t

Extensor carpi ulnaris t

Flexor carpi radialis t
Radial a & vv
Palmaris longus t
Median n
Flexor pollicis longus t
Flexor digitorum
superficialis t
Flexor digitorum profundus t
Pronator quadratus m
Ulnar a
Flexor carpi ulnaris t
Ulnar n
Flexor carpi ulnaris m
Dorsal interosseous n
Interosseous membrane

Ulnar n, dorsal branch
Ulna
Antebrachial fascia

Basilic v

Median antebrachial v
Radial n, superficial branch
Abductor pollicis longus t
Brachioradialis t

Extensor pollicis longus t

Extensor carpi
radialis longus t
Radius
Extensor carpi
radialis brevis t

Cephalic v
Extensor pollicis
longus m & t
Extensor digitorum t
Extensor indicis m & t
Extensor digiti minimi t

Extensor carpi ulnaris t

Flexor carpi radialis t
Radial a & vv
Palmaris longus t
Median n
Flexor pollicis longus t
Flexor digitorum
superficialis t
Flexor digitorum profundus t
Pronator quadratus m
Ulnar a
Flexor carpi ulnaris t
Ulnar n
Flexor carpi ulnaris m
Dorsal interosseous n
Interosseous membrane

Ulnar n, dorsal branch
Ulna
Antebrachial fascia

Basilic v

Forearm, Sagittal

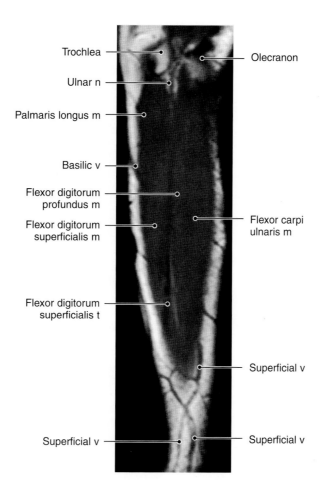

Trochlea

Ulnar n

Palmaris longus m

Basilic v

Flexor digitorum profundus m

Flexor digitorum superficialis m

Flexor digitorum superficialis t

Superficial v

Olecranon

Flexor carpi ulnaris m

Superficial v

Superficial v

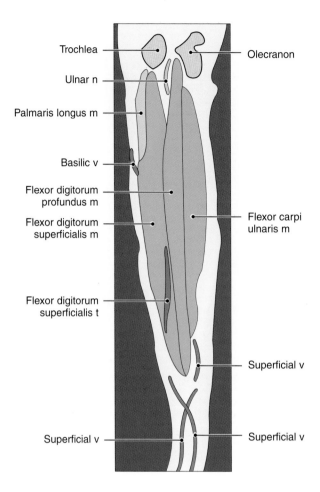

Trochlea

Ulnar n

Palmaris longus m

Basilic v

Flexor digitorum
profundus m

Flexor digitorum
superficialis m

Flexor digitorum
superficialis t

Superficial v

Olecranon

Flexor carpi
ulnaris m

Superficial v

Superficial v

Forearm, Sagittal

Brachialis m
Trochlea
Pronator teres m
Flexor carpi radialis m
Brachialis m
Palmaris longus m
Ulnar n
Flexor digitorum superficialis m
Flexor digitorum profundus m
Flexor digitorum profundus t
Pronator quadratus m
Flexor digitorum superficialis t
Flexor digitorum profundus t

Post fat pad
Triceps m
Olecranon
Trochlear notch
Anconeus m
Coronoid
Flexor digitorum profundus m
Ulna
Extensor digiti minimi t
Triquetrum
Hamate

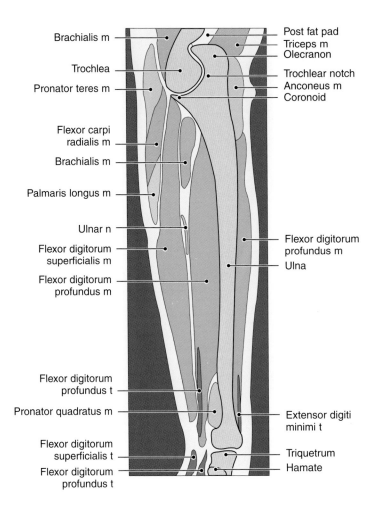

Brachialis m

Trochlea

Pronator teres m

Flexor carpi
radialis m

Brachialis m

Palmaris longus m

Ulnar n

Flexor digitorum
superficialis m

Flexor digitorum
profundus m

Flexor digitorum
profundus t

Pronator quadratus m

Flexor digitorum
superficialis t

Flexor digitorum
profundus t

Post fat pad
Triceps m
Olecranon

Trochlear notch
Anconeus m
Coronoid

Flexor digitorum
profundus m

Ulna

Extensor digiti
minimi t

Triquetrum
Hamate

Forearm, Sagittal

Brachialis m
Brachial a
Brachialis t
Biceps m
Superficial v
Biceps t
Pronator teres m
Brachioradialis m
Supinator m
Flexor carpi radialis m
Radial n, deep branch
Flexor digitorum superficialis m
Flexor pollicis longus m
Pronator quadratus m
Flexor pollicis longus t
Radioscaphocapitate lig

Triceps m
Capitulum
Anconeus m
Radius
Supinator m
Flexor digitorum superficialis m
Extensor digitorum m
Abductor pollicis longus m
Extensor digitorum t
Radius
Scaphoid

Brachialis m

Brachial a

Brachialis t

Biceps m

Superficial v

Biceps t

Pronator teres m

Brachioradialis m

Supinator m

Flexor carpi radialis m

Radial n, deep branch

Flexor digitorum superficialis m

Flexor pollicis longus m

Pronator quadratus m

Flexor pollicis longus t

Radioscaphocapitate lig

Triceps m

Capitulum

Anconeus m

Radius

Supinator m

Flexor digitorum superficialis m

Extensor digitorum m

Abductor pollicis longus m

Extensor digitorum t

Radius

Scaphoid

Forearm, Sagittal

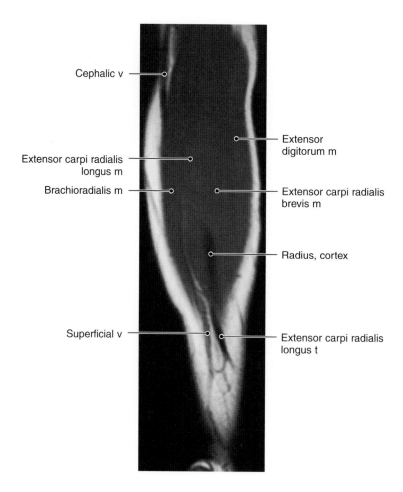

Cephalic v

Extensor digitorum m

Extensor carpi radialis longus m

Brachioradialis m

Extensor carpi radialis brevis m

Radius, cortex

Superficial v

Extensor carpi radialis longus t

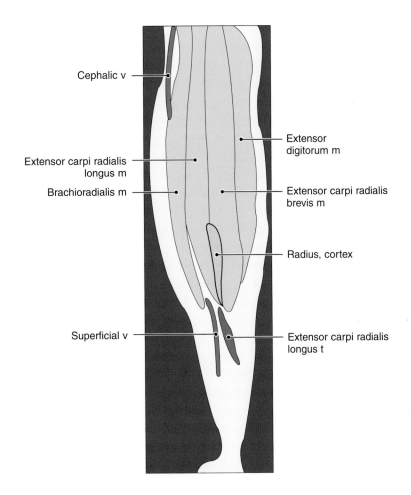

Cephalic v

Extensor carpi radialis longus m

Brachioradialis m

Extensor digitorum m

Extensor carpi radialis brevis m

Radius, cortex

Superficial v

Extensor carpi radialis longus t

5

Wrist and Hand

Wrist and Hand, Coronal

Interosseous mm

3rd Metacarpal

4th Metacarpal

2nd Metacarpal

Trapezoid

Hamate

Extensor carpi
radialis longus t

Capitate

Extensor pollicis
longus t

Triquetrum

Extensor digiti
minimi t

Scaphoid

Lunotriquetral lig

Lunate

Scapholunate lig

Ulna

Radius

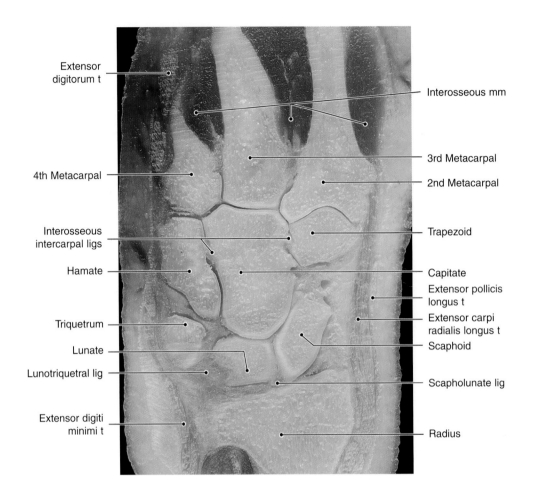

Extensor digitorum t

Interosseous mm

3rd Metacarpal

4th Metacarpal

2nd Metacarpal

Interosseous intercarpal ligs

Trapezoid

Hamate

Capitate

Extensor pollicis longus t

Triquetrum

Extensor carpi radialis longus t

Lunate

Scaphoid

Lunotriquetral lig

Scapholunate lig

Extensor digiti minimi t

Radius

Wrist and Hand, Coronal

Interosseous mm

Extensor digiti
minimi t

3rd Metacarpal

2nd Metacarpal

4th Metacarpal

Extensor carpi
radialis longus t

Hamate

Trapezium

Trapezoid

Capitate

Extensor pollicis
longus t

Triquetrum

Extensor carpi
ulnaris t

Radial collateral lig

Lunate

Scaphoid

Triangular
fibrocartilage &
complex

Scapholunate lig

Ulna

Radius

Interosseous mm

Extensor digiti minimi t

3rd Metacarpal

4th Metacarpal

Extensor digiti minimi t

Hamate

Capitate

Triquetrum

Lunate

Lunotriquetral lig

Extensor carpi ulnaris t

Triangular fibrocartilage & complex

Ulna

2nd Metacarpal

Radial a

Extensor carpi radialis longus t

Trapezium

Extensor pollicis longus t

Trapezoid

Radial collateral lig

Scaphoid

Scapholunate lig

Radius

Extensor carpi radialis longus t

Wrist and Hand, Coronal

Interosseous mm

Adductor pollicis m

Extensor digiti minimi t

4th Metacarpal

5th Metacarpal

3rd Metacarpal

2nd Metacarpal

Trapezoid

Trapezium

Radial a

Hamate

Extensor carpi ulnaris t

Capitate

Triquetrum

Scaphoid

Radial collateral lig

Lunate

Triangular fibrocartilage & complex

Scapholunate lig

Radius

Ulna

Extensor pollicis brevis t

Interosseous mm

Extensor digiti minimi t

Adductor pollicis m

4th Metacarpal

3rd Metacarpal

5th Metacarpal

2nd Metacarpal

Trapezium

Radial a

Hamate

Trapezoid

Extensor carpi ulnaris t

Capitate

Scaphoid

Triquetrum

Radial collateral lig

Lunate

Triangular fibrocartilage & complex

Scapholunate lig

Ulna

Radius

Extensor pollicis brevis t

Wrist and Hand, Coronal

Interosseous mm

Adductor pollicis m

Hypothenar mm

Flexor digitorum
profundus tt

Flexor carpi
radialis t

5th Metacarpal

1st Metacarpal

Hamate, hook

Trapezium

Pisometacarpal lig

Scaphoid

Radial a

Pisiform

Radiolunate lig

Lunate

Triangular
fibrocartilage &
complex

Abductor pollicis
longus & extensor
pollicis brevis tt

Ulna

Radius

Interosseous mm

Adductor pollicis m

Hypothenar mm

5th Metacarpal

Hamate, hook

Pisometacarpal lig

Flexor digitorum profundus tt

Flexor carpi radialis t

1st Metacarpal

Trapezium

Pisiform

Lunate

Triangular fibrocartilage & complex

Ulna

Scaphoid

Radial a

Radiolunate lig

Abductor pollicis longus & extensor pollicis brevis tt

Radius

Pronator quadratus m

Wrist and Hand, Coronal

5th Metacarpal

Hypothenar mm

Hamate, hook

Pisometacarpal lig

Pisohamate lig

Pisiform

Ulna

Interosseous mm

Adductor policis m

Lumbricalis mm

Thenar mm

Flexor pollicis longus t

Flexor digitorum tt

1st Metacarpal

Flexor carpi radialis t

Trapezium

Scaphoid

Radial a

Abductor pollicis longus & extensor pollicis brevis tt

Radius

Pronator quadratus m

5th Metacarpal

Interosseous mm

Lumbricalis mm

Adductor pollicis m

Thenar mm

Flexor pollicis longus t

Hypothenar mm

Flexor digitorum tt

1st Metacarpal

Flexor carpi radialis t

Hamate, hook

Trapezium

Pisometacarpal lig

Pisohamate lig

Scaphoid

Pisiform

Radial a

Abductor pollicis longus & extensor pollicis brevis tt

Radius

Pronator quadratus m

Wrist and Hand, Coronal

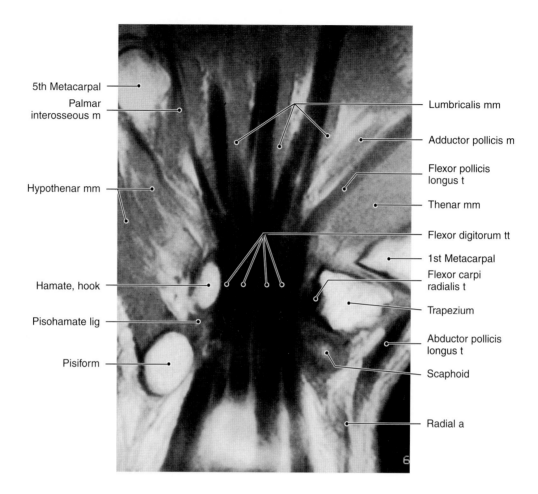

5th Metacarpal

Palmar interosseous m

Hypothenar mm

Hamate, hook

Pisohamate lig

Pisiform

Lumbricalis mm

Adductor pollicis m

Flexor pollicis longus t

Thenar mm

Flexor digitorum tt

1st Metacarpal

Flexor carpi radialis t

Trapezium

Abductor pollicis longus t

Scaphoid

Radial a

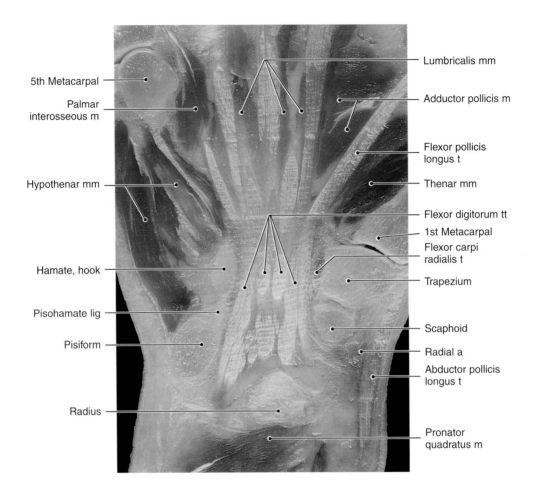

5th Metacarpal

Palmar interosseous m

Hypothenar mm

Hamate, hook

Pisohamate lig

Pisiform

Radius

Lumbricalis mm

Adductor pollicis m

Flexor pollicis longus t

Thenar mm

Flexor digitorum tt

1st Metacarpal

Flexor carpi radialis t

Trapezium

Scaphoid

Radial a

Abductor pollicis longus t

Pronator quadratus m

Wrist and Hand, Coronal

- Lumbricalis mm
- 5th Metacarpal
- Flexor digitorum tt
- Hypothenar mm
- Thenar mm
- Ulnar a
- Flexor retinaculum
- 1st Metacarpal
- Median n
- Trapezium
- Flexor carpi radialis t
- Pisiform
- Flexor pollicis longus t
- Ulnar n
- Flexor digitorum tt

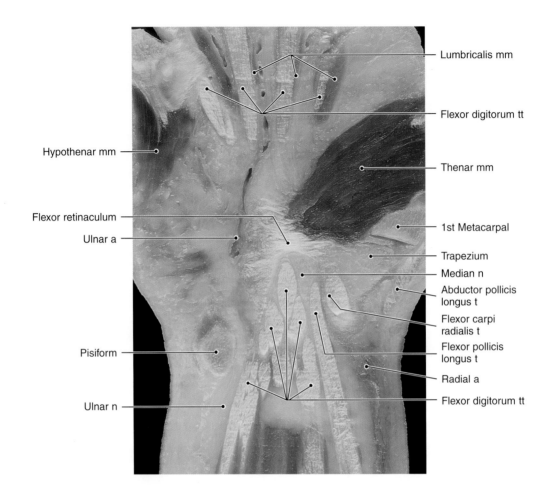

Lumbricalis mm

Flexor digitorum tt

Hypothenar mm

Thenar mm

Flexor retinaculum

Ulnar a

1st Metacarpal

Trapezium

Median n

Abductor pollicis longus t

Flexor carpi radialis t

Pisiform

Flexor pollicis longus t

Radial a

Ulnar n

Flexor digitorum tt

Wrist and Hand, Transverse

Extensor digiti minimi t

Extensor digitorum & indicis tt

Extensor pollicis longus t

Radial tubercle

Extensor carpi radialis brevis t

Extensor carpi radialis longus t

Radius

Extensor pollicis brevis t

Abductor pollicis longus t

Pronator quadratus m

Flexor pollicis longus t

Radial a

Flexor carpi radialis t

Median n

Extensor carpi ulnaris t

Ulna

Distal radioulnar j, articular capsule

Parona space

Flexor digitorum profundus tt

Ulnar n

Ulnar a

Flexor carpi ulnaris m & t

Flexor digitorum superficialis tt

Palmaris longus t

Extensor digiti minimi t

Extensor digitorum & indicis tt

Extensor pollicis longus t

Radial tubercle

Extensor carpi radialis brevis t

Extensor carpi radialis longus t

Radius

Extensor pollicis brevis t

Abductor pollicis longus t

Pronator quadratus m

Flexor pollicis longus t

Radial a

Flexor carpi radialis t

Median n

Extensor carpi ulnaris t

Ulna

Distal radioulnar j, articular capsule

Parona space

Flexor digitorum profundus tt

Ulnar n

Ulnar a

Flexor carpi ulnaris m & t

Flexor digitorum superficialis tt

Palmaris longus t

Extensor retinaculum   Extensor digitorum & indicis tt

Extensor digiti minimi t

Extensor carpi ulnaris t

Ulna

Triangular fibrocartilage & complex

Flexor digitorum profundus tt

Ulnar n

Ulnar a

Flexor carpi ulnaris m & t

Extensor pollicis longus t

Extensor carpi radialis brevis t

Extensor carpi radialis longus t

Radius

Extensor pollicis brevis t

Abductor pollicis longus t

Flexor pollicis longus t

Radial a

Flexor carpi radialis t

Median n

Flexor digitorum superficialis tt   Palmaris longus t

Extensor retinaculum   Extensor digitorum & indicis tt

Extensor digiti minimi t

Extensor carpi ulnaris t

Ulna

Triangular fibrocartilage & complex

Flexor digitorum profundus tt

Ulnar n

Ulnar a

Flexor carpi ulnaris m & t

Extensor pollicis longus t

Extensor carpi radialis brevis t

Extensor carpi radialis longus t

Radius

Extensor pollicis brevis t

Abductor pollicis longus t

Flexor pollicis longus t

Radial a

Flexor carpi radialis t

Median n

Flexor digitorum superficialis tt   Palmaris longus t

Wrist and Hand, Transverse

Extensor retinaculum   Extensor digitorum & indicis tt

Extensor digiti minimi t

Extensor carpi ulnaris t

Triangular fibrocartilage & complex

Lunate

Ulnolunate lig

Flexor digitorum profundus tt

Ulnar n

Ulnar a

Flexor carpi ulnaris m & t

Extensor pollicis longus t

Extensor carpi radialis brevis t

Extensor carpi radialis longus t

Scaphoid

Radius

Extensor pollicis brevis t

Abductor pollicis longus t

Radial a

Flexor pollicis longus t

Flexor carpi radialis t

Median n

Flexor digitorum superficialis tt   Palmaris longus t

Extensor retinaculum   Extensor digitorum & indicis tt

Extensor digiti minimi t

Extensor carpi ulnaris t

Triangular fibrocartilage & complex

Lunate

Ulnolunate lig

Flexor digitorum profundus tt

Ulnar n

Ulnar a

Flexor carpi ulnaris m & t

Extensor pollicis longus t

Extensor carpi radialis brevis t

Extensor carpi radialis longus t

Scaphoid

Radius

Scapholunate lig

Extensor pollicis brevis t

Abductor pollicis longus t

Radial a

Flexor pollicis longus t

Flexor carpi radialis t

Median n

Flexor digitorum superficialis tt   Palmaris longus t

Extensor retinaculum · Extensor digitorum & indicis tt

Extensor digiti minimi t
Dorsal radiocarpal lig
Extensor carpi ulnaris t
Triquetrum
Lunate

Lunotriquetral lig
Flexor digitorum profundus tt
Ulnar n

Ulnar a
Flexor carpi ulnaris t

Scapholunate lig
Extensor pollicis longus t
Extensor carpi radialis brevis t
Extensor carpi radialis longus t
Scaphoid
Radius
Scapholunate lig
Radiolunate lig
Extensor pollicis brevis t
Abductor pollicis longus t
Radial a
Flexor pollicis longus t
Flexor carpi radialis t
Median n

Flexor digitorum superficialis tt · Palmaris longus t

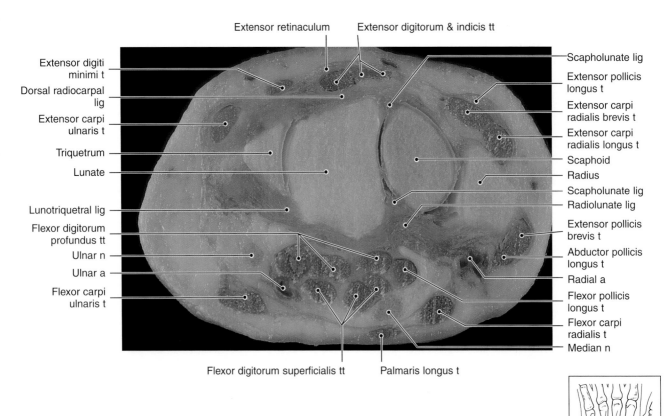

Extensor retinaculum · Extensor digitorum & indicis tt

Extensor digiti minimi t
Dorsal radiocarpal lig
Extensor carpi ulnaris t
Triquetrum
Lunate

Lunotriquetral lig
Flexor digitorum profundus tt
Ulnar n
Ulnar a
Flexor carpi ulnaris t

Scapholunate lig
Extensor pollicis longus t
Extensor carpi radialis brevis t
Extensor carpi radialis longus t
Scaphoid
Radius
Scapholunate lig
Radiolunate lig
Extensor pollicis brevis t
Abductor pollicis longus t
Radial a
Flexor pollicis longus t
Flexor carpi radialis t
Median n

Flexor digitorum superficialis tt · Palmaris longus t

Wrist and Hand, Transverse

Extensor digiti minimi t

Extensor digitorum & indicis tt

Dorsal intercarpal lig

Extensor carpi ulnaris t

Capitate

Triquetrum

Lunate

Lunotriquetral lig

Flexor digitorum profundus tt

Pisiform

Ulnar n

Ulnar a

Flexor carpi ulnaris t

Extensor carpi radialis brevis t

Extensor pollicis longus t

Extensor carpi radialis longus t

Scaphoid

Radial collateral lig

Radial a

Extensor pollicis brevis t

Abductor pollicis longus t

Flexor pollicis longus t

Flexor carpi radialis t

Median n

Flexor digitorum superficialis tt

Palmaris longus t

Extensor digiti minimi t

Extensor digitorum & indicis tt

Dorsal intercarpal lig

Capitate

Extensor carpi radialis brevis t

Extensor pollicis longus t

Extensor carpi radialis longus t

Extensor carpi ulnaris t

Triquetrum

Hamate

Flexor digitorum profundus tt

Pisiform

Ulnar n

Flexor carpi ulnaris t

Ulnar a

Scaphoid

Palmar scaphotriquetral lig

Radial collateral lig

Radial a

Extensor pollicis brevis t

Abductor pollicis longus t

Flexor pollicis longus t

Flexor carpi radialis t

Median n

Flexor digitorum superficialis tt

Palmaris longus t

Extensor digitorum & indicis tt

Extensor digiti minimi t

Extensor carpi ulnaris t

Hamate

Triquetrum

Flexor digitorum profundus tt

Pisiform

Hypothenar mm

Ulnar n

Flexor carpi ulnaris t

Ulnar a

Flexor retinaculum

Dorsal intercarpal lig

Extensor carpi radialis brevis t

Extensor pollicis longus t

Extensor carpi radialis longus t

Capitate

Deltoid (V) lig

Scaphoid

Radial a

Flexor pollicis longus t

Extensor pollicis brevis t

Abductor pollicis longus t

Flexor carpi radialis t

Median n

Flexor digitorum superficialis tt

Palmaris longus t

Extensor digiti minimi t

Extensor digitorum & indicis tt

Extensor carpi ulnaris t

Hamate

Triquetrum

Flexor digitorum profundus tt

Pisiform

Hypothenar mm

Ulnar n

Flexor carpi ulnaris t

Ulnar a

Flexor retinaculum

Dorsal intercarpal lig

Extensor carpi radialis brevis t

Capitate

Extensor carpi radialis longus t

Extensor pollicis longus t

Deltoid (V) lig

Scaphoid

Radial a

Flexor pollicis longus t

Extensor pollicis brevis t

Abductor pollicis longus t

Flexor carpi radialis t

Median n

Flexor digitorum superficialis tt

Palmaris longus t

Wrist and Hand, Transverse

Extensor digitorum & indicis tt

Capitate

Extensor digiti minimi t

Hamate

Extensor carpi ulnaris t

Flexor digitorum profundus tt

Pisometacarpal lig

Hypothenar mm

Pisohamate lig

Ulnar n

Ulnar a

Flexor retinaculum

Extensor carpi radialis brevis t

Extensor carpi radialis longus t

Trapezoid

Extensor pollicis longus t

Radial a

Flexor pollicis longus t

Trapezium

Extensor pollicis brevis t

Abductor pollicis longus t

Flexor carpi radialis t

Thenar mm

Median n

Flexor digitorum superficialis tt   Palmaris longus t

Extensor digitorum & indicis tt

Capitate

Extensor digiti minimi t

Hamate

Extensor carpi ulnaris t

Flexor digitorum profundus tt

Pisohamate lig

Hypothenar mm

Pisometacarpal lig

Ulnar n

Ulnar a

Flexor retinaculum

Extensor carpi radialis brevis t

Extensor carpi radialis longus t

Extensor pollicis longus t

Trapezoid

Radial a

Scaphoid

Deltoid (V) lig

Extensor pollicis brevis t

Abductor pollicis longus t

Trapezium

Flexor carpi radialis t

Thenar mm

Flexor pollicis longus t

Median n

Flexor digitorum superficialis tt   Palmaris longus t

Extensor digitorum & indicis tt

Capitate

Extensor digiti minimi t

Hamate

Extensor carpi ulnaris t

Flexor digitorum profundus tt

Hamate, hook

Hypothenar mm

Ulnar n, deep branch

Ulnar n, superficial branch

Ulnar a

Flexor retinaculum

Extensor carpi radialis brevis t

3rd Metacarpal

Extensor carpi radialis longus t

2nd Metacarpal

Extensor pollicis longus t

Trapezoid

Flexor carpi radialis t

Trapezium

Extensor pollicis brevis t

Abductor pollicis longus t

Flexor pollicis longus t

Thenar mm

Median n

Palmar apon

Flexor digitorum superficialis tt

Extensor digitorum & indicis tt

Capitate

Extensor digiti minimi t

Hamate

Extensor carpi ulnaris t

Flexor digitorum profundus tt

Hamate, hook

Pisometacarpal lig

Hypothenar mm

Pisohamate lig

Ulnar n, deep branch

Ulnar n, superficial branch

Ulnar a

Flexor retinaculum

Extensor carpi radialis brevis t

Extensor carpi radialis longus t

Trapezoid

Extensor pollicis longus t

Radial a

Flexor pollicis longus t

Trapezium

Extensor pollicis brevis t

Abductor pollicis longus t

Flexor carpi radialis t

Thenar mm

Median n

Flexor digitorum superficialis tt

Palmar apon

Wrist and Hand, Transverse

Extensor digitorum & indicis tt

3rd Metacarpal
4th Metacarpal
Extensor digiti minimi t
5th Metacarpal
Flexor digitorum profundus tt
Ulnar n, deep branch
Hypothenar mm
Ulnar n, superficial branch
Palmaris brevis m
Ulnar a

Extensor carpi radialis brevis t
2nd Metacarpal
Extensor carpi radialis longus t
Trapezium
Flexor carpi radialis t
Extensor pollicis longus t
1st Metacarpal
Extensor pollicis brevis t
Flexor pollicis longus t
Abductor pollicis longus t
Thenar mm
Median n

Palmar apon   Flexor digitorum superficialis tt

Extensor digitorum & indicis tt

3rd Metacarpal
4th Metacarpal
Extensor digiti minimi t
5th Metacarpal
Flexor digitorum profundus tt
Hypothenar mm
Ulnar n, deep branch
Ulnar n, superficial branch
Palmaris brevis m
Ulnar a
Flexor retinaculum

Extensor carpi radialis brevis t
2nd Metacarpal
Extensor carpi radialis longus t
Radial a
Extensor pollicis longus t
Trapezium
Flexor carpi radialis t
Extensor pollicis brevis t
1st Metacarpal
Flexor pollicis longus t
Abductor pollicis longus t
Thenar mm
Median n

Flexor digitorum superficialis tt   Palmar apon

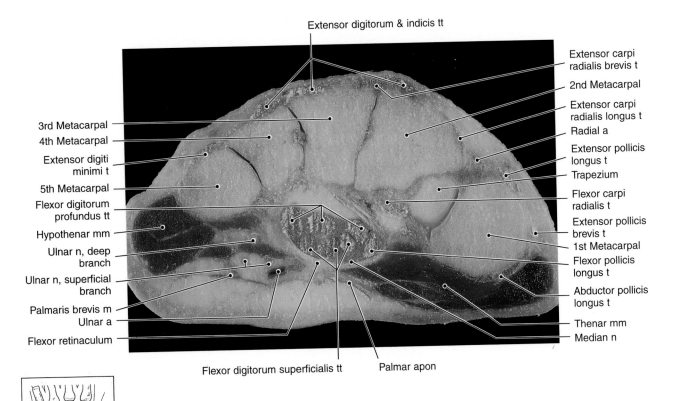

Extensor digitorum & indicis tt

Extensor digiti minimi tt

Flexor digitorum profundus tt

Palmar interosseous m

Hypothenar mm

Ulnar n, superficial branch

Palmaris brevis m

Ulnar a

Dorsal interosseous m

Extensor pollicis longus t

Adductor pollicis m

Extensor pollicis brevis t

Flexor pollicis longus t

Median n

Thenar mm

Flexor digitorum superficialis tt

Palmar apon

1, 2, 3, 4, 5: Metacarpals

Extensor digitorum & indicis tt

Dorsal interosseous mm

Extensor digiti minim t

Flexor digitorum profundus tt

Palmar interosseous m

Hypothenar mm

Ulnar n, superficial branch

Palmaris brevis m

Ulnar a

Dorsal interosseous mm

Extensor pollicis longus t

Adductor pollicis m

Extensor pollicis brevis t

Flexor pollicis longus t

Thenar mm

Median n

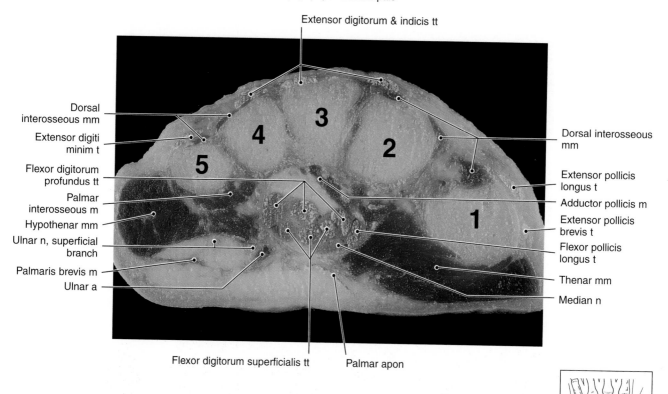

Flexor digitorum superficialis tt

Palmar apon

Wrist and Hand, Transverse

Extensor digitorum & indicis tt

Extensor digiti minimi tt

Flexor digitorum profundus tt

Hypothenar mm

Ulnar a

Radial a

Extensor pollicis longus t

Adductor pollicis m

Flexor pollicis longus t

Thenar mm

Median n

Palmar apon

Flexor digitorum superficialis tt

D: Dorsal interosseous m   P: Palmar interosseous m

Extensor digitorum & indicis tt

Extensor digiti minimi tt

Flexor digitorum profundus tt

Hypothenar mm

Ulnar a

Radial a

Extensor pollicis longus t

Adductor pollicis m

Flexor pollicis longus t

Median n

Thenar mm

Flexor digitorum superficialis tt   Palmar apon

Extensor digitorum & indicis tt

Extensor digiti minimi tt

Flexor digitorum profundus tt

Hypothenar mm

Flexor digitorum superficialis tt

Adductor pollicis m

Extensor pollicis longus t

Flexor pollicis longus t

Thenar mm

Common palmar digital aa & nn

Palmar apon

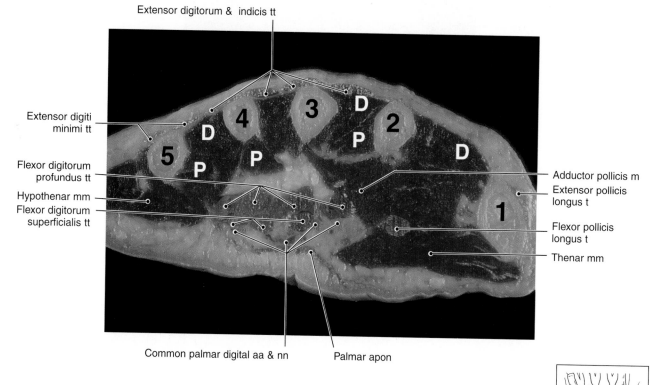

Extensor digitorum & indicis tt

Extensor digiti minimi tt

Flexor digitorum profundus tt

Hypothenar mm

Flexor digitorum superficialis tt

Adductor pollicis m

Extensor pollicis longus t

Flexor pollicis longus t

Thenar mm

Common palmar digital aa & nn

Palmar apon

Wrist and Hand, Sagittal

Hypothenar mm

Triquetrum

Dorsal
interosseous m

5th Metacarpal

Extensor digiti
minimi t

Extensor carpi
ulnaris t

Ulna

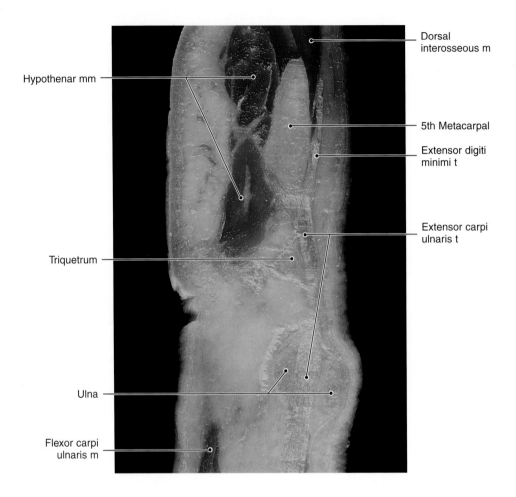

Hypothenar mm

Triquetrum

Ulna

Flexor carpi
ulnaris m

Dorsal
interosseous m

5th Metacarpal

Extensor digiti
minimi t

Extensor carpi
ulnaris t

Wrist and Hand, Sagittal

Palmar interosseous m

Hypothenar mm

Dorsal interosseous m

5th Metacarpal

Hamate

Pisometacarpal lig

Abductor digiti minimi m

Extensor digiti minimi t

Pisiform

Triquetrum

Ulnar collateral lig

Flexor carpi ulnaris m & t

Ulna

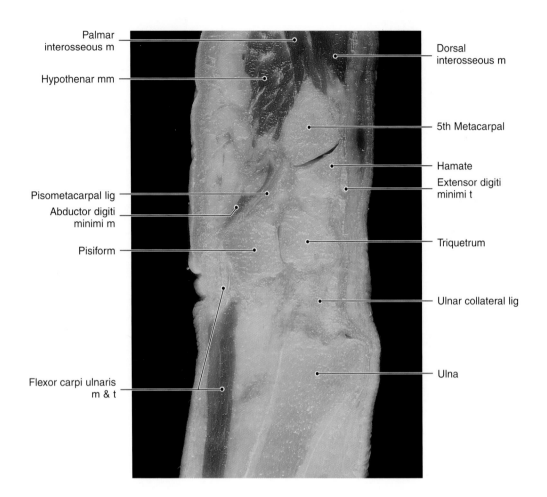

Palmar interosseous m

Hypothenar mm

Pisometacarpal lig

Abductor digiti minimi m

Pisiform

Flexor carpi ulnaris m & t

Dorsal interosseous m

5th Metacarpal

Hamate

Extensor digiti minimi t

Triquetrum

Ulnar collateral lig

Ulna

Wrist and Hand, Sagittal

Palmar interosseous m

Hypothenar mm

5th Metacarpal

Pisohamate & pisometacarpal ligs

Pisiform

Ulnar n

Flexor carpi ulnaris t

Pronator quadratus m

Extensor digitorum t

4th Metacarpal

Hamate

Triquetrum

Extensor digiti minimi t

Triangular fibrocartilage & complex

Ulna

Palmar
interosseous m

Hypothenar mm

5th Metacarpal

Pisohamate &
pisometacarpal ligs

Pisiform

Flexor carpi
ulnaris t

Ulnar n

Pronator quadratus m,
apon

Extensor
digitorum t

4th Metacarpal

Hamate

Triquetrum

Extensor digiti
minimi t

Triangular
fibrocartilage &
complex

Ulna

Wrist and Hand, Sagittal

Hypothenar mm

Ulnar a

Hamate, hook

Pisohamate lig

Ulnar n

Lunotriquetral lig

Ulnar a

Flexor digitorum
profundus t

Flexor carpi
ulnaris t

Palmar
interosseous m

4th Metacarpal

Extensor
digitorum t

Hamate

Triquetrum

Dorsal intercarpal
lig

Lunate

Triangular
fibrocartilage &
complex

Ulna

Extensor indicis
m & t

Pronator
quadratus m

Palmar interosseous m

Superficial palmar
arterial arch

4th Metacarpal

Hypothenar mm

Extensor
digitorum t

Hamate, hook

Ulnar a

Hamate

Pisohamate lig

Ulnar n

Triquetrum

Lunotriquetral lig

Dorsal intercarpal
lig

Lunate

Extensor
digitorum t

Ulnar a

Triangular
fibrocartilage &
complex

Flexor carpi
ulnaris t

Ulna

Flexor digitorum
profundus m & t

Pronator
quadratus m

Extensor indicis
m & t

Wrist and Hand, Sagittal

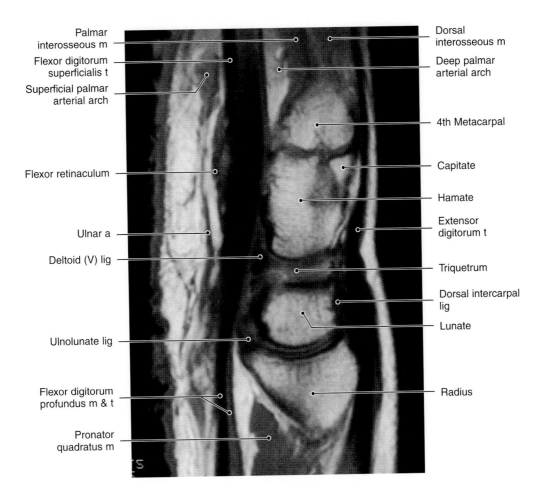

Palmar interosseous m

Flexor digitorum superficialis t

Superficial palmar arterial arch

Flexor retinaculum

Ulnar a

Deltoid (V) lig

Ulnolunate lig

Flexor digitorum profundus m & t

Pronator quadratus m

Dorsal interosseous m

Deep palmar arterial arch

4th Metacarpal

Capitate

Hamate

Extensor digitorum t

Triquetrum

Dorsal intercarpal lig

Lunate

Radius

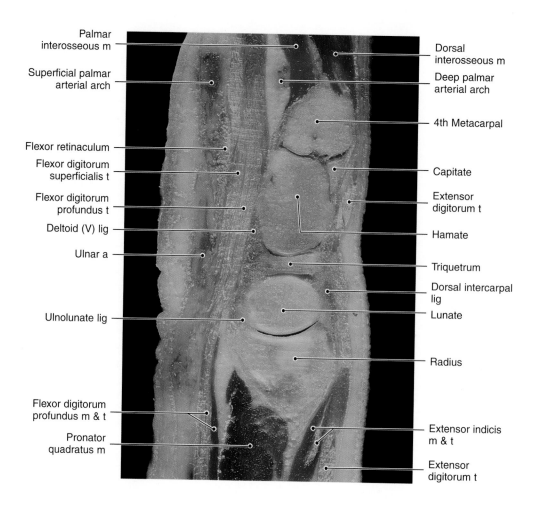

Palmar interosseous m

Superficial palmar arterial arch

Flexor retinaculum

Flexor digitorum superficialis t

Flexor digitorum profundus t

Deltoid (V) lig

Ulnar a

Ulnolunate lig

Flexor digitorum profundus m & t

Pronator quadratus m

Dorsal interosseous m

Deep palmar arterial arch

4th Metacarpal

Capitate

Extensor digitorum t

Hamate

Triquetrum

Dorsal intercarpal lig

Lunate

Radius

Extensor indicis m & t

Extensor digitorum t

Wrist and Hand, Sagittal

Superficial palmar arterial arch

Flexor retinaculum

Flexor digitorum superficialis t

Flexor digitorum profundus t

Deltoid (V) lig

Radiolunate lig

Flexor digitorum superficialis m & t

Flexor digitorum profundus m & t

Pronator quadratus m

Adductor pollicis m

Deep palmar arterial arch

3rd Metacarpal

4th Metacarpal

Extensor digitorum t

Capitate

Dorsal intercarpal lig

Lunate

Dorsal radiocarpal lig

Extensor digitorum t

Radius

Extensor pollicis longus m & t

Superficial palmar arterial arch

Flexor retinaculum

Flexor digitorum profundus t

Flexor digitorum superficialis t

Deltoid (V) lig

Radiolunate lig

Flexor digitorum superficialis m & t

Flexor digitorum profundus m & t

Pronator quadratus m

Adductor pollicis m

Deep palmar arterial arch

3rd Metacarpal

4th Metacarpal

Extensor digitorum t

Capitate

Dorsal intercarpal lig

Lunate

Dorsal radiocarpal lig

Extensor digitorum & indicis tt

Radius

Extensor pollicis longus m

Wrist and Hand, Sagittal

Flexor retinaculum

Palmar apon

Flexor digitorum
superficialis t

Flexor digitorum
profundus t

Deltoid (V) lig

Radiolunate lig

Pronator
quadratus m

Adductor pollicis m

3rd Metacarpal

Extensor
digitorum t

Capitate

Dorsal intercarpal
lig

Lunate

Dorsal radiocarpal
lig

Radius

Extensor pollicis
longus t

Flexor retinaculum

Palmar apon

Flexor digitorum
superficialis t

Flexor digitorum
profundus t

Deltoid (V) lig

Radiolunate lig

Pronator
quadratus m

Flexor digitorum
superficialis m & t

Flexor digitorum
profundus m & t

Adductor pollicis m

3rd Metacarpal

Extensor
digitorum t

Capitate

Dorsal intercarpal
lig

Lunate

Dorsal radiocarpal
lig

Extensor digitorum
& indicis tt

Radius

Extensor pollicis
longus m & t

Wrist and Hand, Sagittal

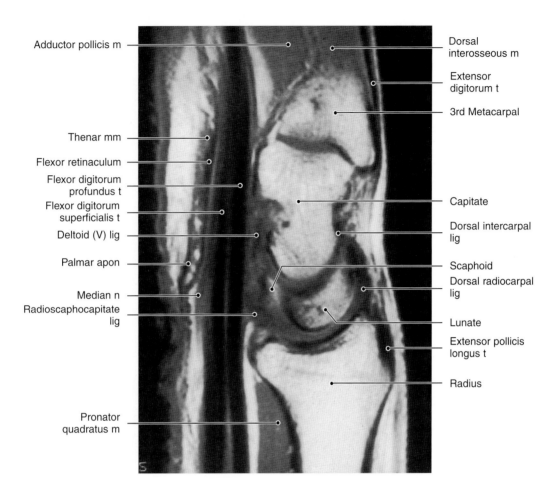

Adductor pollicis m

Thenar mm

Flexor retinaculum

Flexor digitorum profundus t

Flexor digitorum superficialis t

Deltoid (V) lig

Palmar apon

Median n

Radioscaphocapitate lig

Pronator quadratus m

Dorsal interosseous m

Extensor digitorum t

3rd Metacarpal

Capitate

Dorsal intercarpal lig

Scaphoid

Dorsal radiocarpal lig

Lunate

Extensor pollicis longus t

Radius

Adductor pollicis m

Median n

Thenar mm

Flexor retinaculum

Deltoid (V) lig

Flexor digitorum profundus t

Flexor digitorum superficialis t

Palmar apon

Radioscaphocapitate lig

Scapholunate lig

Median n

Flexor digitorum superficialis m & t

Flexor digitorum profundus t

Pronator quadratus m

Dorsal interosseous m

Extensor digitorum t

3rd Metacarpal

Capitate

Dorsal intercarpal lig

Scaphoid

Dorsal radiocarpal lig

Lunate

Extensor pollicis longus t

Radius

Wrist and Hand, Sagittal

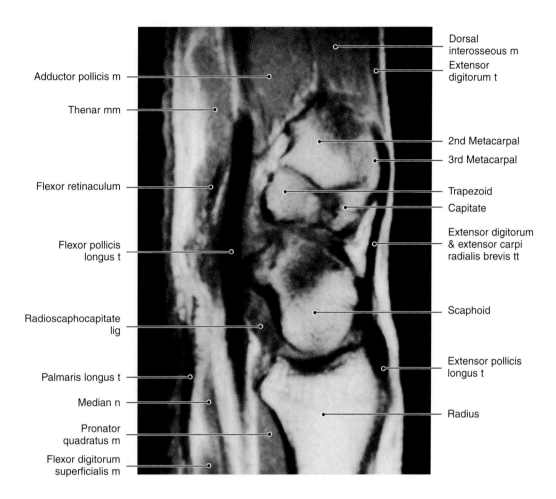

Adductor pollicis m

Thenar mm

Flexor retinaculum

Flexor pollicis longus t

Radioscaphocapitate lig

Palmaris longus t

Median n

Pronator quadratus m

Flexor digitorum superficialis m

Dorsal interosseous m

Extensor digitorum t

2nd Metacarpal

3rd Metacarpal

Trapezoid

Capitate

Extensor digitorum & extensor carpi radialis brevis tt

Scaphoid

Extensor pollicis longus t

Radius

Wrist and Hand, Sagittal

Adductor pollicis m

Flexor pollicis longus t

Thenar mm

Trapezium

Scaphoid

Radioscaphocapitate lig

Radial a

Flexor carpi radialis t

Pronator quadratus m

Dorsal interosseous m

2nd Metacarpal

Trapezoid

Extensor pollicis longus t

Extensor carpi radialis longus t

Radius

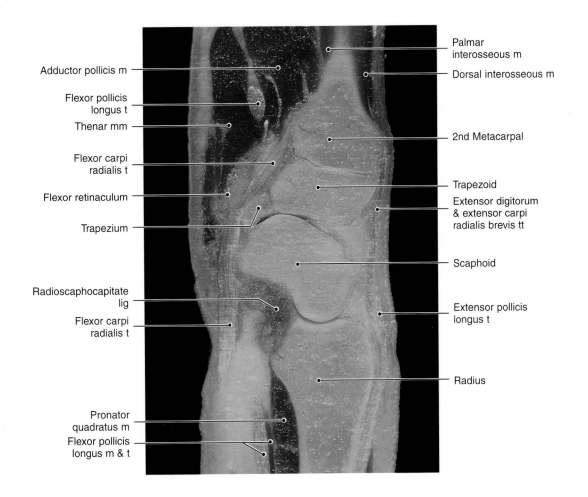

Adductor pollicis m

Flexor pollicis
longus t

Thenar mm

Flexor carpi
radialis t

Flexor retinaculum

Trapezium

Radioscaphocapitate
lig

Flexor carpi
radialis t

Pronator
quadratus m

Flexor pollicis
longus m & t

Palmar
interosseous m

Dorsal interosseous m

2nd Metacarpal

Trapezoid

Extensor digitorum
& extensor carpi
radialis brevis tt

Scaphoid

Extensor pollicis
longus t

Radius

Wrist and Hand, Sagittal

Adductor pollicis m

Flexor pollicis longus t

Thenar mm

Flexor carpi radialis t

Flexor retinaculum

Trapezium

Radioscaphocapitate lig

Flexor carpi radialis t

Pronator quadratus m

Flexor pollicis longus m & t

Dorsal interosseous m

2nd Metacarpal

Trapezoid

Extensor digitorum & extensor carpi radialis brevis tt

Scaphoid

Extensor pollicis longus t

Radius

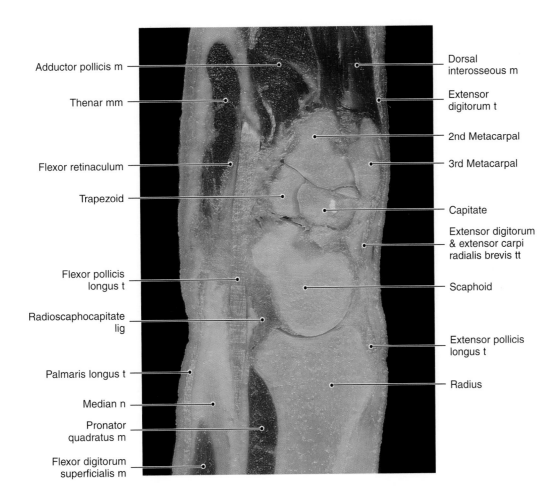

Adductor pollicis m

Thenar mm

Flexor retinaculum

Trapezoid

Flexor pollicis
longus t

Radioscaphocapitate
lig

Palmaris longus t

Median n

Pronator
quadratus m

Flexor digitorum
superficialis m

Dorsal
interosseous m

Extensor
digitorum t

2nd Metacarpal

3rd Metacarpal

Capitate

Extensor digitorum
& extensor carpi
radialis brevis tt

Scaphoid

Extensor pollicis
longus t

Radius

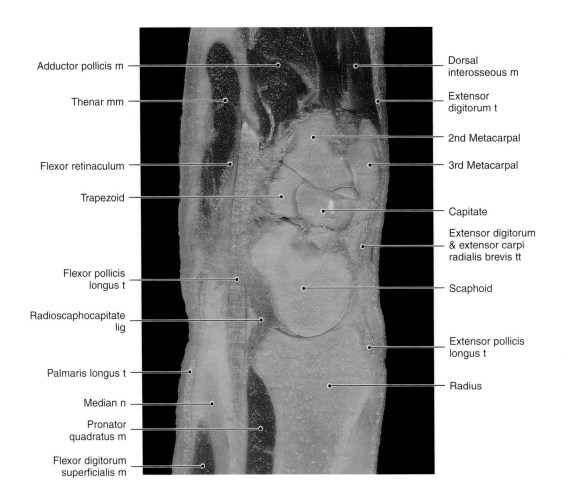

Adductor pollicis m

Thenar mm

Flexor retinaculum

Trapezoid

Flexor pollicis longus t

Radioscaphocapitate lig

Palmaris longus t

Median n

Pronator quadratus m

Flexor digitorum superficialis m

Dorsal interosseous m

Extensor digitorum t

2nd Metacarpal

3rd Metacarpal

Capitate

Extensor digitorum & extensor carpi radialis brevis tt

Scaphoid

Extensor pollicis longus t

Radius

Wrist and Hand, Sagittal

Adductor pollicis m

Flexor pollicis
longus t

Thenar mm

Trapezium

Scaphoid

Radioscaphocapitate
lig

Radial a

Flexor carpi
radialis t

Pronator
quadratus m

Dorsal
interosseous m

2nd Metacarpal

Trapezoid

Extensor pollicis
longus t

Extensor carpi
radialis longus t

Radius

Adductor pollicis m

Flexor pollicis longus t

Thenar mm

Trapezium

Radioscaphocapitate lig

Radial a

Flexor carpi radialis t

Pronator quadratus m

Dorsal interosseous m

2nd Metacarpal

Trapezoid

Scaphoid

Extensor pollicis longus t

Extensor carpi radialis longus t

Radius

Extensor carpi radialis brevis t

Wrist and Hand, Sagittal

Flexor pollicis longus t

Adductor pollicis m

Thenar mm

Carpometacarpal lig

Trapezium

Radial a

Palmar interosseous m

2nd Metacarpal

Extensor carpi radialis longus t

Abductor pollicis longus & extensor pollicis brevis tt

Radius

Adductor pollicis m

Flexor pollicis longus t

Thenar mm

Carpometacarpal lig

Trapezium

Radial a

Abductor pollicis longus t

Palmar interosseous m

2nd Metacarpal

Extensor carpi radialis longus t

Radius

Extensor pollicis brevis m & t

6

Finger

Finger, Coronal

Collateral lig

Middle phalanx

Proximal interphalangeal j

Collateral lig

Extensor (lat band) & interosseous tt

Extensor (lat band) & interosseous tt

Proximal phalanx

Collateral lig

Metacarpophalangeal j

Collateral lig

Interosseous t

Interosseous m

Interosseous t

Metacarpal bone

Middle phalanx

Proximal interphalangeal j

Collateral lig

Collateral lig

Extensor (lat band) & interosseous tt

Extensor (lat band) & interosseous tt

Proximal phalanx

Metacarpophalangeal j

Interosseous t

Collateral lig

Collateral lig

Metacarpal head

Interosseous m

Interosseous t

Interosseous m

Finger, Coronal

Collateral lig

Interosseous t

Collateral lig

Interosseous t

Middle phalanx

Collateral lig

Proximal
interphalangeal j

Flexor digitorum
profundus t

Interosseous t

Proximal phalanx

Metacarpophalangeal j

Interosseous t

Metacarpal head

Middle phalanx

Collateral lig

Proximal
interphalangeal j

Collateral lig

Flexor digitorum
profundus t

Proximal phalanx

Interosseous tt

Collateral lig

Collateral lig

Metacarpophalangeal j

Interosseous t

Metacarpal head

Finger, Transverse

Collateral lig   Extensor digitorum t   Collateral lig

Dorsal digital v

5th MC   4th MC   3rd MC   2nd MC

Interosseous mm & tt

Interosseous mm & tt

Palmar (volar) plate

Deep transverse metacarpal lig

Deep transverse metacarpal lig

Lumbrical m

Palmar digital n & a

Palmar digital n & a

Lumbrical m

Flexor digitorum superficialis & profundus tt

MC: Metacarpal

Collateral lig   Extensor digitorum t   Collateral lig

5th MC   4th MC   3rd MC   2nd MC

Interosseous mm & tt

Interosseous mm & tt

Palmar (volar) plate

Deep transverse metacarpal lig

Deep transverse metacarpal lig

Lumbrical m

Palmar digital n & a

Palmar digital n & a

Lumbrical m

Flexor digitorum superficialis & profundus tt

Flexor tendon sheath

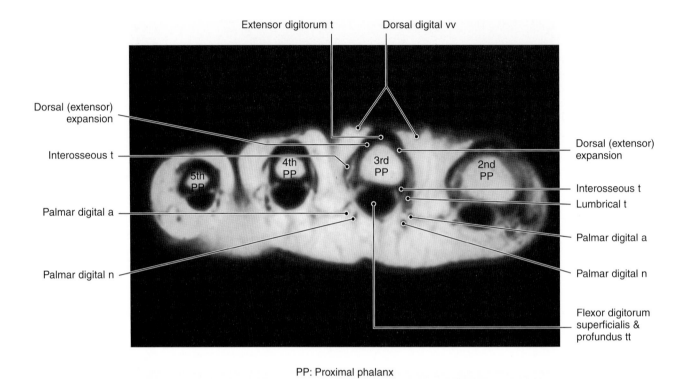

Extensor digitorum t

Dorsal digital vv

Dorsal (extensor) expansion

Interosseous t

Palmar digital a

Palmar digital n

5th PP

4th PP

3rd PP

2nd PP

Dorsal (extensor) expansion

Interosseous t

Lumbrical t

Palmar digital a

Palmar digital n

Flexor digitorum superficialis & profundus tt

PP: Proximal phalanx

Extensor digitorum t

Dorsal digital v

Dorsal (extensor) expansion

5th PP

4th PP

3rd PP

2nd PP

Interosseous t

Palmar digital a

Palmar digital n

Dorsal (extensor) expansion

Interosseous t

Lumbrical t

Palmar digital a

Palmar digital n

Flexor digitorum profundus t

Flexor digitorum superficialis t

Finger, Transverse

5th pp

4th pp

3rd pp

2nd pp

Dorsal (extensor) expansion

Flexor digitorum superficialis t

Palmar digital a

Palmar digital n

Flexor digitorum superficialis t

Palmar digital a

Palmar digital n

Flexor digitorum profundus t

Flexor tendon sheath

PP: Proximal phalanx

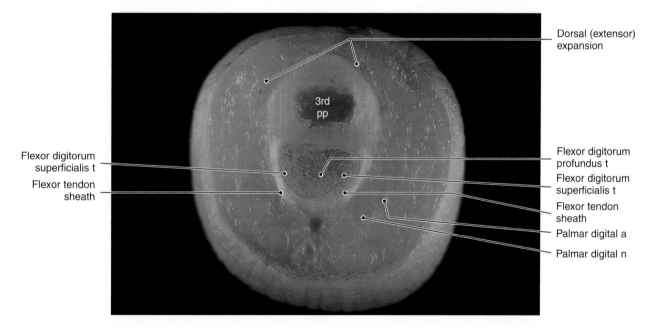

3rd pp

Dorsal (extensor) expansion

Flexor digitorum superficialis t

Flexor tendon sheath

Flexor digitorum profundus t

Flexor digitorum superficialis t

Flexor tendon sheath

Palmar digital a

Palmar digital n

Dorsal (extensor) expansion

5th MP

4th MP

3rd MP

2nd MP

Flexor digitorum superficialis t

Palmar digital a

Palmar digital a

Palmar digital n

Palmar digital n

Flexor digitorum profundus t

MP: Middle phalanx

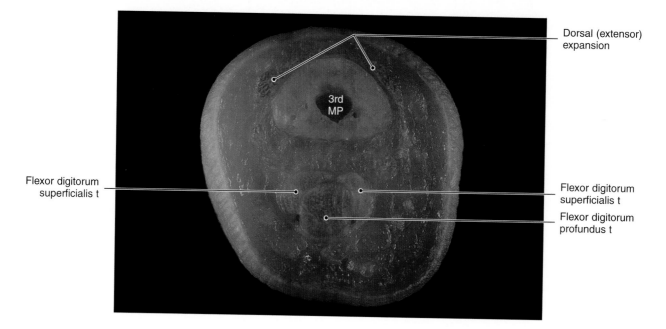

Dorsal (extensor) expansion

3rd MP

Flexor digitorum superficialis t

Flexor digitorum superficialis t

Flexor digitorum profundus t

Finger, Sagittal

Extensor t (central band)

Proximal interphalangeal j

Middle phalanx

Extensor t (common band)

Distal interphalangeal j

Distal phalanx

Palmar (volar) plate

Flexor digitorum profundus t

Palmar (volar) plate

Dorsal (extensor) expansion

Proximal phalanx

Extensor digitorum t

Metacarpophalangeal j

Metacarpal head

Palmar (volar) plate

Flexor digitorum profundus t

Flexor digitorum superficialis t

Flexor digitorum profundus t

Flexor digitorum superficialis t

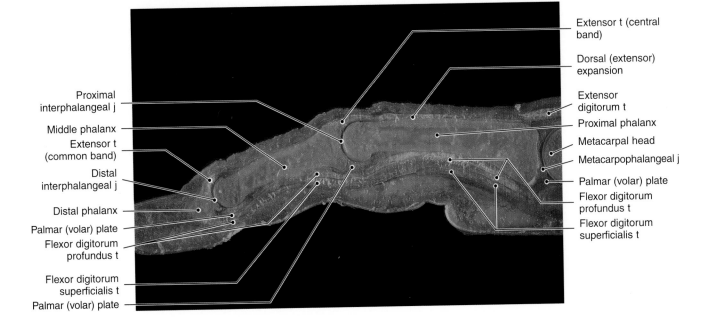

Proximal interphalangeal j

Middle phalanx

Extensor t (common band)

Distal interphalangeal j

Distal phalanx

Palmar (volar) plate

Flexor digitorum profundus t

Flexor digitorum superficialis t

Palmar (volar) plate

Extensor t (central band)

Dorsal (extensor) expansion

Extensor digitorum t

Proximal phalanx

Metacarpal head

Metacarpophalangeal j

Palmar (volar) plate

Flexor digitorum profundus t

Flexor digitorum superficialis t

Hip, Coronal

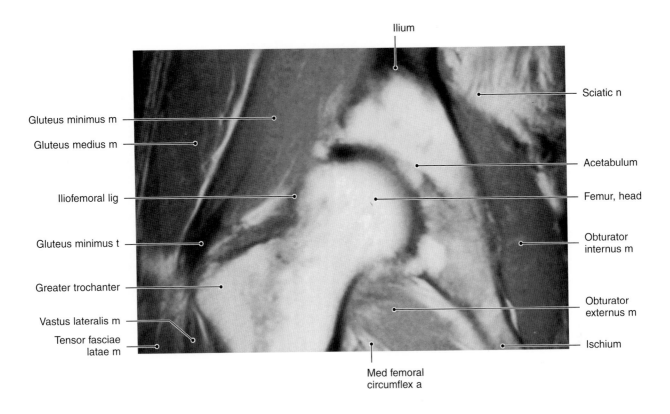

Ilium

Sciatic n

Gluteus minimus m

Gluteus medius m

Acetabulum

Iliofemoral lig

Femur, head

Gluteus minimus t

Obturator internus m

Greater trochanter

Obturator externus m

Vastus lateralis m

Tensor fasciae latae m

Ischium

Med femoral circumflex a

Ilium

Sciatic n

Gluteus minimus m

Gluteus medius m

Sup acetabular labrum

Acetabulum

Iliofemoral lig

Femur, head

Gluteus minimus t

Obturator internus m

Greater trochanter

Obturator externus m

Med femoral circumflex a

Ischium

Iliopsoas t

Quadratus femoris m

Gluteus minimus m

Gluteus medius m

Obturator internus t

Inf gemellus m

Greater trochanter

Obturator externus
m & t

Vastus lateralis m

Piriformis m

Sciatic n

Ischiofemoral lig

Ischium

Obturator
internus m

Quadratus
femoris m

Gluteus minimus m

Gluteus medius m

Obturator internus t

Greater trochanter

Inf gemellus m

Obturator externus
m & t

Vastus lateralis m

Piriformis m

Sciatic n

Ischiofemoral lig

Ischium

Obturator
internus m

Quadratus
femoris m

Sciatic n

Hip, Coronal

Gluteus minimus m

Gluteus medius m

Piriformis t

Greater trochanter

Obturator externus t

Quadratus femoris m

Vastus lateralis m

Piriformis m

Sciatic n

Ischium, spine

Obturator internus t

Inf gemellus m

Obturator internus m

Ischium

Sciatic n

Gluteus minimus m

Gluteus medius m

Piriformis t

Greater trochanter

Obturator externus t

Quadratus femoris m

Piriformis m

Sciatic n

Ischium, spine

Obturator internus t

Inf gemellus m

Obturator internus m

Ischium

Sciatic n

Gluteus minimus m

Gluteus medius m

Iliotibial tract

Piriformis m & t

Coccygeus m

Sciatic n

Ischium, spine

Sup gemellus m

Obturator internus m & t

Greater trochanter

Inf gemellus m

Ischium

Semimembranosus t

Vastus lateralis m

Quadratus femoris m

Sciatic n

Gluteus minimus m

Gluteus medius m

Iliotibial tract

Piriformis m

Sciatic n

Ischium, spine

Sup gemellus m

Inf gemellus m

Obturator internus m & t

Greater trochanter

Gluteus maximus m

Ischium

Vastus lateralis m

Semimembranosus t

Quadratus femoris m

Sciatic n

Hip, Coronal

Gluteus minimus m

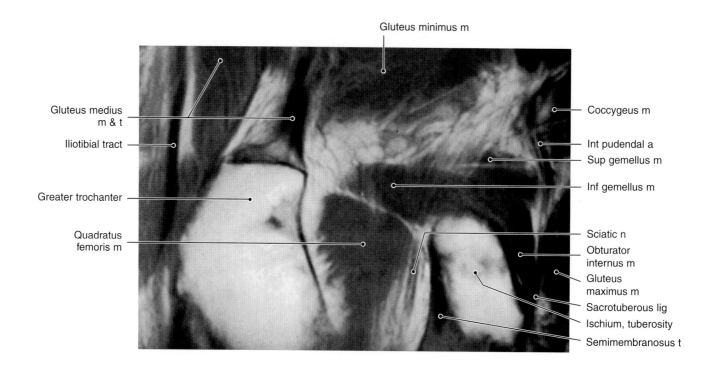

Gluteus medius
m & t

Iliotibial tract

Greater trochanter

Quadratus
femoris m

Coccygeus m

Int pudendal a

Sup gemellus m

Inf gemellus m

Sciatic n

Obturator
internus m

Gluteus
maximus m

Sacrotuberous lig

Ischium, tuberosity

Semimembranosus t

Gluteus minimus m

Gluteus medius
m & t

Inf gemellus m

Greater trochanter

Quadratus
femoris m

Sacrum

Coccygeus m

Sacrospinous lig

Piriformis m

Int pudendal a

Sup gemellus m

Sciatic n

Obturator
internus m

Gluteus
maximus m

Ischium, tuberosity

Sacrotuberous lig

Semimembranosus t

7

Hip

7

Hip

Hip, Coronal

Gluteus minimus m

Gluteus medius m

Piriformis m

Sciatic n

Ischium, spine

Piriformis t

Obturator internus t

Inf gemellus m

Greater trochanter

Obturator externus t

Obturator internus m

Quadratus femoris m

Ischium

Vastus lateralis m

Sciatic n

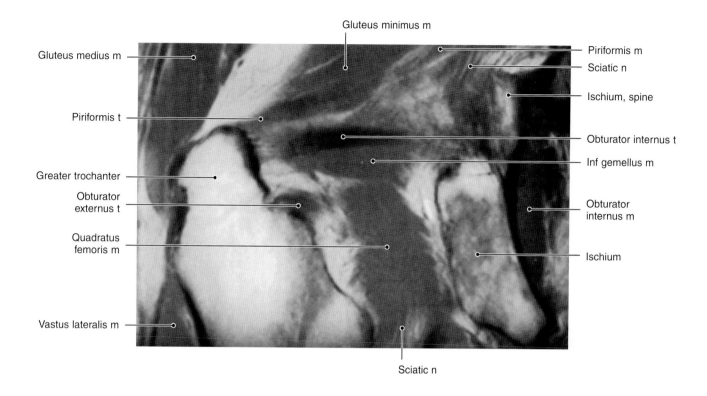

Gluteus minimus m

Gluteus medius m

Piriformis m

Piriformis t

Sciatic n

Ischium, spine

Obturator internus t

Greater trochanter

Inf gemellus m

Obturator externus t

Obturator internus m

Quadratus femoris m

Ischium

Sciatic n

Gluteus minimus m

Gluteus medius m

Obturator internus t

Inf gemellus m

Greater trochanter

Obturator externus
m & t

Vastus lateralis m

Piriformis m

Sciatic n

Ischiofemoral lig

Ischium

Obturator
internus m

Quadratus
femoris m

Gluteus minimus m

Gluteus medius m

Obturator internus t

Greater trochanter

Inf gemellus m

Obturator externus
m & t

Vastus lateralis m

Piriformis m

Sciatic n

Ischiofemoral lig

Ischium

Obturator
internus m

Quadratus
femoris m

Sciatic n

Hip, Coronal

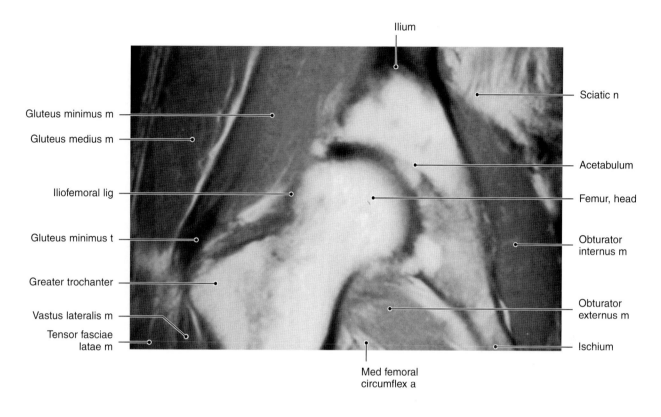

Ilium

Gluteus minimus m

Gluteus medius m

Iliofemoral lig

Gluteus minimus t

Greater trochanter

Vastus lateralis m

Tensor fasciae latae m

Med femoral circumflex a

Sciatic n

Acetabulum

Femur, head

Obturator internus m

Obturator externus m

Ischium

Ilium

Gluteus minimus m

Gluteus medius m

Sup acetabular labrum

Iliofemoral lig

Gluteus minimus t

Greater trochanter

Med femoral circumflex a

Iliopsoas t

Quadratus femoris m

Sciatic n

Acetabulum

Femur, head

Obturator internus m

Obturator externus m

Ischium

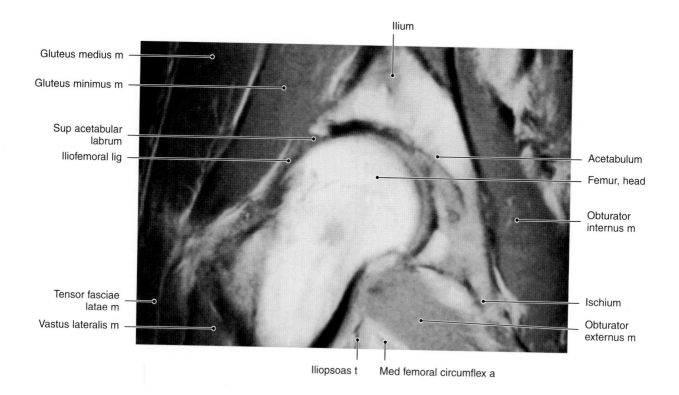

Ilium

Gluteus medius m

Gluteus minimus m

Sup acetabular labrum

Iliofemoral lig

Acetabulum

Femur, head

Obturator internus m

Tensor fasciae latae m

Vastus lateralis m

Ischium

Obturator externus m

Iliopsoas t

Med femoral circumflex a

Iliofemoral lig

Sup acetabular labrum

Gluteus medius m

Gluteus minimus m & t

Ilium

Acetabulum

Femur, head

Obturator internus m

Tensor fasciae latae m

Vastus lateralis m

Ischium

Obturator externus m

Iliopsoas t

Med femoral circumflex a

Hip, Coronal

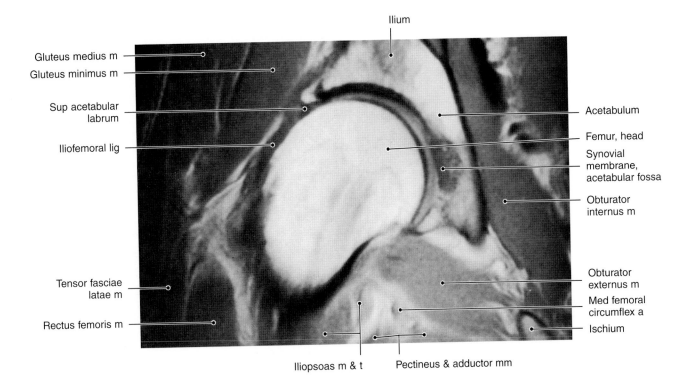

Ilium

Gluteus medius m

Gluteus minimus m

Sup acetabular labrum

Iliofemoral lig

Acetabulum

Femur, head

Synovial membrane, acetabular fossa

Obturator internus m

Tensor fasciae latae m

Rectus femoris m

Obturator externus m

Med femoral circumflex a

Ischium

Iliopsoas m & t

Pectineus & adductor mm

Sup acetabular labrum

Gluteus medius m

Gluteus minimus m

Iliofemoral lig

Acetabulum

Femur, head

Synovial membrane, acetabular fossa

Obturator internus m

Inf acetabular labrum

Tensor fasciae latae m

Rectus femoris m

Vastus lateralis m

Obturator externus m

Med femoral circumflex a

Iliopsoas m & t

Pectineus & adductor mm

Ilium

Gluteus medius m

Gluteus minimus m

Sup acetabular labrum

Iliofemoral lig

Tensor fasciae latae m

Lat femoral circumflex a

Rectus femoris m

Acetabulum

Lig teres & synovial membrane

Femur, head

Obturator internus m

Obturator externus m

Med femoral circumflex a

Ischium

Iliopsoas m & t

Pectineus & adductor mm

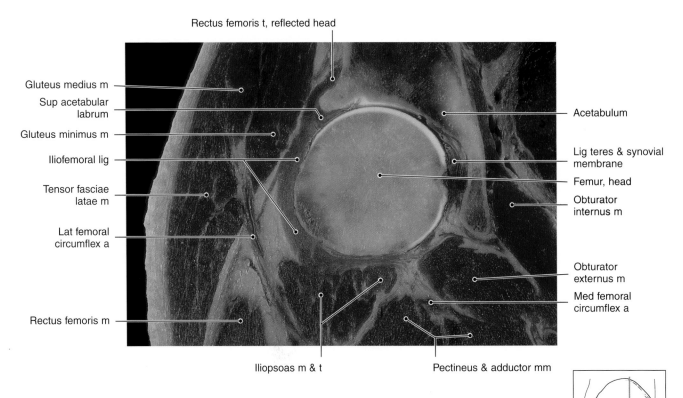

Rectus femoris t, reflected head

Gluteus medius m

Sup acetabular labrum

Gluteus minimus m

Iliofemoral lig

Tensor fasciae latae m

Lat femoral circumflex a

Rectus femoris m

Acetabulum

Lig teres & synovial membrane

Femur, head

Obturator internus m

Obturator externus m

Med femoral circumflex a

Iliopsoas m & t

Pectineus & adductor mm

Hip, Coronal

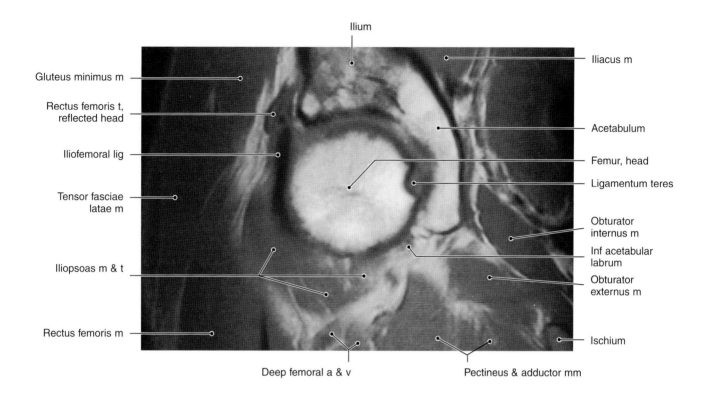

Ilium

Iliacus m

Gluteus minimus m

Rectus femoris t, reflected head

Acetabulum

Iliofemoral lig

Femur, head

Ligamentum teres

Tensor fasciae latae m

Obturator internus m

Inf acetabular labrum

Iliopsoas m & t

Obturator externus m

Rectus femoris m

Ischium

Deep femoral a & v

Pectineus & adductor mm

Ilium

Gluteus minimus m

Rectus femoris t,
reflected head

Sup acetabular
labrum

Iliofemoral lig

Tensor fasciae
latae m

Rectus femoris m

Iliacus m

Acetabulum

Femur, head

Ligamentum teres

Synovial
membrane,
acetabular fossa

Obturator
internus m

Inf acetabular
labrum

Obturator
externus m

Iliopsoas m & t

Pectineus m

Hip, Coronal

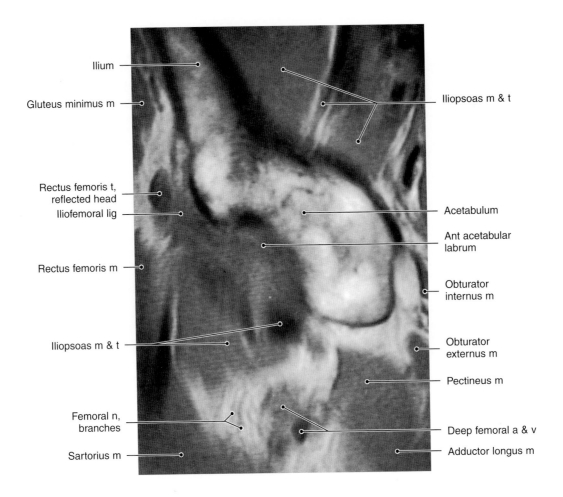

Ilium

Gluteus minimus m

Iliopsoas m & t

Rectus femoris t, reflected head

Iliofemoral lig

Acetabulum

Ant acetabular labrum

Rectus femoris m

Obturator internus m

Iliopsoas m & t

Obturator externus m

Pectineus m

Femoral n, branches

Deep femoral a & v

Sartorius m

Adductor longus m

Ilium

Gluteus minimus m

Rectus femoris t,
reflected head

Iliofemoral lig

Rectus femoris m

Iliopsoas m & t

Femoral n,
branches

Sartorius m

Iliopsoas m & t

Acetabulum

Ant acetabular
labrum

Pectineus m

Deep femoral a & v

Adductor longus m

Femoral a & v

Hip, Coronal

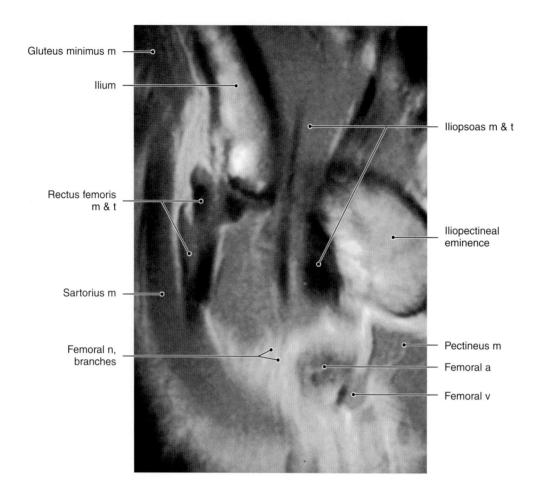

Gluteus minimus m

Ilium

Rectus femoris m & t

Sartorius m

Femoral n, branches

Iliopsoas m & t

Iliopectineal eminence

Pectineus m

Femoral a

Femoral v

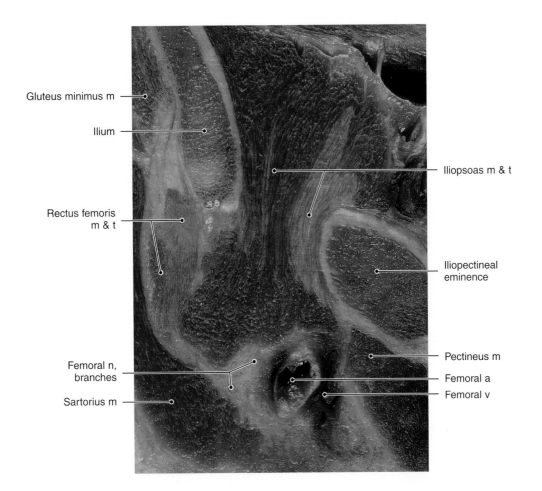

Gluteus minimus m

Ilium

Rectus femoris
m & t

Femoral n,
branches

Sartorius m

Iliopsoas m & t

Iliopectineal
eminence

Pectineus m

Femoral a

Femoral v

Hip, Transverse

Iliopsoas m & t Femoral n

Rectus femoris t

Sartorius m

Ant inf iliac spine

Femoral a & v

Tensor fasciae latae m

Iliofemoral lig

Acetabulum

Gluteus minimus m

Obturator internus m

Gluteus medius m & t

Sciatic n

Iliotibial tract

Piriformis m

Gluteus maximus m

Iliopsoas m & t Femoral n

Rectus femoris t

Sartorius m

Ant inf iliac spine

Femoral a & v

Tensor fasciae latae m

Iliofemoral lig

Acetabulum

Gluteus minimus m

Obturator internus m

Gluteus medius m & t

Sciatic n

Iliotibial tract

Piriformis m

Gluteus maximus m

Iliopsoas m & t

Femoral n

Rectus femoris t

Sartorius m

Ant inf iliac spine

Rectus femoris t, reflected head

Iliofemoral lig

Tensor fasciae latae m

Gluteus minimus m

Gluteus medius m & t

Iliotibial tract

Gluteus maximus m

Femoral a & v

Femur, head

Obturator internus m

Sciatic n

Piriformis m

Iliopsoas m & t

Femoral n

Rectus femoris t

Sartorius m

Ant inf iliac spine

Iliofemoral lig

Tensor fasciae latae m

Rectus femoris t, reflected head

Gluteus minimus m

Gluteus medius m

Femoral a & v

Femur, head

Obturator internus m

Hip, Transverse

Iliopsoas m & t

Femoral n

Rectus femoris t

Sartorius m

Iliofemoral lig

Rectus femoris t, reflected head

Tensor fasciae latae m

Gluteus minimus m

Gluteus medius m & t

Iliotibial tract

Femoral a & v

Pubis

Femur, head

Obturator internus m

Sciatic n

Ischium, spine

Sacrotuberous lig

Gluteus maximus m

Piriformis m & t

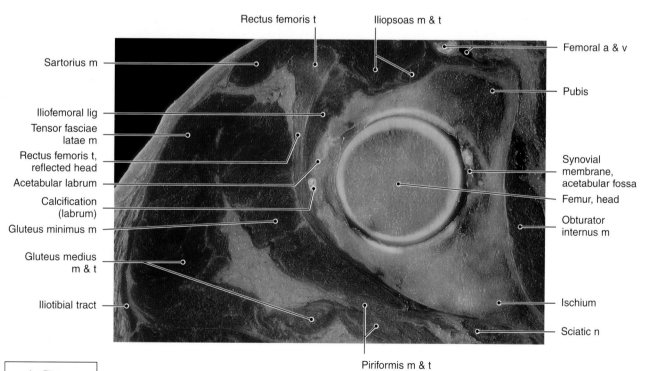

Rectus femoris t

Iliopsoas m & t

Sartorius m

Iliofemoral lig

Tensor fasciae latae m

Rectus femoris t, reflected head

Acetabular labrum

Calcification (labrum)

Gluteus minimus m

Gluteus medius m & t

Iliotibial tract

Femoral a & v

Pubis

Synovial membrane, acetabular fossa

Femur, head

Obturator internus m

Ischium

Sciatic n

Piriformis m & t

Iliopsoas m & t   Femoral n

Rectus femoris t

Sartorius m

Iliofemoral lig

Tensor fasciae
latae m

Gluteus minimus m

Gluteus medius
m & t

Iliotibial tract

Femoral a & v

Pubis

Ant acetabular
labrum

Femur, head

Obturator
internus m

Post acetabular
labrum

Ischium

Sciatic n

Sacrotuberous lig

Gluteus maximus m   Piriformis m & t

Iliopsoas m & t   Femoral n

Sartorius m

Rectus femoris t

Ant acetabular
labrum

Iliofemoral lig

Tensor fasciae
latae m

Rectus femoris t,
reflected head

Gluteus minimus m

Gluteus medius
m & t

Iliotibial tract

Femoral a & v

Pubis

Synovial membrane,
acetabular fossa

Femur, head

Post acetabular
labrum

Obturator
internus m

Ischium

Sciatic n

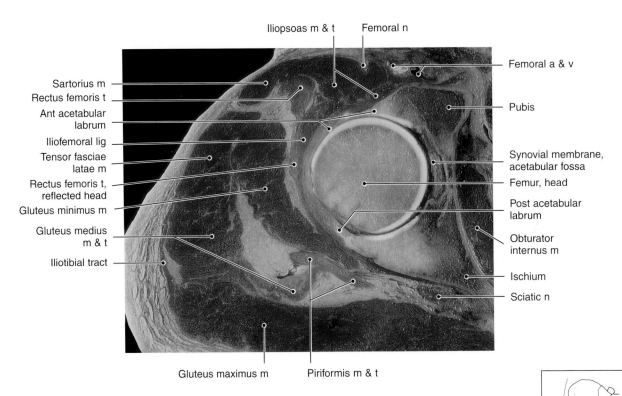

Gluteus maximus m   Piriformis m & t

Hip, Transverse

Iliopsoas m & t   Femoral n

Rectus femoris t
Sartorius m

Iliofemoral lig

Tensor fasciae
latae m

Gluteus minimus m

Gluteus medius
m & t

Iliotibial tract

Gluteus maximus m   Piriformis t

Femoral a & v
Pubis
Ant acetabular
labrum

Femur, head
Synovial
membrane,
acetabular fossa
Obturator
internus m
Ischiofemoral lig
Post acetabular
labrum

Ischium
Sciatic n
Inf gluteal a
Sacrotuberous lig

Iliopsoas m & t   Femoral n

Sartorius m
Rectus femoris t
Iliofemoral lig
Tensor fasciae
latae m
Gluteus minimus m

Gluteus medius
m & t

Iliotibial tract

Gluteus maximus m   Piriformis t

Femoral a & v
Pubis
Ant acetabular
labrum
Femur, head
Synovial
membrane,
acetabular fossa
Obturator
internus m
Ischiofemoral lig
Post acetabular
labrum
Ischium
Sciatic n
Inf gluteal a

Iliopsoas m & t
Femoral n
Femoral a & v
Pectineus m
Sartorius m
Rectus femoris m & t
Pubis
Ant acetabular labrum
Iliofemoral lig
Tensor fasciae latae m
Gluteus minimus m & t
Lig teres & synovial membrane
Femur, head
Gluteus medius m & t
Obturator internus m
Post acetabular labrum
Ischiofemoral lig
Ischium
Sciatic n
Inf gluteal a
Gluteus maximus m
Sacrotuberous lig
Greater trochanter
Obturator internus t

Iliopsoas m & t
Femoral n
Femoral a & v
Pectineus m
Sartorius m
Rectus femoris m & t
Pubis
Ant acetabular labrum
Iliofemoral lig
Tensor fasciae latae m
Lig teres & synovial membrane
Femur, head
Gluteus minimus m & t
Obturator internus m
Gluteus medius m & t
Post acetabular labrum
Ischiofemoral lig
Iliotibial tract
Ischium
Sciatic n
Inf gluteal a
Gluteus maximus m
Greater trochanter
Obturator internus t

Hip, Transverse

Iliopsoas m & t · Femoral n

Sartorius m

Rectus femoris m & t

Iliofemoral lig

Tensor fasciae latae m

Gluteus minimus m & t

Gluteus medius m & t

Iliotibial tract

Gluteus maximus m

Greater trochanter · Inf gemellus m

Pubis

Lig teres & synovial membrane

Femur, head

Obturator internus m

Post acetabular labrum

Ischiofemoral lig

Ischium

Obturator internus t

Sciatic n

Sacrotuberous lig

Iliopsoas m & t · Femoral n

Sartorius m

Rectus femoris m & t

Iliofemoral lig

Tensor fasciae latae m

Gluteus minimus m & t

Gluteus medius m & t

Iliotibial tract

Gluteus maximus m

Greater trochanter · Inf gemellus m

Femoral a & v

Pectineus m

Pubis

Ant acetabular labrum

Lig teres & synovial membrane

Femur, head

Obturator internus m

Post acetabular labrum

Ischiofemoral lig

Ischium

Obturator internus t

Sciatic n

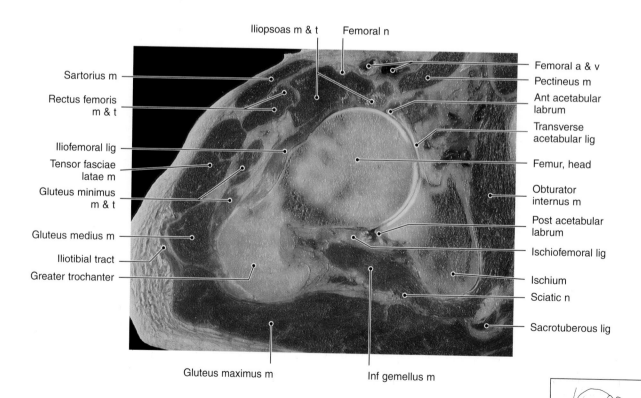

Iliopsoas m & t   Femoral n

Sartorius m

Rectus femoris m & t

Iliofemoral lig

Tensor fasciae latae m

Gluteus minimus m & t

Gluteus medius m

Iliotibial tract

Greater trochanter

Femoral a & v

Transverse acetabular lig

Femur, head

Obturator internus m

Ischiofemoral lig

Ischium

Sciatic n

Sacrotuberous lig

Gluteus maximus m

Inf gemellus m

Iliopsoas m & t   Femoral n

Sartorius m

Rectus femoris m & t

Iliofemoral lig

Tensor fasciae latae m

Gluteus minimus m & t

Gluteus medius m

Iliotibial tract

Greater trochanter

Femoral a & v

Pectineus m

Ant acetabular labrum

Transverse acetabular lig

Femur, head

Obturator internus m

Post acetabular labrum

Ischiofemoral lig

Ischium

Sciatic n

Sacrotuberous lig

Gluteus maximus m

Inf gemellus m

Hip, Transverse

Iliopsoas m & t
Femoral n
Femoral a & v
Pectineus m
Obturator externus m
Sartorius m
Rectus femoris m & t
Iliofemoral lig
Lat femoral circumflex a
Tensor fasciae latae m
Gluteus minimus m & t
Gluteus medius m
Iliotibial tract
Greater trochanter
Gluteus maximus m
Femur, head
Obturator internus m
Ischiofemoral lig
Ischium
Inf gemellus m
Sciatic n
Sacrotuberous lig
Obturator externus t
Quadratus femoris m

Iliopsoas m & t
Femoral n
Femoral a & v
Pectineus m
Sartorius m
Rectus femoris m & t
Iliofemoral lig
Lat femoral circumflex a
Tensor fasciae latae m
Gluteus minimus m & t
Gluteus medius m
Iliotibial tract
Greater trochanter
Gluteus maximus m
Obturator externus m
Transverse acetabular lig
Femur, head
Obturator internus m
Ischiofemoral lig
Inf gemellus m
Ischium
Sciatic n
Sacrotuberous lig
Obturator externus t
Quadratus femoris m

Iliopsoas m & t
Femoral n
Sartorius m
Rectus femoris m & t
Iliofemoral lig
Lat femoral circumflex a
Tensor fasciae latae m
Gluteus minimus t
Gluteus medius m
Iliotibial tract
Greater trochanter
Gluteus maximus m
Femoral a & v
Pectineus m
Obturator externus m
Femur, head
Obturator internus m
Ischium, tuberosity
Sciatic n
Semimembranosus t
Biceps femoris & semitendinosus tt
Sacrotuberous lig
Obturator externus t
Quadratus femoris m

Iliopsoas m & t
Femoral n
Sartorius m
Rectus femoris m & t
Iliofemoral lig
Lat femoral circumflex a
Tensor fasciae latae m
Gluteus minimus t
Gluteus medius m
Iliotibial tract
Greater trochanter
Gluteus maximus m
Femoral a & v
Pectineus m
Obturator externus m
Femur, head
Obturator internus m
Ischiofemoral lig
Ischium, tuberosity
Sciatic n
Semimembranosus t
Biceps femoris & semitendinosus tt
Obturator externus t
Quadratus femoris m

Hip, Transverse

Iliopsoas m & t · Femoral n

Sartorius m

Rectus femoris m & t

Iliofemoral lig

Lat femoral circumflex a

Tensor fasciae latae m

Gluteus minimus t

Iliotibial tract

Greater trochanter

Gluteus maximus m

Femoral a & v

Adductor longus m

Pectineus m

Obturator externus m

Femur, neck

Quadratus femoris m

Ischium, tuberosity

Sciatic n

Semimembranosus t

Biceps femoris & semitendinosus tt

Iliopsoas m & t · Femoral n

Sartorius m

Rectus femoris m & t

Iliofemoral lig

Lat femoral circumflex a

Tensor fasciae latae m

Gluteus minimus t

Iliotibial tract

Greater trochanter

Gluteus maximus m

Femoral a & v

Pectineus m

Adductor longus m

Obturator externus m

Femur, neck

Quadratus femoris m

Ischium, tuberosity

Sciatic n

Semimembranosus t

Biceps femoris & semitendinosus tt

Sacrotuberous lig

Femoral n, branches

Femoral a & v

Sartorius m

Rectus femoris m

Iliofemoral lig

Lat femoral circumflex a

Vastus lateralis m

Tensor fasciae latae m

Femur

Iliotibial tract

Pectineus m

Adductor longus m

Adductor brevis m

Iliopsoas m & t

Med femoral circumflex a

Obturator externus m

Quadratus femoris m

Ischium, tuberosity

Semimembranosus t

Biceps femoris & semitendinosus tt

Gluteus maximus m

Sciatic n

Femoral n, branches

Femoral a & v

Sartorius m

Rectus femoris m

Lat femoral circumflex a

Iliofemoral lig

Vastus lateralis m

Tensor fasciae latae m

Femur

Iliotibial tract

Pectineus m

Adductor longus m

Iliopsoas m & t

Adductor brevis m

Med femoral circumflex a

Obturator externus m

Quadratus femoris m

Ischium, tuberosity

Semimembranosus t

Biceps femoris & semitendinosus tt

Gluteus maximus m

Sciatic n

Hip, Transverse

Femoral n, branches

Femoral a & v

Sartorius m

Deep femoral a & v

Rectus femoris m

Lat femoral circumflex a

Iliofemoral lig

Vastus lateralis m

Tensor fasciae latae m

Femur, calcar

Femur

Iliotibial tract

Pectineus m

Adductor longus m

Adductor brevis m

Iliopsoas m & t

Med femoral circumflex a

Quadratus femoris m

Ischium

Sciatic n

Semimembranosus t

Biceps femoris & semitendinosus tt

Vastus lateralis t

Gluteus maximus m

Femoral n, branches

Femoral a & v

Sartorius m

Deep femoral a & v

Rectus femoris m

Lat femoral circumflex a

Iliofemoral lig

Vastus lateralis m

Tensor fasciae latae m

Femur, calcar

Femur

Iliotibial tract

Pectineus m

Adductor longus m

Adductor brevis m

Iliopsoas m & t

Med femoral circumflex a

Quadratus femoris m

Sciatic n

Semimembranosus t

Biceps femoris & semitendinosus tt

Vastus lateralis t

Gluteus maximus m

Femoral n, branches

Femoral a & v

Sartorius m

Rectus femoris m

Deep femoral a & v

Vastus intermedius m

Tensor fasciae latae m

Femur, calcar

Vastus lateralis m

Femur

Iliotibial tract

Adductor longus m

Pectineus m

Adductor brevis m

Iliopsoas m & t

Quadratus femoris m

Semimembranosus t

Biceps femoris & semitendinosus tt

Gluteus maximus m

Sciatic n

Femoral n, branches

Femoral a & v

Sartorius m

Rectus femoris m

Deep femoral a & v

Vastus intermedius m

Femur,calcar

Tensor fasciae latae m

Vastus lateralis m

Femur

Iliotibial tract

Adductor longus m

Pectineus m

Adductor brevis m

Iliopsoas m & t

Quadratus femoris m

Semimembranosus t

Biceps femoris & semitendinosus tt

Gluteus maximus m

Sciatic n

Hip, Sagittal

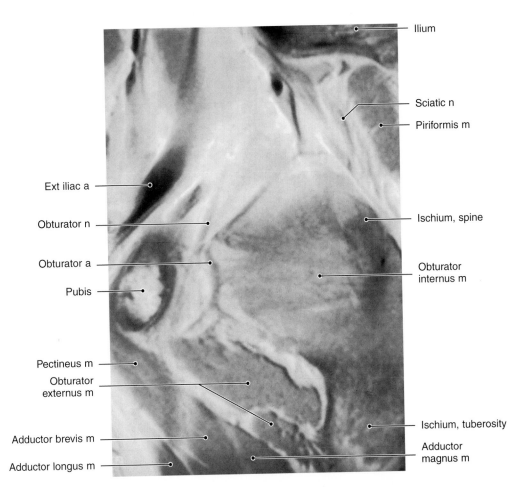

Ilium

Sciatic n

Piriformis m

Ext iliac a

Obturator n

Ischium, spine

Obturator a

Obturator
internus m

Pubis

Pectineus m

Obturator
externus m

Ischium, tuberosity

Adductor brevis m

Adductor longus m

Adductor
magnus m

Sciatic n

Piriformis m

Ext iliac a

Obturator n

Inf gluteal a

Ischium, spine

Obturator a

Pubis

Obturator
internus m

Obturator
externus m

Inf gemellus m

Pectineus m

Ischium, tuberosity

Adductor brevis m

Adductor
magnus m

Adductor longus m

Semimembranosus t

Hip, Sagittal

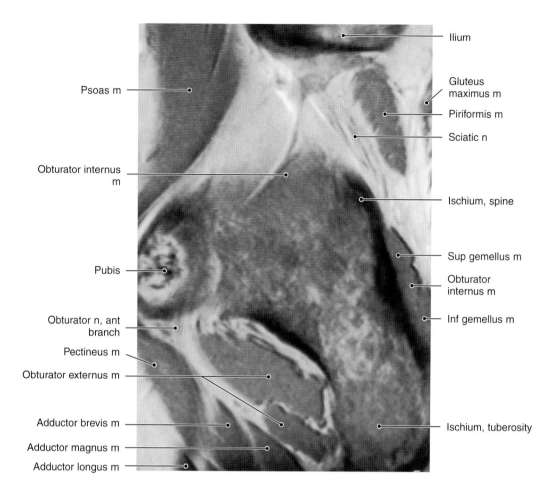

Psoas m

Obturator internus m

Pubis

Obturator n, ant branch

Pectineus m

Obturator externus m

Adductor brevis m

Adductor magnus m

Adductor longus m

Ilium

Gluteus maximus m

Piriformis m

Sciatic n

Ischium, spine

Sup gemellus m

Obturator internus m

Inf gemellus m

Ischium, tuberosity

Psoas m

Obturator internus m

Pubis

Obturator n, ant branch

Obturator externus m

Pectineus m

Adductor magnus m

Adductor brevis m

Adductor longus m

Piriformis m

Sciatic n

Gluteus maximus m

Ischium, spine

Inf gluteal a

Sup gemellus m

Obturator internus m

Inf gemellus m

Ischium, tuberosity

Quadratus femoris m

Semimembranosus t

Hip, Sagittal

Ilium

Iliopsoas m

Acetabular fossa

Obturator
externus m

Pectineus m

Adductor
magnus m

Adductor brevis m

Piriformis m

Gluteus
maximus m

Sciatic n

Sup gemellus m

Obturator internus t

Inf gemellus m

Ischium, tuberosity

Quadratus
femoris m

Ilium

Iliopsoas m

Ligamentum teres

Obturator
externus m

Pectineus m

Adductor
magnus m

Adductor brevis m

Adductor longus m

Piriformis m

Gluteus
maximus m

Sciatic n

Inf gluteal a

Sup gemellus m

Obturator internus t

Inf gemellus m

Ischium, tuberosity

Biceps femoris &
semitendinosus mm

Quadratus
femoris m

Semimembranosus t

Hip, Sagittal

Ilium

Iliopsoas m & t

Femur, head

Femoral a

Pectineus m

Femoral v

Adductor brevis m

Adductor magnus m

Gluteus medius m

Gluteus minimus m

Piriformis m

Sciatic n

Sup gemellus m

Obturator internus t

Inf gemellus m

Post acetabular labrum

Obturator externus m

Semimembranosus t

Quadratus femoris m

Ilium

Iliopsoas m & t

Femur, head

Ant acetabular labrum

Femoral a

Pectineus m

Adductor brevis m

Femoral v

Gluteus medius m

Gluteus minimus m

Piriformis m

Gluteus maximus m

Sciatic n

Sup gemellus m

Obturator internus t

Inf gemellus m

Post acetabular labrum

Obturator externus m

Semimembranosus t

Quadratus femoris m

Adductor magnus m

Biceps femoris & semitendinosus mm

Hip, Sagittal

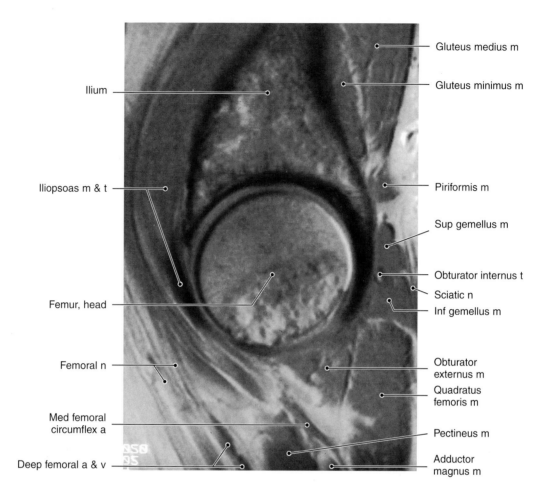

Ilium

Iliopsoas m & t

Femur, head

Femoral n

Med femoral circumflex a

Deep femoral a & v

Gluteus medius m

Gluteus minimus m

Piriformis m

Sup gemellus m

Obturator internus t

Sciatic n

Inf gemellus m

Obturator externus m

Quadratus femoris m

Pectineus m

Adductor magnus m

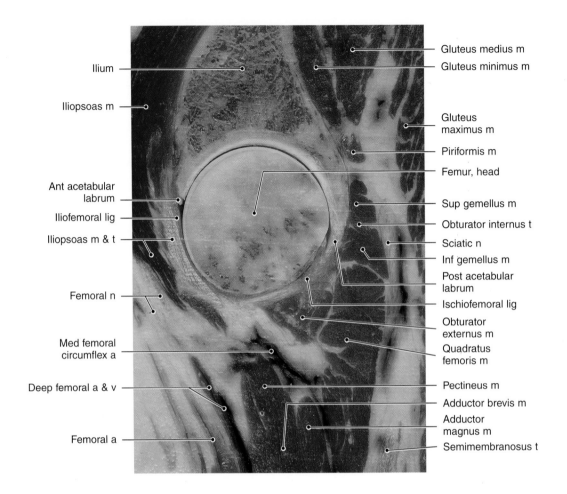

Ilium

Iliopsoas m

Ant acetabular labrum

Iliofemoral lig

Iliopsoas m & t

Femoral n

Med femoral circumflex a

Deep femoral a & v

Femoral a

Gluteus medius m

Gluteus minimus m

Gluteus maximus m

Piriformis m

Femur, head

Sup gemellus m

Obturator internus t

Sciatic n

Inf gemellus m

Post acetabular labrum

Ischiofemoral lig

Obturator externus m

Quadratus femoris m

Pectineus m

Adductor brevis m

Adductor magnus m

Semimembranosus t

Hip, Sagittal

Ilium

Ant inf iliac spine

Iliofemoral lig

Femur, head

Iliopsoas m & t

Sartorius m

Lat femoral circumflex a

Gluteus medius m

Gluteus minimus m

Gluteus maximus m

Piriformis t

Sup gemellus m

Obturator internus t

Inf gemellus m

Ischiofemoral lig

Obturator externus t

Sciatic n

Quadratus femoris m

Pectineus m

Ilium

Ant inf iliac spine

Ant acetabular labrum

Iliofemoral lig

Femur, head

Iliopsoas m & t

Sartorius m

Lat femoral circumflex a

Gluteus medius m

Gluteus maximus m

Gluteus minimus m

Piriformis t

Post acetabular labrum

Sup gemellus m

Obturator internus t

Inf gemellus m

Ischiofemoral lig

Obturator externus t

Quadratus femoris m

Sciatic n

Pectineus m

Adductor magnus m

Hip, Sagittal

Ilium

Gluteus medius m

Gluteus minimus m

Rectus femoris t

Sup acetabular labrum

Iliofemoral lig

Piriformis t

Sup gemellus m

Obturator internus t

Femur

Inf gemellus m

Iliopsoas m

Obturator externus t

Quadratus femoris m

Sartorius m

Rectus femoris m

Lesser trochanter

Lat femoral circumflex a

Ilium

Gluteus medius m

Gluteus minimus m

Rectus femoris t, reflected head

Sup acetabular labrum

Rectus femoris t

Piriformis t

Iliofemoral lig

Sup gemellus m

Iliopsoas m

Obturator internus t

Inf gemellus m

Femur

Obturator externus t

Iliofemoral lig

Quadratus femoris m

Sartorius m

Lat femoral circumflex a

Iliopsoas t

Rectus femoris m

Pectineus m

Hip, Sagittal

Gluteus minimus m

Iliofemoral lig

Rectus femoris m

Vastus intermedius m

Gluteus maximus m

Gluteus medius m & t

Piriformis t

Greater trochanter

Obturator externus t

Gluteus maximus m

Quadratus femoris m

Femur

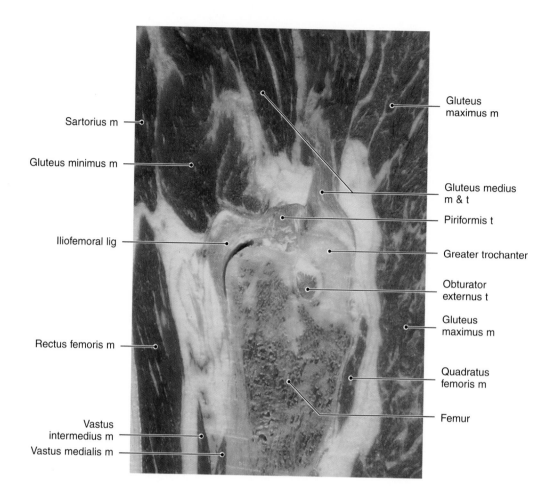

Sartorius m

Gluteus minimus m

Iliofemoral lig

Rectus femoris m

Vastus
intermedius m

Vastus medialis m

Gluteus
maximus m

Gluteus medius
m & t

Piriformis t

Greater trochanter

Obturator
externus t

Gluteus
maximus m

Quadratus
femoris m

Femur

8

Upper Leg (Thigh)

Thigh, Coronal

Gluteus maximus m

Semitendinosus m

Vastus lateralis m

Adductor magnus m

Semimembranosus m

Biceps femoris m, short head

Sciatic n

Biceps femoris m, long head

Gracilis m

Popliteal a

Sartorius m

Lat femoral condyle

Gracilis t

Fabella

Semitendinosus t

Sartorius t

Gastrocnemius m, lat head

Gastrocnemius m, med head

Gluteus maximus m

Semitendinosus m

Vastus lateralis m

Adductor magnus m

Semimembranosus m

Biceps femoris m,
short head

Sciatic n

Biceps femoris m,
long head

Gracilis m

Popliteal a

Sartorius m
Lat femoral condyle
Gracilis t
Fabella
Semitendinosus t
Sartorius t
Gastrocnemius m,
lat head

Gastrocnemius m,
med head

Thigh, Coronal

Gluteus minimus m

Gluteus medius m

Femur, head

Femoral triangle

Femoral v

Deep femoral a

Vastus lateralis m

Femoral v

Vastus intermedius m

Adductor canal

Femur

Prefemoral fat body

Vastus lateralis t &
lat patellar retinaculum

Iliotibial tract

Tibia

Ilium

Obturator internus m

Obturator externus m

Inf pubic ramus

Femoral a

Pectineus m

Adductor brevis m

Deep femoral v

Adductor longus m

Femoral a

Gracilis m

Adductor magnus m

Femoral a

Greater saphenous v

Sartorius m

Vastus medialis m

Med meniscus

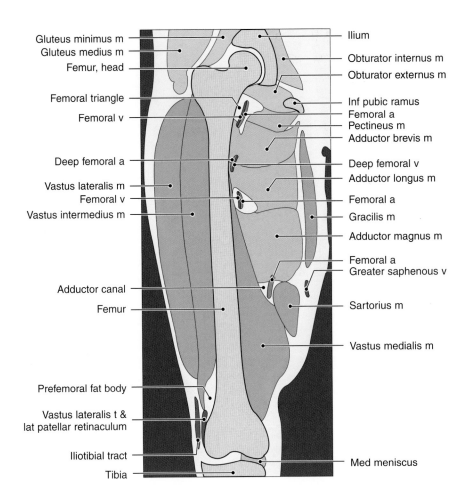

Gluteus minimus m
Gluteus medius m
Femur, head

Femoral triangle
Femoral v

Deep femoral a

Vastus lateralis m
Femoral v
Vastus intermedius m

Adductor canal

Femur

Prefemoral fat body

Vastus lateralis t &
lat patellar retinaculum

Iliotibial tract
Tibia

Ilium
Obturator internus m
Obturator externus m

Inf pubic ramus
Femoral a
Pectineus m
Adductor brevis m

Deep femoral v
Adductor longus m

Femoral a
Gracilis m

Adductor magnus m

Femoral a
Greater saphenous v

Sartorius m

Vastus medialis m

Med meniscus

Thigh, Coronal

Gluteus minimus m —
Gluteus medius m —
Femur, head —
Obturator externus m —
Iliopsoas m —
Tensor fasciae latae m —

Femoral v —
Femoral a —

Vastus intermedius m —

Vastus lateralis m —

Quadriceps t —

Patellar lig —

— Acetabulum
— Urinary bladder
— Sup pubic ramus
— Corpus cavernosum
— Corpus spongiosum

— Pectineus m
— Adductor longus m
— Gracilis m

— Adductor magnus m

— Femoral v
— Femoral a

— Sartorius m

— Vastus medialis m

— Patella

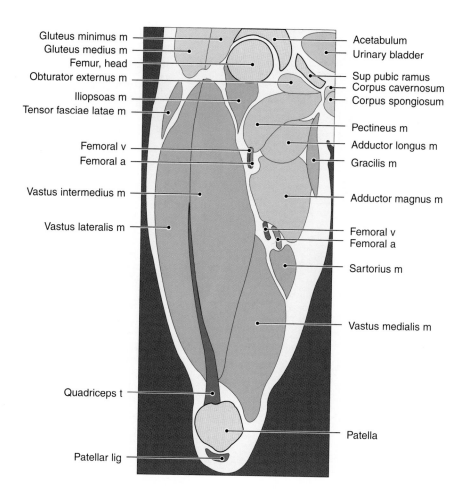

Gluteus minimus m

Gluteus medius m

Femur, head

Obturator externus m

Iliopsoas m

Tensor fasciae latae m

Femoral v

Femoral a

Vastus intermedius m

Vastus lateralis m

Quadriceps t

Patellar lig

Acetabulum

Urinary bladder

Sup pubic ramus

Corpus cavernosum

Corpus spongiosum

Pectineus m

Adductor longus m

Gracilis m

Adductor magnus m

Femoral v

Femoral a

Sartorius m

Vastus medialis m

Patella

Thigh, Coronal

Iliopsoas m

Tensor fasciae latae m

Inguinal lymph node

Rectus femoris m

Vastus lateralis m

Femoral a

Femoral v

Urinary bladder

Pectineus m

Corpus cavernosum

Corpus spongiosum

Inguinal lymph node

Adductor longus m

Testis

Sartorius m

Vastus medialis m

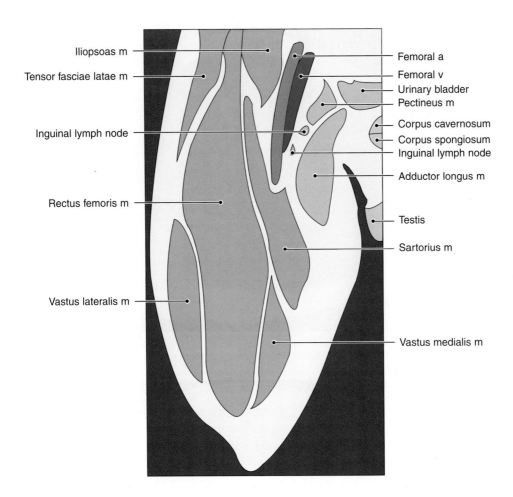

Iliopsoas m

Tensor fasciae latae m

Inguinal lymph node

Rectus femoris m

Vastus lateralis m

Femoral a

Femoral v

Urinary bladder

Pectineus m

Corpus cavernosum

Corpus spongiosum

Inguinal lymph node

Adductor longus m

Testis

Sartorius m

Vastus medialis m

Thigh, Transverse

Fascia lata
Rectus femoris m & t
Tensor fasciae latae m
Vastus intermedius m
Vastus medialis m
Vastus lateralis m
Femur
Iliotibial tract
Vastus lateralis t
Lat intermuscular septum
Sciatic n
Gluteus maximus m

Greater saphenous v
Sartorius m
Femoral a
Femoral n
Femoral v
Adductor longus m & t
Deep femoral a & v
Gracilis m
Adductor brevis m
Adductor magnus m
Semimembranosus t
Semitendinosus m
Biceps femoris t, long head

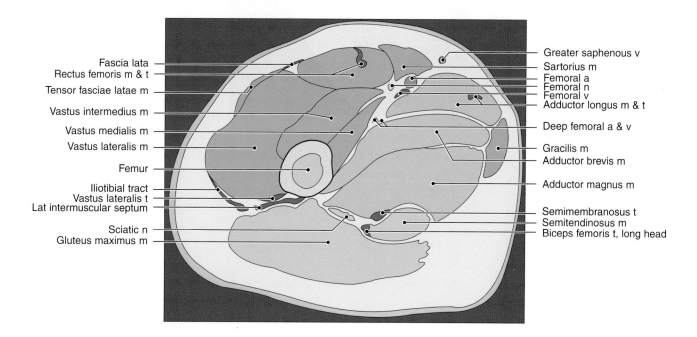

Fascia lata
Rectus femoris m & t
Tensor fasciae latae m
Vastus intermedius m
Vastus medialis m
Vastus lateralis m
Femur
Iliotibial tract
Vastus lateralis t
Lat intermuscular septum
Sciatic n
Gluteus maximus m

Greater saphenous v
Sartorius m
Femoral a
Femoral n
Femoral v
Adductor longus m & t
Deep femoral a & v
Gracilis m
Adductor brevis m
Adductor magnus m
Semimembranosus t
Semitendinosus m
Biceps femoris t, long head

Rectus femoris m & t

Femoral a & v
Vastus intermedius m

Vastus medialis m
Vastus lateralis m
Femur

Linea aspera

Sciatic n
Biceps femoris m,
long head
Gluteus maximus m

Sartorius m
Greater saphenous v
Femoral n
Femoral n,
ant cutaneous branch
Adductor longus m
Superficial fascia
Adductor brevis m
Deep femoral a & v
Gracilis m
Adductor magnus m
Fascia lata
Semimembranosus t
Biceps femoris t,
long head
Semitendinosus m

Rectus femoris m & t

Femoral a & v
Vastus intermedius m

Vastus medialis m
Vastus lateralis m
Femur

Linea aspera

Sciatic n
Biceps femoris m,
long head
Gluteus maximus m

Sartorius m
Greater saphenous v
Femoral n
Femoral n,
ant cutaneous branch
Adductor longus m
Superficial fascia
Adductor brevis m
Deep femoral a & v
Gracilis m
Adductor magnus m
Fascia lata
Semimembranosus t
Biceps femoris t,
long head
Semitendinosus m

Thigh, Transverse

Rectus femoris m & t
Vastus medialis m
Vastus intermedius m
Femur
Vastus lateralis m
Linea aspera
Lat intermuscular septum
Sciatic n
Perforating a & v
Biceps femoris m & t, long head
Fascia lata

Sartorius m
Greater saphenous v
Femoral n
Femoral a & v
Femoral n, ant cutaneous branch
Superficial fascia
Adductor longus m
Deep femoral a & v
Gracilis m
Adductor magnus m
Semimembranosus t
Semitendinosus m
Superficial fascia
Semimembranosus m

Rectus femoris m & t
Vastus medialis m
Vastus intermedius m
Femur
Vastus lateralis m
Linea aspera
Lat intermuscular septum
Sciatic n
Perforating a & v
Biceps femoris m & t, long head
Fascia lata

Sartorius m
Greater saphenous v
Femoral n
Femoral a & v
Femoral n, ant cutaneous branch
Superficial fascia
Adductor longus m
Deep femoral a & v
Gracilis m
Adductor magnus m
Semimembranosus t
Semitendinosus m
Superficial fascia
Semimembranosus m

Rectus femoris m
Vastus lateralis m
Vastus intermedius m
Femur
Linea aspera
Biceps femoris m, short head
Perforating a & v
Sciatic n
Lat intermuscular septum
Fascia lata
Biceps femoris m, long head

Vastus medialis m
Intermediate cutaneous n
Sartorius m
Femoral a & v
Saphenous n
Greater saphenous v
Adductor longus m
Superficial fascia
Adductor magnus m
Gracilis m
Semimembranosus t
Semitendinosus m
Semimembranosus m

Rectus femoris m
Vastus lateralis m
Vastus intermedius m
Femur
Linea aspera
Biceps femoris m, short head
Perforating a & v
Sciatic n
Lat intermuscular septum
Fascia lata
Biceps femoris m, long head

Vastus medialis m
Intermediate cutaneous n
Sartorius m
Femoral a & v
Saphenous n
Greater saphenous v
Adductor longus m
Superficial fascia
Adductor magnus m
Gracilis m
Semimembranosus t
Semitendinosus m
Semimembranosus m

Thigh, Transverse

Vastus lateralis m & t

Vastus intermedius m

Femur

Vastus lateralis t

Adductor magnus m

Biceps femoris m, short head

Common peroneal n

Tibial n

Biceps femoris m, long head

Fascia lata

Rectus femoris m & t

Vastus intermedius t

Vastus medialis m

Popliteal a & v

Saphenous n

Greater saphenous v

Sartorius m

Adductor magnus m & t

Superficial fascia

Semimembranosus m

Gracilis m

Gracilis t

Semitendinosus m & t

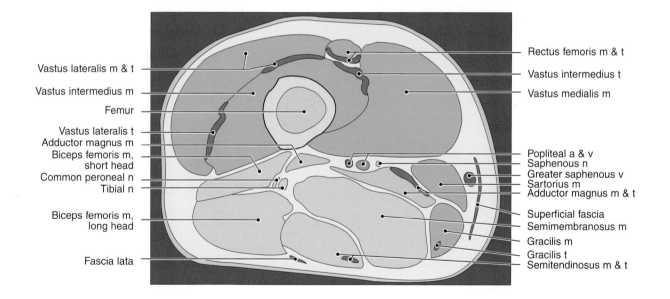

Vastus lateralis m & t

Vastus intermedius m

Femur

Vastus lateralis t

Adductor magnus m

Biceps femoris m, short head

Common peroneal n

Tibial n

Biceps femoris m, long head

Fascia lata

Rectus femoris m & t

Vastus intermedius t

Vastus medialis m

Popliteal a & v

Saphenous n

Greater saphenous v

Sartorius m

Adductor magnus m & t

Superficial fascia

Semimembranosus m

Gracilis m

Gracilis t

Semitendinosus m & t

Rectus femoris t
Fascia lata
Vastus lateralis m & t
Vastus intermedius m
Femur
Iliotibial tract
Popliteal v
Biceps femoris m, short head
Common peroneal n
Tibial n
Biceps femoris m, long head
Semitendinosus m & tt
Fascia lata

Vastus intermedius t
Suprapatellar bursa
Vastus intermedius m
Vastus medialis m
Fascia lata
Popliteal a
Adductor magnus m & t
Greater saphenous v
Sartorius m
Semimembranosus m
Gracilis m & t
Fascia lata

Rectus femoris t
Fascia lata
Vastus lateralis m & t
Vastus intermedius m
Femur
Iliotibial tract
Popliteal v
Biceps femoris m, short head
Common peroneal n
Tibial n
Biceps femoris m, long head
Semitendinosus m & tt
Fascia lata

Vastus intermedius t
Suprapatellar bursa
Vastus intermedius m
Vastus medialis m
Fascia lata
Popliteal a
Adductor magnus m & t
Greater saphenous v
Sartorius m
Semimembranosus m
Gracilis m & t
Fascia lata

Thigh, Sagittal

Sup pubic ramus

Pectineus m

Adductor brevis m

Adductor longus m

Sartorius m

Vastus medialis m

Med femoral condyle

Med meniscus

Tibia

Piriformis m

Ilium

Obturator internus m

Gluteus maximus m

Sciatic n

Adductor magnus m

Semimembranosus m

Semitendinosus m

Gracilis m

Semimembranosus t

Gastrocnemius m, med head

Sup pubic ramus

Pectineus m

Adductor brevis m

Adductor longus m

Sartorius m

Vastus medialis m

Med femoral condyle

Med meniscus

Tibia

Piriformis m

Ilium

Obturator internus m

Gluteus maximus m

Sciatic n

Adductor magnus m

Semimembranosus m

Semitendinosus m

Gracilis m

Semimembranosus t

Gastrocnemius m,
med head

Thigh, Sagittal

Iliopsoas m
Femur, head
Femoral v
Femoral a
Sartorius m
Adductor longus m
Vastus medialis m
Prefemoral fat body
Patella
Infrapatellar fat body
Patellar lig
Ant cruciate lig
Tibia

Piriformis m
Sup & inf gemellus mm
Gluteus maximus m
Quadratus femoris m
Obturator externus m
Adductor magnus m
Semitendinosus m
Popliteal v
Popliteal a
Semimembranosus m
Gastrocnemius m, med head
Post cruciate lig

Iliopsoas m

Femur, head

Femoral v

Femoral a

Sartorius m

Adductor longus m

Vastus medialis m

Prefemoral fat body

Patella

Infrapatellar fat body

Patellar lig

Ant cruciate lig

Tibia

Piriformis m

Sup & inf gemellus mm

Gluteus maximus m

Quadratus femoris m

Obturator externus m

Adductor magnus m

Semitendinosus m

Popliteal v

Popliteal a

Semimembranosus m

Gastrocnemius m, med head

Post cruciate lig

Thigh, Sagittal

Gluteus medius m

Sartorius m

Tensor fasciae latae m

Lat femoral circumflex a

Rectus femoris m

Vastus intermedius m

Prefemoral fat body

Quadriceps t

Patella

Patellar lig

Infrapatellar fat body

Tibia

Gluteus maximus m

Quadratus femoris m

Adductor magnus m

Femur

Biceps femoris m, long head

Biceps femoris m, short head

Lat femoral condyle

Gastrocnemius m, lat head

Lat meniscus

Gluteus medius m

Sartorius m

Tensor fasciae latae m

Lat femoral
circumflex a

Rectus femoris m

Vastus intermedius m

Prefemoral fat body

Quadriceps t

Patella

Patellar lig

Infrapatellar fat body

Tibia

Gluteus maximus m

Quadratus femoris m

Adductor magnus m

Femur

Biceps femoris m,
long head

Biceps femoris m,
short head

Lat femoral condyle

Gastrocnemius m,
lat head

Lat meniscus

Thigh, Sagittal

Gluteus medius m

Tensor fasciae latae m

Lat femoral circumflex a

Greater trochanter

Gluteus maximus m

Rectus femoris m

Vastus lateralis m

Biceps femoris m, long head

Vastus lateralis t

Biceps femoris m, short head

Knee, Coronal

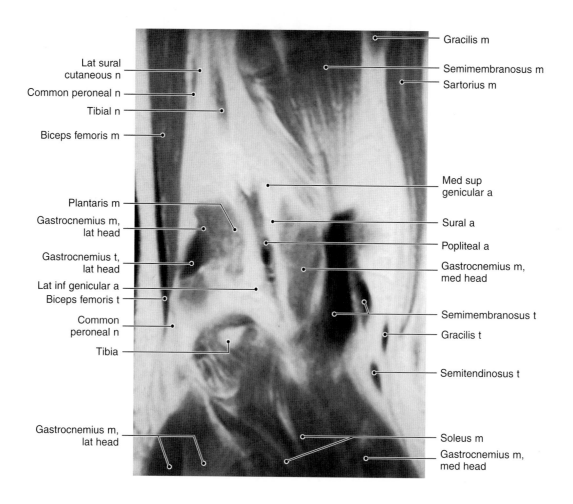

Gracilis m

Lat sural
cutaneous n

Common peroneal n

Tibial n

Biceps femoris m

Semimembranosus m

Sartorius m

Med sup
genicular a

Plantaris m

Gastrocnemius m,
lat head

Sural a

Popliteal a

Gastrocnemius t,
lat head

Gastrocnemius m,
med head

Lat inf genicular a

Biceps femoris t

Common
peroneal n

Tibia

Semimembranosus t

Gracilis t

Semitendinosus t

Gastrocnemius m,
lat head

Soleus m

Gastrocnemius m,
med head

9
Knee

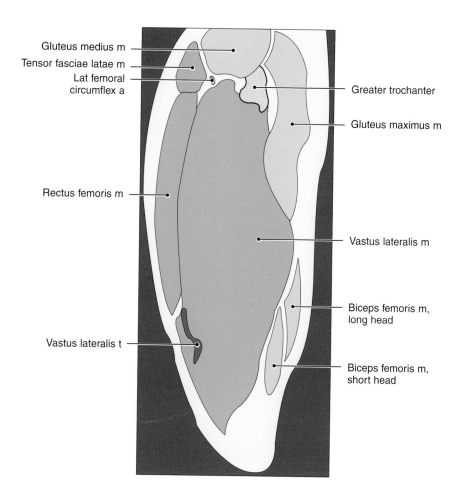

Gluteus medius m

Tensor fasciae latae m

Lat femoral circumflex a

Greater trochanter

Gluteus maximus m

Rectus femoris m

Vastus lateralis m

Biceps femoris m, long head

Vastus lateralis t

Biceps femoris m, short head

Biceps femoris m

Lat sural
cutaneous n

Common
peroneal n

Tibial n

Biceps femoris t

Gastrocnemius t,
lat head

Plantaris m

Gastrocnemius m,
lat head

Gracilis m

Semimembranosus m

Sartorius m

Popliteal a & v

Gastrocnemius m,
med head

Semimembranosus t

Gracilis t

Semitendinosus t

Soleus m

Gastrocnemius m,
med head

Knee, Coronal

Common peroneal n

Tibial n

Biceps femoris m

Perforating a

Gastrocnemius m & t, lat head

Lat femoral condyle

Popliteus t

Biceps femoris t

Post meniscofemoral lig of Wrisberg

Lat tibial plateau

Fibula

Soleus m & t

Semimembranosus m

Sartorius m

Saphenous n

Med inf genicular a

Joint capsule

Popliteal a

Med femoral condyle

Gastrocnemius m, med head

Sartorius t

Med tibial plateau

Post cruciate lig

Gracilis t

Semimembranosus t

Semitendinosus t

Gastrocnemius m, med head

Common peroneal n

Tibial n

Perforating a

Biceps femoris m

Popliteal a

Gastrocnemius m & t, lat head

Lat femoral condyle

Popliteus t

Biceps femoris t

Arcuate popliteal lig & joint capsule

Lat tibial plateau

Fibula

Soleus m & t

Semimembranosus m

Sartorius m

Saphenous n

Gastrocnemius m & t, med head

Joint capsule

Med femoral condyle

Oblique popliteal lig & tibial collateral lig

Sartorius t

Med tibial plateau

Post cruciate lig

Gracilis t

Semimembranosus t

Semitendinosus t

Gastrocnemius m, med head

Knee, Coronal

Lat sup genicular a

Biceps femoris m

Gastrocnemius
m & t, lat head

Lat femoral condyle

Popliteus t

Lat meniscus, post horn

Biceps femoris t

Fibular collateral lig

Sup tibiofibular joint

Fibula

Popliteus m

Peroneus longus m

Sartorius m

Saphenous n

Med sup
genicular a

Popliteal a

Gastrocnemius
m & t, med head

Med femoral condyle

Lat inf genicular a

Med inf genicular a

Sartorius t

Med meniscus, post horn

Post cruciate lig

Tibia

Semimembranosus t

Sartorius t

Gracilis t

Semitendinosus t

Gastrocnemius m,
med head

Biceps femoris m

Gastrocnemius
m & t, lat head

Lat femoral condyle
Lat inf genicular a

Lat meniscus, post horn
Popliteus t
Biceps femoris t
Fibular collateral lig

Sup tibiofibular joint

Fibula

Popliteus m

Semimembranosus m

Sartorius m

Med sup
genicular a
Popliteal a

Gastrocnemius
m & t, med head

Med femoral condyle

Med inf genicular a

Sartorius t
Med meniscus, post horn

Post cruciate lig

Tibia

Semimembranosus t

Gracilis t

Semitendinosus t

Gastrocnemius m,
med head

Knee, Coronal

Vastus lateralis m
Biceps femoris m
Iliotibial tract

Popliteal a

Gastrocnemius m & t, med head

Gastrocnemius m & t, lat head

Lat inf genicular a
Ant cruciate lig
Lat femoral condyle
Popliteus t
Fibular collateral lig
Lat meniscus

Med femoral condyle

Post cruciate lig
Med meniscus

Inf fascicle, lat meniscus
Biceps femoris t

Sartorius t
Tibia
Semimembranosus t

Sup tibiofibular joint

Fibula

Gracilis t
Med inf genicular a
Semitendinosus t
Popliteus m

Peroneus longus m

Vastus lateralis m

Biceps femoris m

Iliotibial tract

Gastrocnemius
m & t, lat head

Lat inf genicular a

Ant cruciate lig

Lat femoral condyle

Lat meniscus

Popliteus t

Inf fascicle,
lat meniscus

Fibular collateral lig

Biceps femoris t

Sup tibiofibular joint

Fibula

Peroneus longus m

Popliteal a

Gastrocnemius
m & t, med head

Med femoral condyle

Post cruciate lig

Med meniscus

Tibia

Semimembranosus t

Sartorius t

Gracilis t

Semitendinosus t

Popliteus m

Knee, Coronal

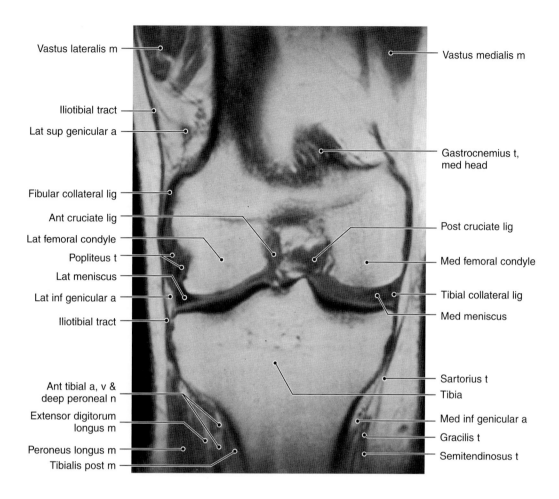

Vastus lateralis m

Iliotibial tract

Lat sup genicular a

Fibular collateral lig

Ant cruciate lig

Lat femoral condyle

Popliteus t

Lat meniscus

Lat inf genicular a

Iliotibial tract

Ant tibial a, v & deep peroneal n

Extensor digitorum longus m

Peroneus longus m

Tibialis post m

Vastus medialis m

Gastrocnemius t, med head

Post cruciate lig

Med femoral condyle

Tibial collateral lig

Med meniscus

Sartorius t

Tibia

Med inf genicular a

Gracilis t

Semitendinosus t

Vastus medialis m

Vastus lateralis m

Lat sup genicular a

Iliotibial tract

Ant cruciate lig

Gastrocnemius t,
med head

Fibular collateral lig

Lat femoral condyle

Med femoral condyle

Popliteus t

Post cruciate lig

Med meniscus

Iliotibial tract

Tibial collateral lig

Lat meniscus

Sartorius t

Ant tibial a, v &
deep peroneal n

Tibia

Extensor digitorum
longus m

Med inf genicular a

Peroneus longus m

Gracilis t

Semitendinosus t

Tibialis post m

Knee, Coronal

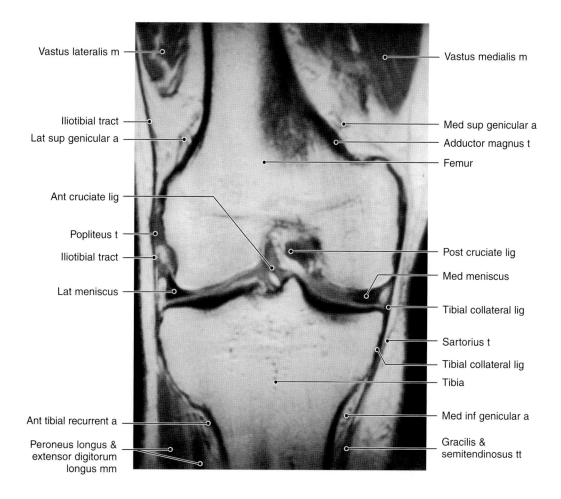

Vastus lateralis m

Vastus medialis m

Iliotibial tract

Lat sup genicular a

Med sup genicular a

Adductor magnus t

Femur

Ant cruciate lig

Popliteus t

Iliotibial tract

Lat meniscus

Post cruciate lig

Med meniscus

Tibial collateral lig

Sartorius t

Tibial collateral lig

Tibia

Ant tibial recurrent a

Med inf genicular a

Peroneus longus &
extensor digitorum
longus mm

Gracilis &
semitendinosus tt

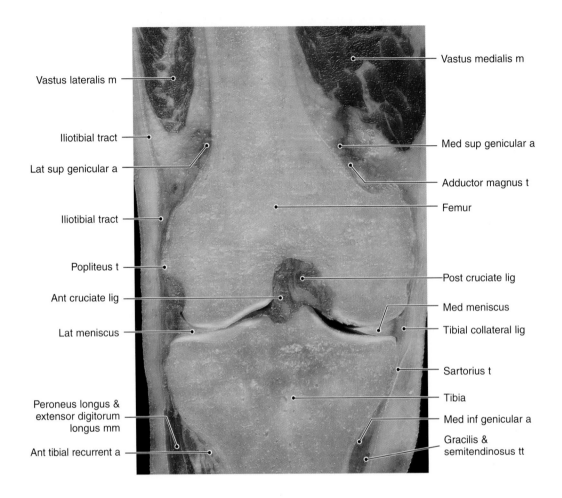

Vastus lateralis m

Vastus medialis m

Iliotibial tract

Lat sup genicular a

Med sup genicular a

Adductor magnus t

Iliotibial tract

Femur

Popliteus t

Post cruciate lig

Ant cruciate lig

Med meniscus

Lat meniscus

Tibial collateral lig

Sartorius t

Peroneus longus & extensor digitorum longus mm

Tibia

Med inf genicular a

Ant tibial recurrent a

Gracilis & semitendinosus tt

Knee, Coronal

Vastus lateralis m

Lat sup genicular a

Iliotibial tract

Femur

Ant cruciate lig

Iliotibial tract

Lat meniscus

Extensor digitorum longus m

Ant tibial recurrent a

Vastus medialis m

Med sup genicular a

Tibial collateral lig

Post cruciate lig

Med meniscus

Tibial collateral lig

Tibia

Med inf genicular a

Sartorius, gracilis & semitendinosus tt

Vastus lateralis m

Lat sup genicular a

Femur

Ant cruciate lig

Infrapatellar fat body

Lat meniscus,
ant horn

Iliotibial tract

Extensor digitorum
longus m

Ant tibial recurrent a

Vastus medialis m

Med sup
genicular a

Post cruciate lig

Med meniscus

Tibial collateral lig

Tibia

Med inf genicular a

Sartorius, gracilis &
semitendinosus tt

Knee, Coronal

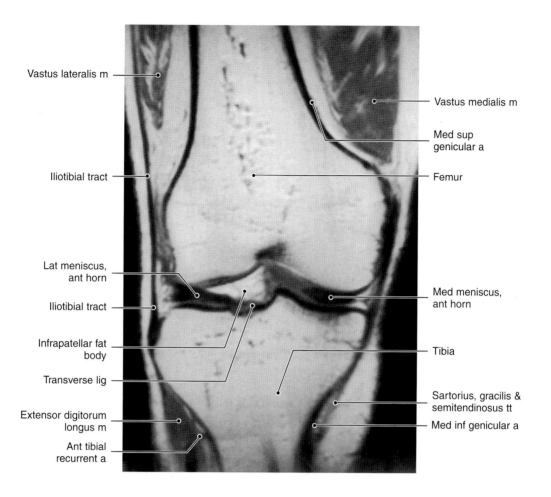

Vastus lateralis m

Iliotibial tract

Lat meniscus, ant horn

Iliotibial tract

Infrapatellar fat body

Transverse lig

Extensor digitorum longus m

Ant tibial recurrent a

Vastus medialis m

Med sup genicular a

Femur

Med meniscus, ant horn

Tibia

Sartorius, gracilis & semitendinosus tt

Med inf genicular a

Vastus lateralis m

Lat sup genicular a

Infrapatellar fat body

Iliotibial tract

Transverse lig

Lat meniscus, ant horn

Iliotibial tract

Extensor digitorum longus m

Vastus medialis m

Med sup genicular a

Femur

Med meniscus, ant horn

Tibia

Sartorius, gracilis & semitendinosus tt

Med inf genicular a

Knee, Coronal

Vastus lateralis m

Iliotibial tract

Infrapatellar fat body

Iliotibial tract

Ant tibial recurrent a

Extensor digitorum longus m

Tibialis ant m

Med sup genicular a

Vastus medialis m & t (apon)

Femur

Med meniscus, ant horn

Tibia

Sartorius, gracilis & semitendinosus tt

Vastus lateralis m

Med sup genicular a

Vastus medialis m & t (apon)

Femur

Iliotibial tract

Infrapatellar fat body

Med meniscus, ant horn

Iliotibial tract

Tibia

Sartorius, gracilis & semitendinosus tt

Tibialis ant m

Knee, Coronal

Vastus lateralis m

Vastus medialis m & t (apon)

Femur

Iliotibial tract, vastus lateralis t (apon) & lat patellar retinaculum

Med meniscus, ant horn

Lat inf genicular a

Med inf genicular a

Infrapatellar fat body

Sartorius, gracilis & semitendinosus tt & med patellar retinaculum

Tibia

Lat patellar retinaculum

Vastus lateralis m

Vastus medialis
m & t (apon)

Femur

Iliotibial tract,
vastus lateralis t
(apon) & lat patellar
retinaculum

Infrapatellar fat body

Med meniscus,
ant horn

Tibia

Sartorius, gracilis &
semitendinosus tt &
med patellar retinaculum

Lat patellar
retinaculum

Knee, Coronal

Vastus lateralis t

Iliotibial tract, vastus lateralis t (apon) & lat patellar retinaculum

Lat inf genicular a

Infrapatellar fat body

Patellar lig

Vastus intermedius m & t (apon)

Prefemoral fat body

Vastus medialis m & t (apon)

Femur

Med inf genicular a

Med patellar retinaculum

Vastus lateralis t

Vastus intermedius m & t (apon)

Vastus medialis m & t (apon)

Prefemoral fat body

Iliotibial tract, vastus lateralis t (apon) & lat patellar retinaculum

Femur

Lat inf genicular a

Med inf genicular a

Med patellar retinaculum

Infrapatellar fat body

Patellar lig

Knee, Transverse

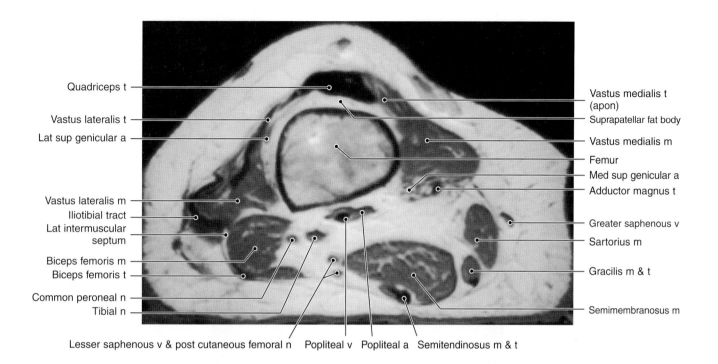

Quadriceps t

Vastus lateralis t

Lat sup genicular a

Vastus lateralis m

Iliotibial tract

Lat intermuscular septum

Biceps femoris m

Biceps femoris t

Common peroneal n

Tibial n

Vastus medialis t (apon)

Suprapatellar fat body

Vastus medialis m

Femur

Med sup genicular a

Adductor magnus t

Greater saphenous v

Sartorius m

Gracilis m & t

Semimembranosus m

Lesser saphenous v & post cutaneous femoral n   Popliteal v   Popliteal a   Semitendinosus m & t

Quadriceps t

Vastus lateralis t

Lat sup genicular a

Vastus lateralis m

Iliotibial tract

Lat intermuscular septum

Biceps femoris m

Biceps femoris t

Common peroneal n

Tibial n

Vastus medialis t (apon)

Suprapatellar fat body

Vastus medialis m

Femur

Adductor magnus t

Med sup genicular a

Greater saphenous v

Sartorius m

Gracilis m & t

Semimembranosus m

Popliteal v   Lesser saphenous v   Popliteal a   Semitendinosus m & t

Quadriceps t

Vastus lateralis t

Vastus medialis t (apon)

Suprapatellar fat body

Vastus medialis m

Femur

Med sup genicular a

Adductor magnus t

Greater saphenous v

Sartorius m

Gracilis m & t

Semimembranosus m

Semitendinosus t

Vastus lateralis m

Iliotibial tract

Lat intermuscular septum

Lat sup genicular a

Biceps femoris m & t

Common peroneal n

Tibial n

Lesser saphenous v

Popliteal v

Popliteal a

Quadriceps t

Vastus lateralis t

Vastus medialis t (apon)

Suprapatellar fat body

Vastus medialis m

Femur

Med sup genicular a

Adductor magnus t

Greater saphenous v

Sartorius m

Gracilis m & t

Semimembranosus m

Semitendinosus t

Vastus lateralis m

Iliotibial tract

Lat intermuscular septum

Lat sup genicular a

Biceps femoris m & t

Common peroneal n

Tibial n

Lesser saphenous v

Popliteal v

Popliteal a

Knee, Transverse

Quadriceps t • Suprapatellar bursa • Suprapatellar fat body

Vastus lateralis t
Prefemoral fat body

Vastus medialis m & t (apon)
Femur

Med sup genicular a
Adductor magnus t
Gastrocnemius m & t, med head
Greater saphenous v

Iliotibial tract

Lat sup genicular a

Biceps femoris m & t
Common peroneal n
Lat sural cutaneous n

Sartorius m
Gracilis t
Semimembranosus m & t
Semitendinosus t

Tibial n • Lesser saphenous v • Popliteal a & v

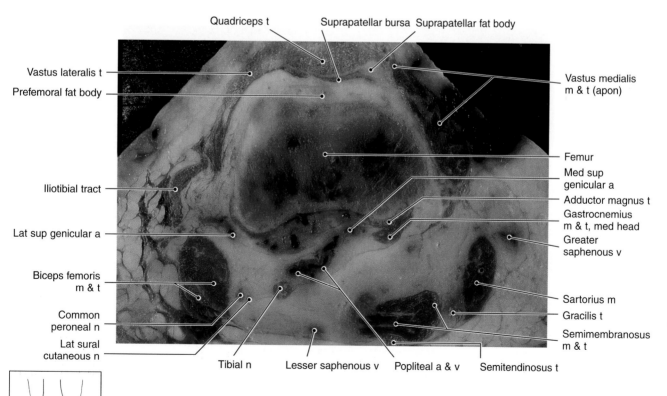

Quadriceps t • Suprapatellar bursa • Suprapatellar fat body

Vastus lateralis t
Prefemoral fat body

Vastus medialis m & t (apon)

Iliotibial tract

Femur
Med sup genicular a
Adductor magnus t
Gastrocnemius m & t, med head
Greater saphenous v

Lat sup genicular a

Biceps femoris m & t
Common peroneal n
Lat sural cutaneous n

Sartorius m
Gracilis t
Semimembranosus m & t

Tibial n • Lesser saphenous v • Popliteal a & v • Semitendinosus t

Quadriceps t Patella Suprapatellar fat body

Lat patellar retinaculum

Vastus lateralis t

Prefemoral fat body

Iliotibial tract
Med sup genicular a
Plantaris t

Lat sup genicular a
Biceps femoris m & t

Common peroneal n
Lat sural cutaneous n

Vastus medialis t (apon)

Suprapatellar bursa

Vastus medialis m
Femur

Gastrocnemius m & t, med head

Greater saphenous v

Sartorius m

Gracilis t
Semimembranosus m & t
Semitendinosus t

Tibial n Lesser saphenous v Popliteal a & v

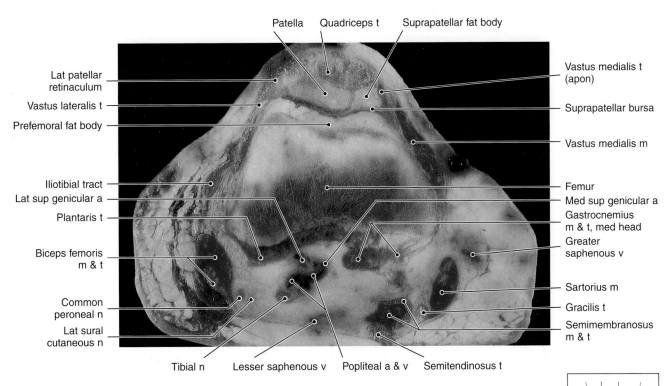

Patella Quadriceps t Suprapatellar fat body

Lat patellar retinaculum

Vastus lateralis t

Prefemoral fat body

Iliotibial tract
Lat sup genicular a
Plantaris t

Biceps femoris m & t

Common peroneal n

Lat sural cutaneous n

Vastus medialis t (apon)

Suprapatellar bursa

Vastus medialis m

Femur
Med sup genicular a
Gastrocnemius m & t, med head
Greater saphenous v

Sartorius m

Gracilis t
Semimembranosus m & t

Tibial n Lesser saphenous v Popliteal a & v Semitendinosus t

Knee, Transverse

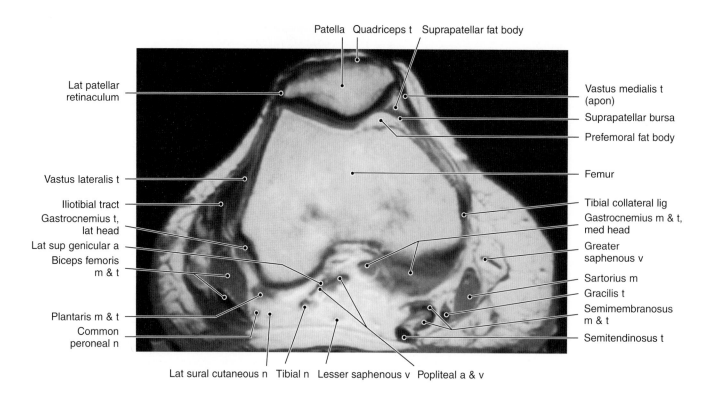

Patella   Quadriceps t   Suprapatellar fat body

Lat patellar retinaculum

Vastus medialis t (apon)

Suprapatellar bursa

Prefemoral fat body

Femur

Vastus lateralis t

Iliotibial tract

Gastrocnemius t, lat head

Lat sup genicular a

Biceps femoris m & t

Plantaris m & t

Common peroneal n

Tibial collateral lig

Gastrocnemius m & t, med head

Greater saphenous v

Sartorius m

Gracilis t

Semimembranosus m & t

Semitendinosus t

Lat sural cutaneous n   Tibial n   Lesser saphenous v   Popliteal a & v

Patella   Quadriceps t   Suprapatellar fat body

Lat patellar retinaculum

Vastus medialis t (apon)

Suprapatellar bursa

Prefemoral fat body

Femur

Vastus lateralis t

Iliotibial tract

Lat sup genicular a

Gastrocnemius t, lat head

Biceps femoris m & t

Plantaris m & t

Common peroneal n

Lat sural cutaneous n

Tibial collateral lig

Gastrocnemius m & t, med head

Greater saphenous v

Sartorius m

Gracilis t

Semimembranosus m & t

Tibial n   Lesser saphenous v   Popliteal a & v   Semitendinosus t

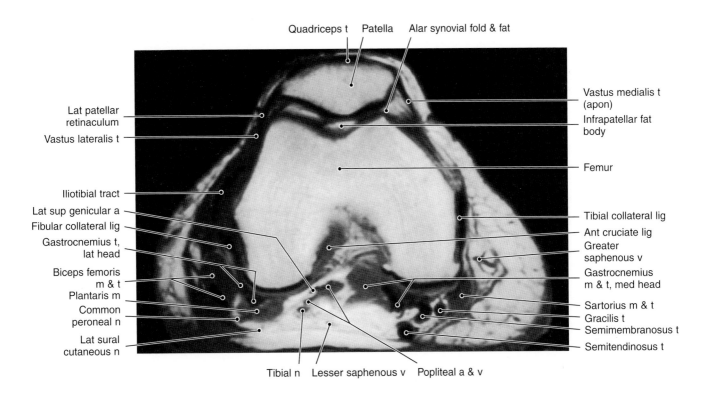

Quadriceps t   Patella   Alar synovial fold & fat

Lat patellar retinaculum

Vastus lateralis t

Iliotibial tract

Lat sup genicular a

Fibular collateral lig

Gastrocnemius t, lat head

Biceps femoris m & t

Plantaris m

Common peroneal n

Lat sural cutaneous n

Vastus medialis t (apon)

Infrapatellar fat body

Femur

Tibial collateral lig

Ant cruciate lig

Greater saphenous v

Gastrocnemius m & t, med head

Sartorius m & t

Gracilis t

Semimembranosus t

Semitendinosus t

Tibial n   Lesser saphenous v   Popliteal a & v

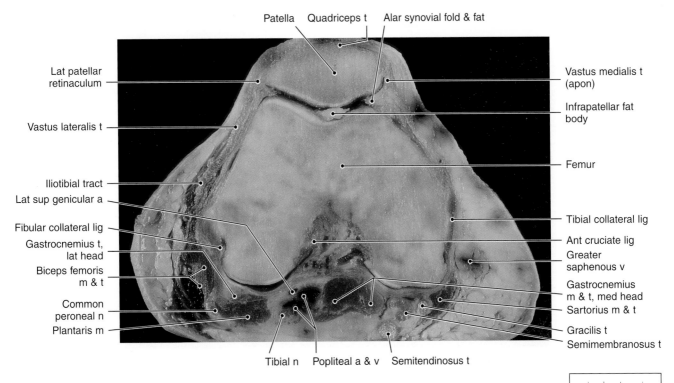

Patella   Quadriceps t   Alar synovial fold & fat

Lat patellar retinaculum

Vastus lateralis t

Iliotibial tract

Lat sup genicular a

Fibular collateral lig

Gastrocnemius t, lat head

Biceps femoris m & t

Common peroneal n

Plantaris m

Vastus medialis t (apon)

Infrapatellar fat body

Femur

Tibial collateral lig

Ant cruciate lig

Greater saphenous v

Gastrocnemius m & t, med head

Sartorius m & t

Gracilis t

Semimembranosus t

Tibial n   Popliteal a & v   Semitendinosus t

Knee, Transverse

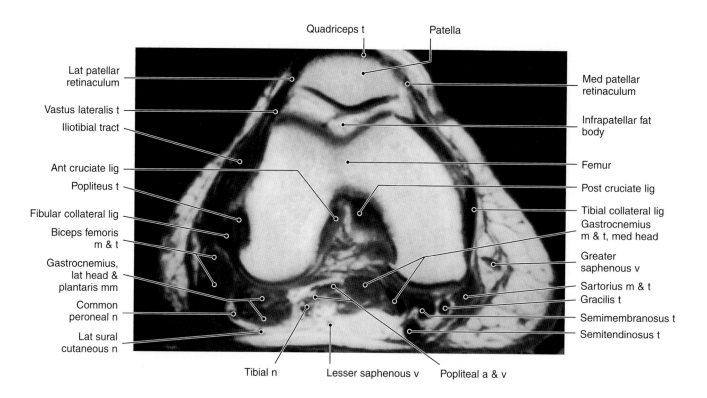

Quadriceps t · Patella

Lat patellar retinaculum · Med patellar retinaculum

Vastus lateralis t · Infrapatellar fat body

Iliotibial tract

Ant cruciate lig · Femur

Popliteus t · Post cruciate lig

Fibular collateral lig · Tibial collateral lig

Biceps femoris m & t · Gastrocnemius m & t, med head

Gastrocnemius, lat head & plantaris mm · Greater saphenous v

Common peroneal n · Sartorius m & t · Gracilis t

Lat sural cutaneous n · Semimembranosus t · Semitendinosus t

Tibial n · Lesser saphenous v · Popliteal a & v

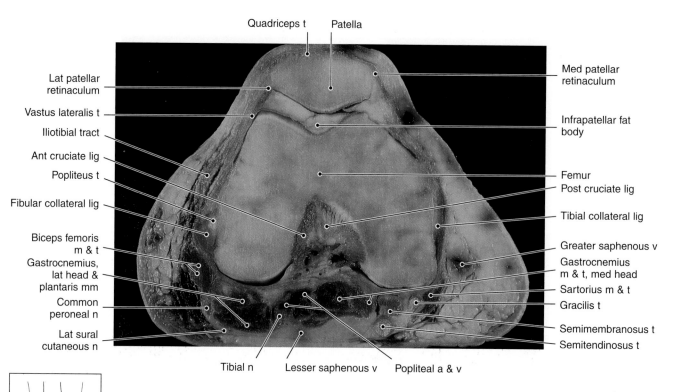

Quadriceps t · Patella

Lat patellar retinaculum · Med patellar retinaculum

Vastus lateralis t · Infrapatellar fat body

Iliotibial tract

Ant cruciate lig · Femur

Popliteus t · Post cruciate lig

Fibular collateral lig · Tibial collateral lig

Biceps femoris m & t · Greater saphenous v

Gastrocnemius, lat head & plantaris mm · Gastrocnemius m & t, med head

Common peroneal n · Sartorius m & t · Gracilis t

Lat sural cutaneous n · Semimembranosus t · Semitendinosus t

Tibial n · Lesser saphenous v · Popliteal a & v

Infrapatellar fat body Patellar lig

Lat patellar retinaculum

Vastus lateralis t

Iliotibial tract

Lat femoral condyle
Ant cruciate lig
Popliteus t
Fibular collateral lig
Biceps femoris m & t

Gastrocnemius, lat head & plantaris mm

Common peroneal n

Lat sural cutaneous n

Med patellar retinaculum

Tibial collateral lig

Med femoral condyle

Post cruciate lig

Greater saphenous v

Sartorius m & t

Gracilis t

Semimembranosus t

Semitendinosus t

Gastrocnemius m & t, med head

Oblique popliteal lig & joint capsule Tibial n Lesser saphenous v Popliteal a & v

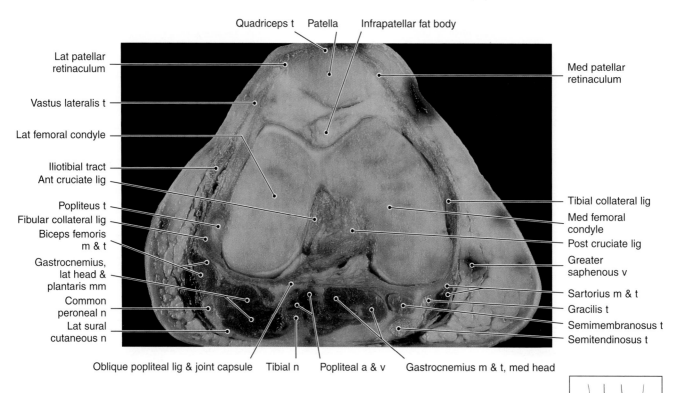

Quadriceps t Patella Infrapatellar fat body

Lat patellar retinaculum

Vastus lateralis t

Lat femoral condyle

Iliotibial tract
Ant cruciate lig

Popliteus t
Fibular collateral lig
Biceps femoris m & t

Gastrocnemius, lat head & plantaris mm

Common peroneal n

Lat sural cutaneous n

Med patellar retinaculum

Tibial collateral lig

Med femoral condyle

Post cruciate lig

Greater saphenous v

Sartorius m & t

Gracilis t

Semimembranosus t

Semitendinosus t

Oblique popliteal lig & joint capsule Tibial n Popliteal a & v Gastrocnemius m & t, med head

Knee, Transverse

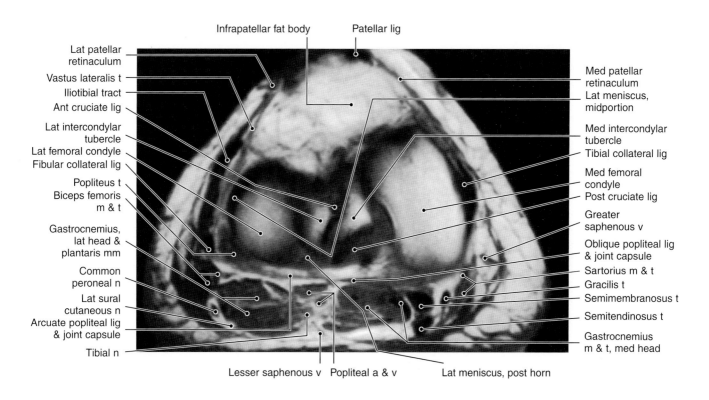

Infrapatellar fat body
Patellar lig
Lat patellar retinaculum
Vastus lateralis t
Iliotibial tract
Ant cruciate lig
Lat intercondylar tubercle
Lat femoral condyle
Fibular collateral lig
Popliteus t
Biceps femoris m & t
Gastrocnemius, lat head & plantaris mm
Common peroneal n
Lat sural cutaneous n
Arcuate popliteal lig & joint capsule
Tibial n
Med patellar retinaculum
Lat meniscus, midportion
Med intercondylar tubercle
Tibial collateral lig
Med femoral condyle
Post cruciate lig
Greater saphenous v
Oblique popliteal lig & joint capsule
Sartorius m & t
Gracilis t
Semimembranosus t
Semitendinosus t
Gastrocnemius m & t, med head
Lesser saphenous v
Popliteal a & v
Lat meniscus, post horn

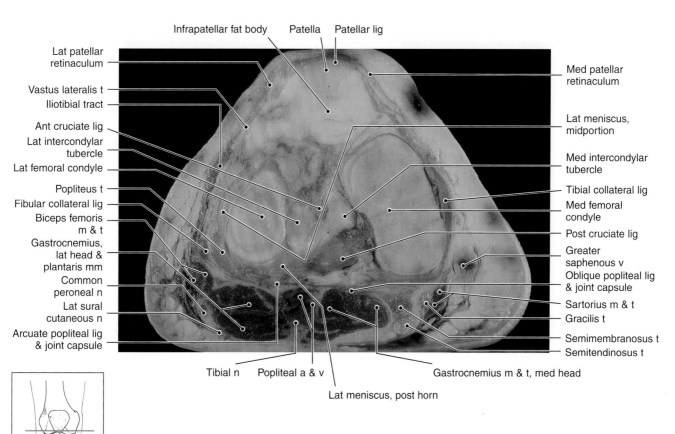

Infrapatellar fat body
Patella
Patellar lig
Lat patellar retinaculum
Vastus lateralis t
Iliotibial tract
Ant cruciate lig
Lat intercondylar tubercle
Lat femoral condyle
Popliteus t
Fibular collateral lig
Biceps femoris m & t
Gastrocnemius, lat head & plantaris mm
Common peroneal n
Lat sural cutaneous n
Arcuate popliteal lig & joint capsule
Med patellar retinaculum
Lat meniscus, midportion
Med intercondylar tubercle
Tibial collateral lig
Med femoral condyle
Post cruciate lig
Greater saphenous v
Oblique popliteal lig & joint capsule
Sartorius m & t
Gracilis t
Semimembranosus t
Semitendinosus t
Tibial n
Popliteal a & v
Gastrocnemius m & t, med head
Lat meniscus, post horn

Infrapatellar fat body

Patellar lig

Iliotibial tract &
vastus lateralis t

Lat meniscus,
ant horn

Ant cruciate lig

Lat meniscus,
midportion

Lat meniscus,
post horn

Fibular collateral lig

Popliteus t

Biceps femoris t

Gastrocnemius,
lat head &
plantaris mm

Common
peroneal n

Lat sural
cutaneous n

Arcuate popliteal lig
& joint capsule

Med meniscus,
ant horn

Med femoral
condyle

Tibial collateral lig

Med meniscus,
midportion

Tibia, intercondylar
area

Med meniscus,
post horn

Greater
saphenous v

Sartorius m & t

Gracilis t

Semimembranosus t

Semitendinosus t

Gastrocnemius
m & t, med head

Oblique popliteal lig
& joint capsule

Tibial n

Post cruciate lig

Lesser saphenous v

Popliteal a & v

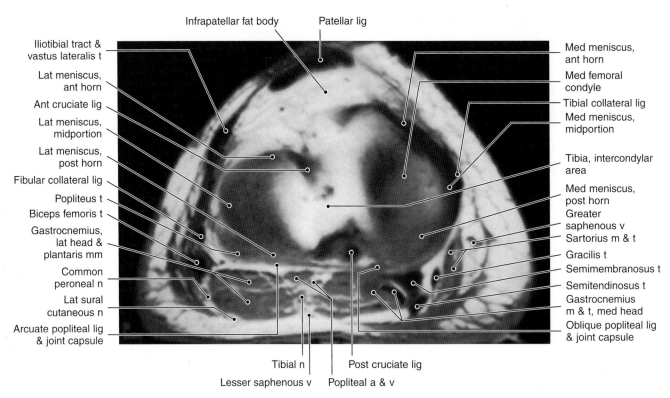

Iliotibial tract & vastus lateralis t

Patellar lig

Infrapatellar fat body

Lat meniscus,
ant horn

Ant cruciate lig

Lat tibial plateau,
articular cartilage

Post cruciate lig

Lat meniscus,
post horn

Popliteus t

Fibular collateral lig

Arcuate popliteal lig
& joint capsule

Biceps femoris t

Common
peroneal n

Gastrocnemius,
lat head &
plantaris mm

Med meniscus,
ant horn

Med femoral
condyle

Med meniscus,
midportion

Tibial collateral lig

Tibia, intercondylar
area

Med meniscus,
post horn

Oblique popliteal lig
& joint capsule

Greater
saphenous v

Sartorius m & t

Gracilis t

Semimembranosus t

Semitendinosus t

Lat sural cutaneous n

Lesser saphenous v

Tibial n

Popliteal a & v

Gastrocnemius m & t,
med head

Knee, Transverse

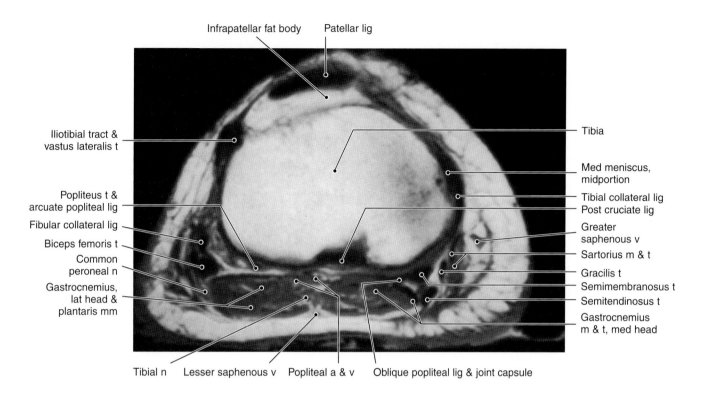

Infrapatellar fat body — Patellar lig

Iliotibial tract & vastus lateralis t

Popliteus t & arcuate popliteal lig

Fibular collateral lig

Biceps femoris t

Common peroneal n

Gastrocnemius, lat head & plantaris mm

Tibia

Med meniscus, midportion

Tibial collateral lig

Post cruciate lig

Greater saphenous v

Sartorius m & t

Gracilis t

Semimembranosus t

Semitendinosus t

Gastrocnemius m & t, med head

Tibial n   Lesser saphenous v   Popliteal a & v   Oblique popliteal lig & joint capsule

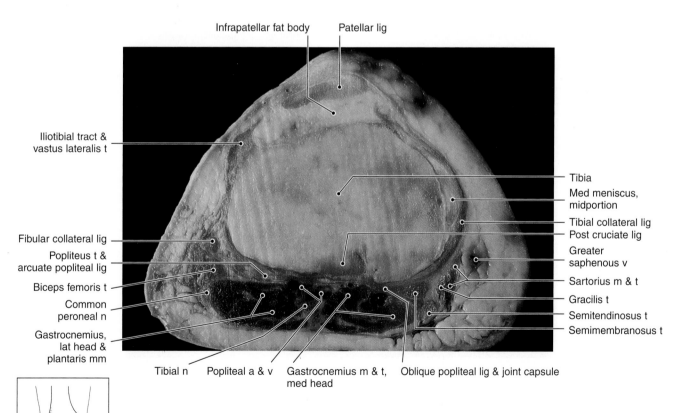

Infrapatellar fat body — Patellar lig

Iliotibial tract & vastus lateralis t

Fibular collateral lig

Popliteus t & arcuate popliteal lig

Biceps femoris t

Common peroneal n

Gastrocnemius, lat head & plantaris mm

Tibia

Med meniscus, midportion

Tibial collateral lig

Post cruciate lig

Greater saphenous v

Sartorius m & t

Gracilis t

Semitendinosus t

Semimembranosus t

Tibial n   Popliteal a & v   Gastrocnemius m & t, med head   Oblique popliteal lig & joint capsule

Patellar lig

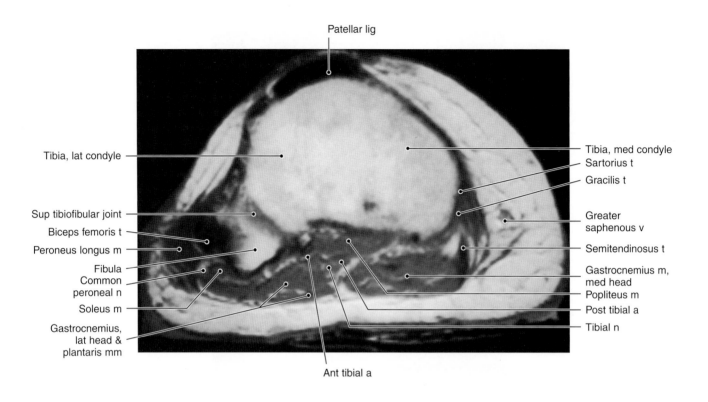

Tibia, lat condyle

Sup tibiofibular joint

Biceps femoris t

Peroneus longus m

Fibula

Common peroneal n

Soleus m

Gastrocnemius, lat head & plantaris mm

Tibia, med condyle

Sartorius t

Gracilis t

Greater saphenous v

Semitendinosus t

Gastrocnemius m, med head

Popliteus m

Post tibial a

Tibial n

Ant tibial a

Patellar lig

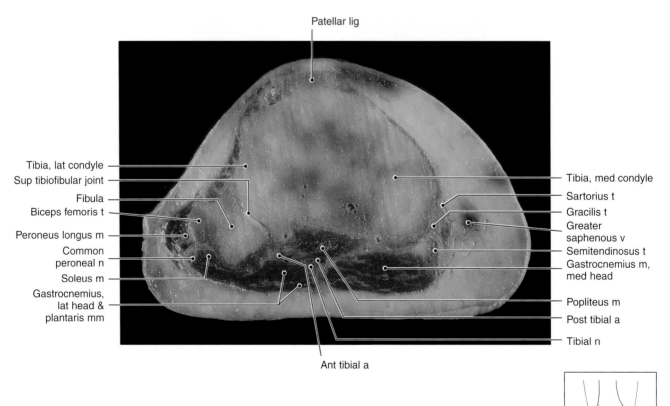

Tibia, lat condyle

Sup tibiofibular joint

Fibula

Biceps femoris t

Peroneus longus m

Common peroneal n

Soleus m

Gastrocnemius, lat head & plantaris mm

Tibia, med condyle

Sartorius t

Gracilis t

Greater saphenous v

Semitendinosus t

Gastrocnemius m, med head

Popliteus m

Post tibial a

Tibial n

Ant tibial a

Knee, Sagittal

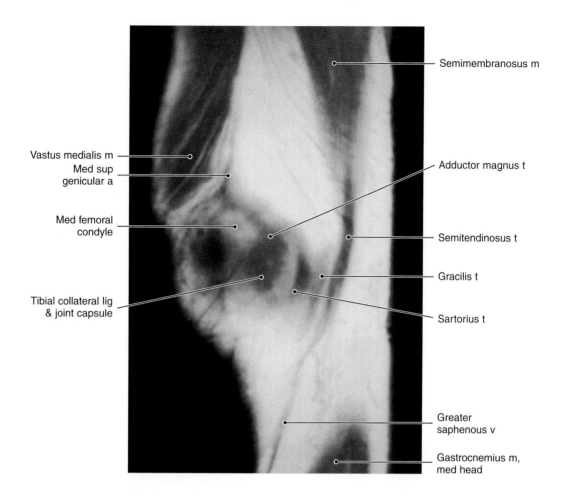

Semimembranosus m

Vastus medialis m

Med sup genicular a

Adductor magnus t

Med femoral condyle

Semitendinosus t

Gracilis t

Tibial collateral lig & joint capsule

Sartorius t

Greater saphenous v

Gastrocnemius m, med head

Vastus medialis m

Semimembranosus m & t

Med sup genicular a

Adductor magnus t

Med femoral condyle

Med patellar retinaculum

Semitendinosus t

Gracilis t

Sartorius t

Tibial collateral lig & joint capsule

Greater saphenous v

Gastrocnemius m, med head

Knee, Sagittal

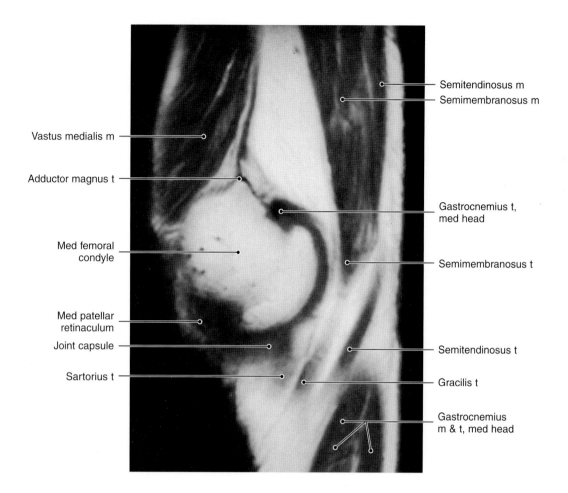

Semitendinosus m

Semimembranosus m

Vastus medialis m

Adductor magnus t

Gastrocnemius t, med head

Med femoral condyle

Semimembranosus t

Med patellar retinaculum

Joint capsule

Semitendinosus t

Sartorius t

Gracilis t

Gastrocnemius m & t, med head

Semitendinosus m

Semimembranosus m

Vastus medialis m

Adductor magnus t

Gastrocnemius t, med head

Med femoral condyle

Semimembranosus t

Med patellar retinaculum

Gracilis t

Joint capsule

Semitendinosus t

Sartorius t

Gastrocnemius m & t, med head

Knee, Sagittal

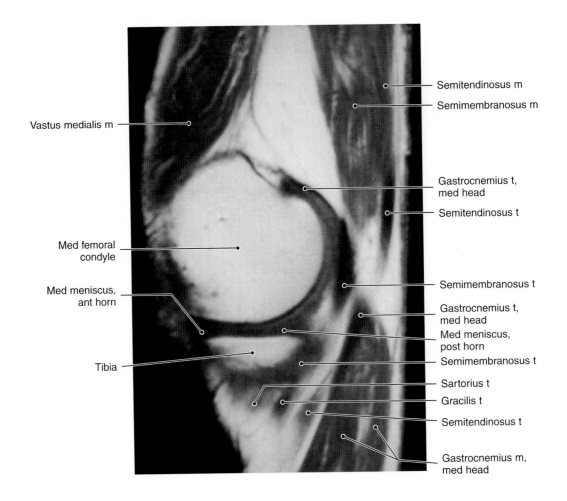

Vastus medialis m

Med femoral condyle

Med meniscus, ant horn

Tibia

Semitendinosus m

Semimembranosus m

Gastrocnemius t, med head

Semitendinosus t

Semimembranosus t

Gastrocnemius t, med head

Med meniscus, post horn

Semimembranosus t

Sartorius t

Gracilis t

Semitendinosus t

Gastrocnemius m, med head

Semitendinosus m

Vastus medialis m

Semimembranosus m

Semitendinosus t

Gastrocnemius t, med head

Med femoral condyle

Med patellar retinaculum

Semimembranosus t

Gastrocnemius t, med head

Med meniscus, ant horn

Med meniscus, post horn

Tibia

Semimembranosus t

Gracilis t

Sartorius t

Semitendinosus t

Gastrocnemius m, med head

Knee, Sagittal

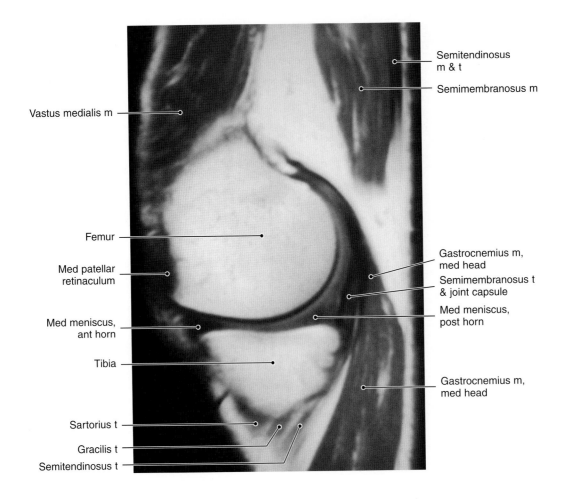

Semitendinosus m & t

Semimembranosus m

Vastus medialis m

Femur

Med patellar retinaculum

Med meniscus, ant horn

Tibia

Sartorius t

Gracilis t

Semitendinosus t

Gastrocnemius m, med head

Semimembranosus t & joint capsule

Med meniscus, post horn

Gastrocnemius m, med head

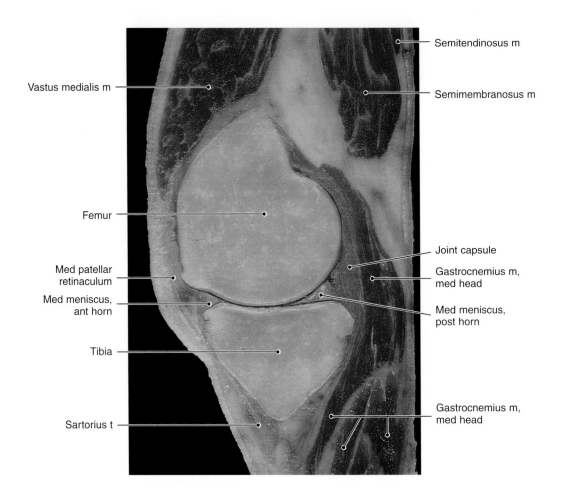

Semitendinosus m

Vastus medialis m

Semimembranosus m

Femur

Joint capsule

Med patellar
retinaculum

Gastrocnemius m,
med head

Med meniscus,
ant horn

Med meniscus,
post horn

Tibia

Sartorius t

Gastrocnemius m,
med head

Knee, Sagittal

Vastus medialis m

Suprapatellar fat body

Vastus medialis t (apon)

Femur

Med patellar retinaculum

Med inf genicular a

Med meniscus, ant horn

Tibia

Sartorius t

Semitendinosus m

Popliteal a

Semimembranosus m

Joint capsule

Gastrocnemius m, med head

Med meniscus, post horn

Gastrocnemius m, med head

Vastus medialis m

Suprapatellar fat body

Vastus medialis t (apon)

Femur

Med patellar retinaculum

Med inf genicular a

Med meniscus, ant horn

Tibia

Sartorius t

Popliteal a

Semimembranosus m

Gastrocnemius m, med head

Joint capsule

Med meniscus, post horn

Gastrocnemius m, med head

Knee, Sagittal

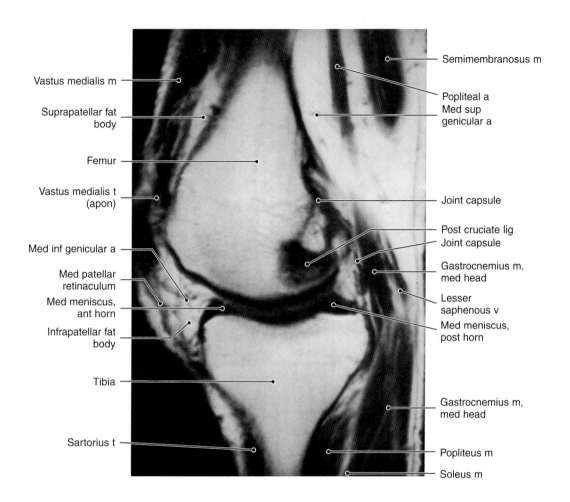

Vastus medialis m

Suprapatellar fat body

Femur

Vastus medialis t (apon)

Med inf genicular a

Med patellar retinaculum

Med meniscus, ant horn

Infrapatellar fat body

Tibia

Sartorius t

Semimembranosus m

Popliteal a
Med sup genicular a

Joint capsule

Post cruciate lig
Joint capsule

Gastrocnemius m, med head

Lesser saphenous v

Med meniscus, post horn

Gastrocnemius m, med head

Popliteus m

Soleus m

Vastus medialis m

Suprapatellar fat body

Femur

Vastus medialis t (apon)

Med patellar retinaculum

Med inf genicular a

Med meniscus, ant horn

Infrapatellar fat body

Tibia

Sartorius t

Popliteal a

Semimembranosus m

Med sup genicular a

Lesser saphenous v

Gastrocnemius m, med head

Joint capsule

Post cruciate lig

Med meniscus, post horn

Gastrocnemius m, med head

Popliteus m

Soleus m

Knee, Sagittal

Rectus femoris m

Femur

Prefemoral fat body

Quadriceps t

Suprapatellar bursa

Suprapatellar fat body

Patella

Med inf genicular a

Patellar lig

Infrapatellar fat body

Tibia

Lesser saphenous v

Semimembranosus m

Popliteal a & v

Med sup genicular a

Joint capsule

Post meniscofemoral lig of Wrisberg

Post cruciate lig

Gastrocnemius m, med head

Popliteal a & v

Popliteus m

Soleus m

Rectus femoris m

Femur

Prefemoral fat body

Quadriceps t

Suprapatellar bursa

Suprapatellar fat body

Patella

Patellar lig

Med inf genicular a

Infrapatellar fat body

Patellar lig

Tibia

Lesser saphenous v

Semimembranosus m

Med sup genicular a

Popliteal a & v

Joint capsule

Post meniscofemoral lig of Wrisberg

Post cruciate lig

Popliteal a & v

Gastrocnemius m, med head

Popliteus m

Soleus m

Knee, Sagittal

Rectus femoris m

Prefemoral fat body

Quadriceps t
Suprapatellar bursa
Suprapatellar fat body

Patella

Ant cruciate lig
Med inf genicular a

Patellar lig
Infrapatellar fat body

Tibia

Femur
Popliteal v

Med sup genicular a

Popliteal a & v

Joint capsule
Post cruciate lig

Post meniscofemoral lig of Wrisberg

Post cruciate lig

Gastrocnemius m, med head

Popliteal v
Popliteus m
Soleus m

Rectus femoris m

Femur

Prefemoral fat body

Suprapatellar bursa

Quadriceps t

Suprapatellar fat body

Patella

Infrapatellar synovial fold

Med inf genicular a

Ant cruciate lig

Infrapatellar fat body

Patellar lig

Tibia

Popliteal v

Lesser saphenous v

Med sup genicular a

Popliteal a & v

Joint capsule

Post cruciate lig

Post meniscofemoral lig of Wrisberg

Post cruciate lig

Gastrocnemius m, med head

Popliteus m

Popliteal v & tibial n

Soleus m

Knee, Sagittal

Rectus femoris m

Prefemoral fat body

Quadriceps t

Suprapatellar bursa

Suprapatellar fat body

Patella

Transverse lig

Lat inf genicular a

Infrapatellar fat body

Patellar lig

Tibia

Tibial n

Femur

Lat sup genicular a

Tibial n

Ant cruciate lig

Oblique popliteal lig & joint capsule

Post meniscofemoral lig of Wrisberg

Post cruciate lig

Popliteus m

Gastrocnemius, lat head & plantaris mm

Popliteal v & tibial n

Soleus m

Rectus femoris m

Prefemoral fat body
Quadriceps t
Suprapatellar bursa
Suprapatellar fat body

Patella

Transverse lig
Lat inf genicular a
Infrapatellar fat body
Patellar lig

Tibia

Tibial n

Lat sup genicular a
Tibial n
Femur

Oblique popliteal lig & joint capsule
Ant cruciate lig
Post meniscofemoral lig of Wrisberg
Post cruciate lig
Gastrocnemius, lat head & plantaris mm
Popliteal v & tibial n
Popliteus m
Soleus m

Knee, Sagittal

Biceps femoris m

Common peroneal n

Femur

Lat sup genicular a

Prefemoral fat body

Quadriceps t

Suprapatellar bursa

Suprapatellar fat body

Patella

Plantaris m

Gastrocnemius m, lat head

Lat inf genicular a

Infrapatellar fat body

Patellar lig

Lat inf genicular a

Lat meniscus, post horn

Popliteus t

Tibia

Popliteus m

Gastrocnemius, lat head & soleus mm

Biceps femoris m

Common peroneal n

Prefemoral fat body

Quadriceps t

Suprapatellar bursa

Suprapatellar fat body

Lat sup genicular a

Femur

Patella

Gastrocnemius m, lat head

Plantaris m

Lat inf genicular a

Lat meniscus, ant horn

Infrapatellar fat body

Patellar lig

Tibia

Lat inf genicular a

Lat meniscus, post horn

Popliteus t

Popliteus m

Gastrocnemius, lat head & soleus mm

Knee, Sagittal

Biceps femoris m

Prefemoral fat body

Quadriceps t

Suprapatellar bursa

Suprapatellar fat body

Lat sup genicular a

Femur

Common peroneal n

Gastrocnemius, lat head & plantaris tt

Patella

Fabella

Gastrocnemius m, lat head

Lat inf genicular a

Lat meniscus, ant horn

Lat sural cutaneous n

Patellar lig

Infrapatellar fat body

Tibia

Lat meniscus, post horn

Popliteus t

Sup tibiofibular joint

Fibula

Ant tibial a

Tibialis ant m

Soleus m

Extensor digitorum longus m

Interosseous membrane

Prefemoral fat body

Quadriceps t

Suprapatellar bursa

Suprapatellar fat body

Patella

Lat meniscus, ant horn

Lat inf genicular a

Infrapatellar fat body

Patellar lig

Tibia

Extensor digitorum longus m

Tibialis ant m

Biceps femoris m

Lat sup genicular a

Femur

Gastrocnemius, lat head & plantaris tt

Common peroneal n

Fabella

Lat meniscus, post horn

Gastrocnemius m, lat head

Lat sural cutaneous n

Popliteus t

Sup tibiofibular joint

Fibula

Soleus m

Ant tibial a

Interosseous membrane

Knee, Sagittal

Vastus lateralis m

Vastus lateralis t

Patella

Lat inf genicular a

Infrapatellar fat body

Extensor digitorum longus m

Tibialis ant m

Lat sup genicular a

Biceps femoris m

Lat femoral condyle

Gastrocnemius, lat head & plantaris tt

Popliteus t

Lat femoral condyle

Lat meniscus, midportion

Popliteus t

Tibia

Sup tibiofibular joint

Fibula

Soleus m

Vastus lateralis m

Vastus lateralis t

Patella

Lat inf genicular a

Infrapatellar fat body

Extensor digitorum longus m

Tibialis ant m

Biceps femoris m

Lat sup genicular a

Gastrocnemius, lat head & plantaris tt

Lat femoral condyle

Popliteus t

Lat femoral condyle

Lat meniscus, midportion

Popliteus t

Tibia

Sup tibiofibular joint

Fibula

Soleus m

Knee, Sagittal

Vastus lateralis m

Vastus lateralis t

Lat patellar retinaculum

Tibia

Peroneus longus & extensor digitorum longus mm

Tibialis ant m

Biceps femoris m

Lat femoral epicondyle

Fibular collateral lig

Biceps femoris t

Biceps femoris t

Fibula

Peroneus longus m

Vastus lateralis m

Vastus lateralis t

Lat patellar
retinaculum

Tibia

Tibialis ant m

Peroneus longus &
extensor digitorum
longus mm

Biceps femoris m

Biceps femoris t

Lat femoral
epicondyle

Fibular collateral lig

Popliteus t

Biceps femoris t

Sup tibiofibular joint

Fibula

Peroneus longus m

10

Lower Leg

Lower Leg, Coronal

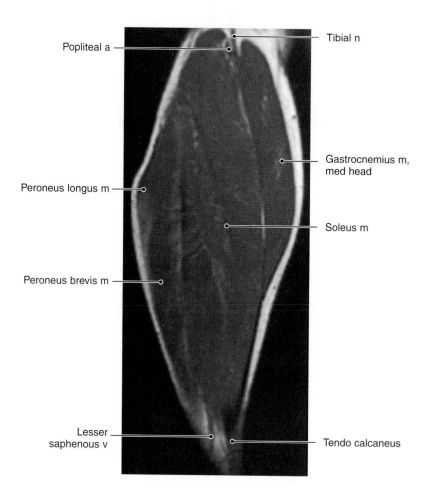

Popliteal a

Tibial n

Gastrocnemius m, med head

Peroneus longus m

Soleus m

Peroneus brevis m

Lesser saphenous v

Tendo calcaneus

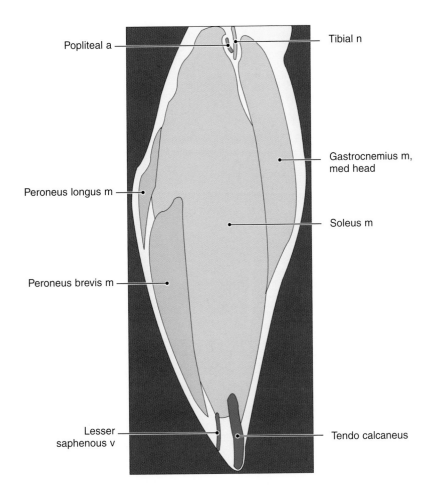

Popliteal a

Tibial n

Gastrocnemius m, med head

Peroneus longus m

Soleus m

Peroneus brevis m

Lesser saphenous v

Tendo calcaneus

Lower Leg, Coronal

Popliteal a
Lat femoral condyle
Biceps femoris m
Lat meniscus
Tibia
Fibular collateral lig

Popliteal v

Peroneus longus m

Peroneus brevis m

Fibula

Peroneal a

Peroneus longus &
brevis tt

Lesser
saphenous v

Gastrocnemius m, med head
Med femoral condyle

Sartorius m
Gracilis t
Popliteus m

Tibial n
Popliteal a
Gastrocnemius m,
med head

Soleus m

Post tibial a

Flexor hallucis
longus m

Tendo calcaneus
Calcaneus

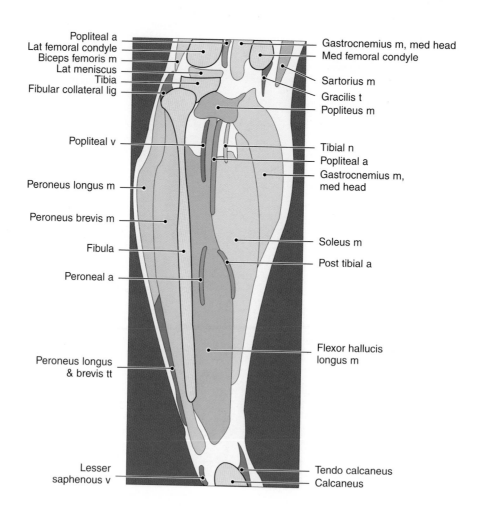

Popliteal a
Lat femoral condyle
Biceps femoris m
Lat meniscus
Tibia
Fibular collateral lig

Gastrocnemius m, med head
Med femoral condyle

Sartorius m
Gracilis t
Popliteus m

Popliteal v

Tibial n
Popliteal a
Gastrocnemius m,
med head

Peroneus longus m

Peroneus brevis m

Soleus m

Fibula

Post tibial a

Peroneal a

Flexor hallucis
longus m

Peroneus longus
& brevis tt

Lesser
saphenous v

Tendo calcaneus
Calcaneus

Lower Leg, Coronal

Fibular collateral lig
Lat femoral condyle
Iliotibial tract
Lat meniscus

Fibula, head

Extensor digitorum
longus m

Extensor hallucis
longus m

Lat malleolus

Med femoral condyle
Post cruciate lig
Ant cruciate lig
Sartorius m
Semimembranosus t
Tibia

Popliteus m

Gastrocnemius m,
med head

Soleus m
Flexor digitorum
longus m

Tibialis post m

Flexor hallucis
longus m
Tibia

Calcaneus

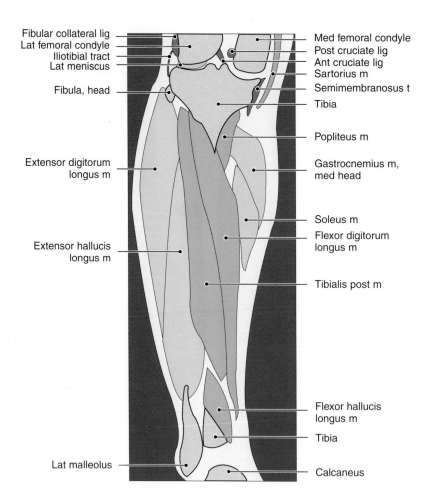

Fibular collateral lig

Lat femoral condyle

Iliotibial tract

Lat meniscus

Fibula, head

Extensor digitorum
longus m

Extensor hallucis
longus m

Lat malleolus

Med femoral condyle

Post cruciate lig

Ant cruciate lig

Sartorius m

Semimembranosus t

Tibia

Popliteus m

Gastrocnemius m,
med head

Soleus m

Flexor digitorum
longus m

Tibialis post m

Flexor hallucis
longus m

Tibia

Calcaneus

Lower Leg, Coronal

Iliotibial tract
Lat meniscus

Extensor digitorum
longus m

Tibialis ant m

Extensor hallucis
longus m

Extensor retinaculum

Femur
Tibial collateral lig
Med meniscus

Superficial v
Flexor digitorum
longus m

Superficial v

Tibia

Greater saphenous v

Talus
Calcaneus

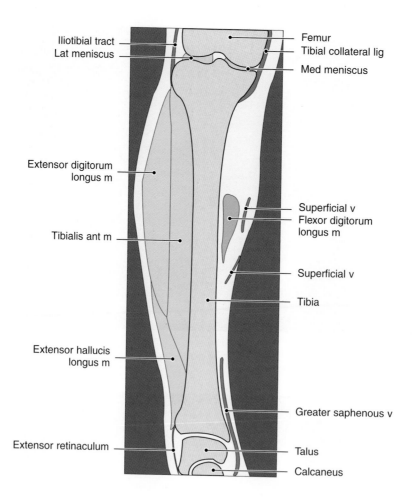

Iliotibial tract

Lat meniscus

Extensor digitorum
longus m

Tibialis ant m

Extensor hallucis
longus m

Extensor retinaculum

Femur

Tibial collateral lig

Med meniscus

Superficial v

Flexor digitorum
longus m

Superficial v

Tibia

Greater saphenous v

Talus

Calcaneus

Lower Leg, Transverse

Tibialis ant m

Extensor digitorum longus m

Peroneus longus m & t

Tibialis post m

Deep peroneal n

Superficial peroneal n

Tibialis post m

Post intermuscular septum

Fibula

Crural fascia

Gastrocnemius m, lat head

Med sural cutaneous n

Superficial fascia

Tibia

Crural fascia

Popliteus m

Popliteal a

Popliteal v

Greater saphenous v

Tibial n

Soleus m & t

Plantaris t

Gastrocnemius m, med head

Lesser saphenous v

Tibialis ant m

Extensor digitorum longus m

Peroneus longus m & t

Tibialis post m

Deep peroneal n

Superficial peroneal n

Tibialis post m

Post intermuscular septum

Fibula

Crural fascia

Gastrocnemius m, lat head

Med sural cutaneous n

Superficial fascia

Tibia

Crural fascia

Popliteus m

Popliteal a

Popliteal v

Greater saphenous v

Tibial n

Soleus m & t

Plantaris t

Gastrocnemius m, med head

Lesser saphenous v

Tibialis ant m

Extensor digitorum longus m

Peroneus brevis m & t
Interosseous membrane
Peroneus longus m & t
Deep peroneal n
Superficial peroneal n
Popliteal a
Post intermuscular septum
Fibula
Crural fascia

Gastrocnemius m, lat head

Lesser saphenous v

Tibia
Crural fascia
Popliteus m
Tibialis post m
Greater saphenous v
Popliteal v
Tibial n
Soleus m
Plantaris t

Gastrocnemius m, med head

Med sural cutaneous n
Crural fascia

Tibialis ant m

Extensor digitorum longus m

Peroneus brevis m & t
Interosseous membrane
Peroneus longus m & t
Deep peroneal n
Superficial peroneal n
Popliteal a
Post intermuscular septum
Fibula
Crural fascia

Gastrocnemius m, lat head

Lesser saphenous v

Tibia
Crural fascia
Popliteus m
Tibialis post m
Greater saphenous v
Popliteal v
Tibial n
Soleus m
Plantaris t

Gastrocnemius m, med head

Med sural cutaneous n
Crural fascia

Lower Leg, Transverse

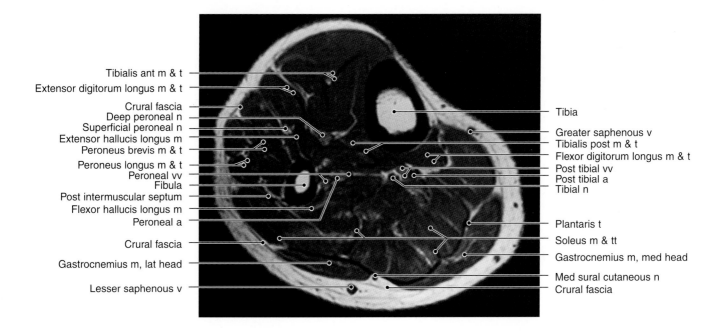

Tibialis ant m & t
Extensor digitorum longus m & t
Crural fascia
Deep peroneal n
Superficial peroneal n
Extensor hallucis longus m
Peroneus brevis m & t
Peroneus longus m & t
Peroneal vv
Fibula
Post intermuscular septum
Flexor hallucis longus m
Peroneal a
Crural fascia
Gastrocnemius m, lat head
Lesser saphenous v

Tibia
Greater saphenous v
Tibialis post m & t
Flexor digitorum longus m & t
Post tibial vv
Post tibial a
Tibial n
Plantaris t
Soleus m & tt
Gastrocnemius m, med head
Med sural cutaneous n
Crural fascia

Tibialis ant m & t
Extensor digitorum longus m & t
Crural fascia
Deep peroneal n
Superficial peroneal n
Extensor hallucis longus m
Peroneus brevis m & t
Peroneus longus m & t
Peroneal vv
Fibula
Post intermuscular septum
Flexor hallucis longus m
Peroneal a
Crural fascia
Gastrocnemius m, lat head
Lesser saphenous v

Tibia
Greater saphenous v
Tibialis post m & t
Flexor digitorum longus m & t
Post tibial vv
Post tibial a
Tibial n
Plantaris t
Soleus m & tt
Gastrocnemius m, med head
Med sural cutaneous n
Crural fascia

Tibialis ant m & t
Crural fascia
Extensor digitorum longus m & t
Extensor hallucis longus m & tt
Med dorsal cutaneous n
Intermediate dorsal cutaneous n
Peroneus brevis m & t
Crural fascia
Interosseous membrane
Peroneus longus m & t
Peroneal vv
Peroneal a
Fibula
Flexor hallucis longus m & t
Lesser saphenous v

Tibia
Ant tibial v
Deep peroneal n
Ant tibial a
Greater saphenous v
Tibialis post m & t
Flexor digitorum longus m & t
Post tibial vv
Post tibial a
Tibial n
Soleus t
Plantaris t
Soleus m & tt
Sural n

Tibialis ant m & t
Crural fascia
Extensor digitorum longus m & t
Extensor hallucis longus m & tt
Med dorsal cutaneous n
Intermediate dorsal cutaneous n
Peroneus brevis m & t
Crural fascia
Interosseous membrane
Peroneus longus m & t
Peroneal vv
Peroneal a
Fibula
Flexor hallucis longus m & t
Lesser saphenous v

Tibia
Ant tibial v
Deep peroneal n
Ant tibial a
Greater saphenous v
Tibialis post m & t
Flexor digitorum longus m & t
Post tibial vv
Post tibial a
Tibial n
Soleus t
Plantaris t
Soleus m & tt
Sural n

Lower Leg, Transverse

Crural fascia
Extensor digitorum longus tt
Extensor hallucis longus t
Extensor hallucis longus m
Extensor digitorum longus m
Ant intermuscular septum
Interosseous membrane
Peroneus brevis t
Peroneal a
Peroneal vv
Fibula
Peroneus longus m & t
Peroneus brevis m

Lesser saphenous v

Tibialis ant m & t

Tibia
Ant tibial a
Ant tibial v
Deep peroneal n
Crural fascia
Greater saphenous v
Flexor digitorum longus m & tt
Tibialis post m & t
Post tibial vv
Post tibial a
Tibial n
Flexor hallucis longus m & t
Plantaris t

Tendo calcaneus
Soleus m & t

Sural n

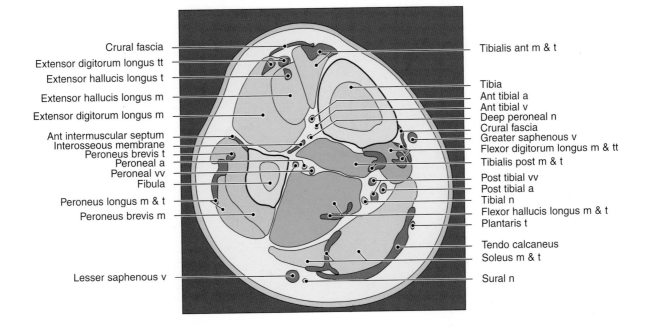

Crural fascia
Extensor digitorum longus tt
Extensor hallucis longus t
Extensor hallucis longus m
Extensor digitorum longus m
Ant intermuscular septum
Interosseous membrane
Peroneus brevis t
Peroneal a
Peroneal vv
Fibula
Peroneus longus m & t
Peroneus brevis m

Lesser saphenous v

Tibialis ant m & t

Tibia
Ant tibial a
Ant tibial v
Deep peroneal n
Crural fascia
Greater saphenous v
Flexor digitorum longus m & tt
Tibialis post m & t
Post tibial vv
Post tibial a
Tibial n
Flexor hallucis longus m & t
Plantaris t

Tendo calcaneus
Soleus m & t

Sural n

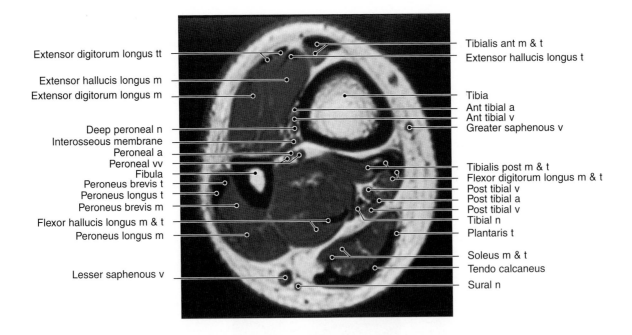

Extensor digitorum longus tt
Extensor hallucis longus m
Extensor digitorum longus m
Deep peroneal n
Interosseous membrane
Peroneal a
Peroneal vv
Fibula
Peroneus brevis t
Peroneus longus t
Peroneus brevis m
Flexor hallucis longus m & t
Peroneus longus m
Lesser saphenous v

Tibialis ant m & t
Extensor hallucis longus t
Tibia
Ant tibial a
Ant tibial v
Greater saphenous v
Tibialis post m & t
Flexor digitorum longus m & t
Post tibial v
Post tibial a
Post tibial v
Tibial n
Plantaris t
Soleus m & t
Tendo calcaneus
Sural n

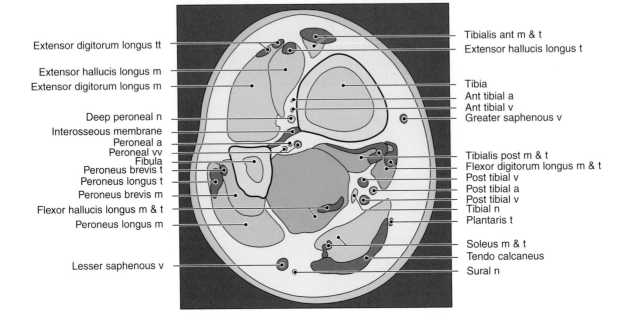

Extensor digitorum longus tt
Extensor hallucis longus m
Extensor digitorum longus m
Deep peroneal n
Interosseous membrane
Peroneal a
Peroneal vv
Fibula
Peroneus brevis t
Peroneus longus t
Peroneus brevis m
Flexor hallucis longus m & t
Peroneus longus m
Lesser saphenous v

Tibialis ant m & t
Extensor hallucis longus t
Tibia
Ant tibial a
Ant tibial v
Greater saphenous v
Tibialis post m & t
Flexor digitorum longus m & t
Post tibial v
Post tibial a
Post tibial v
Tibial n
Plantaris t
Soleus m & t
Tendo calcaneus
Sural n

Lower Leg, Sagittal

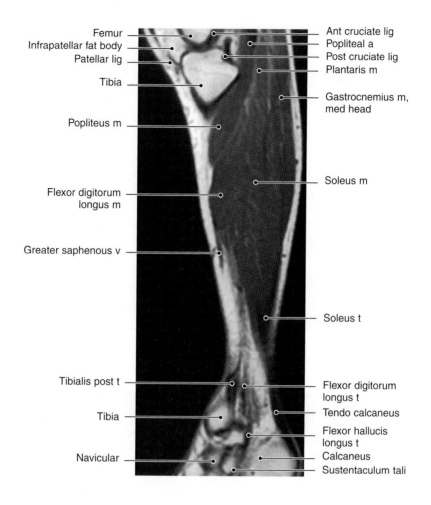

Femur
Infrapatellar fat body
Patellar lig
Tibia
Popliteus m
Flexor digitorum longus m
Greater saphenous v
Tibialis post t
Tibia
Navicular

Ant cruciate lig
Popliteal a
Post cruciate lig
Plantaris m
Gastrocnemius m, med head
Soleus m
Soleus t
Flexor digitorum longus t
Tendo calcaneus
Flexor hallucis longus t
Calcaneus
Sustentaculum tali

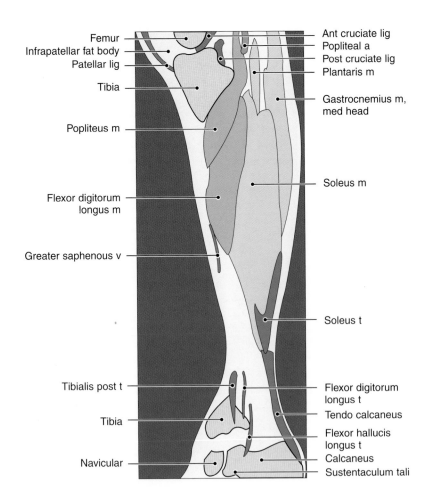

Femur

Infrapatellar fat body

Patellar lig

Tibia

Popliteus m

Flexor digitorum longus m

Greater saphenous v

Tibialis post t

Tibia

Navicular

Ant cruciate lig

Popliteal a

Post cruciate lig

Plantaris m

Gastrocnemius m, med head

Soleus m

Soleus t

Flexor digitorum longus t

Tendo calcaneus

Flexor hallucis longus t

Calcaneus

Sustentaculum tali

Lower Leg, Sagittal

Femur
Infrapatellar fat body
Med meniscus
Patellar lig
Tibia
Popliteus m
Tibialis post m
Flexor digitorum
longus m
Tibia
Talus
Navicular
Intermediate cuneiform

Plantaris m
Popliteal a
Gastrocnemius m,
med head
Soleus m
Flexor hallucis longus m
Flexor hallucis longus t
Soleus t
Post talofibular lig
Tarsal sinus
Calcaneus

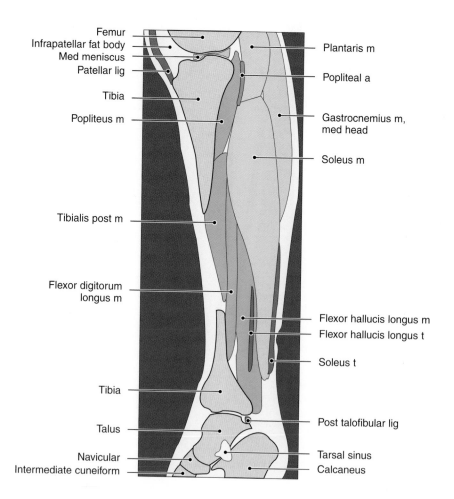

Femur

Infrapatellar fat body

Med meniscus

Patellar lig

Tibia

Popliteus m

Tibialis post m

Flexor digitorum longus m

Tibia

Talus

Navicular

Intermediate cuneiform

Plantaris m

Popliteal a

Gastrocnemius m, med head

Soleus m

Flexor hallucis longus m

Flexor hallucis longus t

Soleus t

Post talofibular lig

Tarsal sinus

Calcaneus

Lower Leg, Sagittal

Tibia
Infrapatellar fat body
Patellar lig
Tibialis post m
Tibia
Tibialis ant t
Extensor hallucis longus m & t
Extensor digitorum longus t
Navicular

Lat meniscus
Popliteus m
Gastrocnemius m, lat head
Popliteal a
Flexor digitorum longus m
Soleus m
Flexor hallucis longus m
Peroneus brevis m
Talus
Peroneus brevis t
Peroneus longus t
Calcaneus

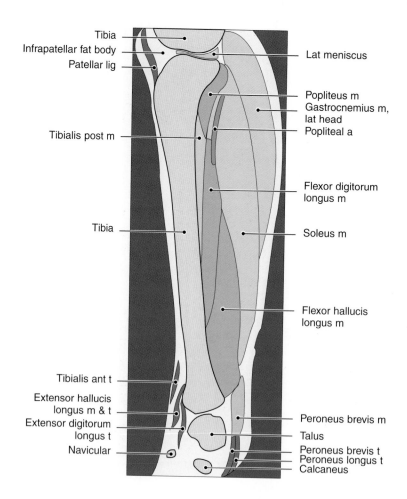

Tibia

Infrapatellar fat body

Patellar lig

Lat meniscus

Popliteus m

Gastrocnemius m, lat head

Popliteal a

Tibialis post m

Flexor digitorum longus m

Tibia

Soleus m

Flexor hallucis longus m

Tibialis ant t

Extensor hallucis longus m & t

Extensor digitorum longus t

Navicular

Peroneus brevis m

Talus

Peroneus brevis t

Peroneus longus t

Calcaneus

Lower Leg, Sagittal

Biceps femoris t

Ant tibial a

Tibialis ant m

Fibula

Gastrocnemius m, lat head

Soleus m

Tibialis ant t

Extensor hallucis longus & extensor digitorum longus mm

Peroneus longus m

Ankle and Foot, Coronal

Peroneus brevis m

Flexor hallucis longus m & t

Sural n

Lesser saphenous v

Calcaneus

11

Ankle and Foot

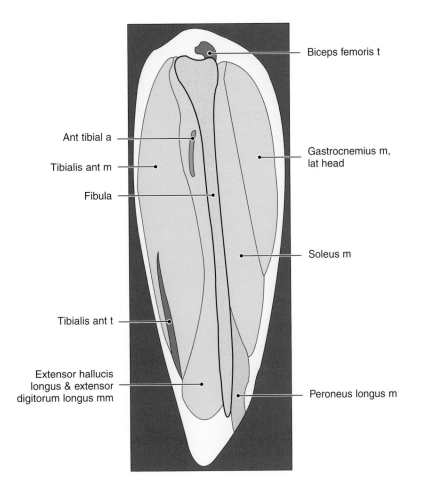

Biceps femoris t

Ant tibial a

Tibialis ant m

Fibula

Gastrocnemius m, lat head

Soleus m

Tibialis ant t

Extensor hallucis longus & extensor digitorum longus mm

Peroneus longus m

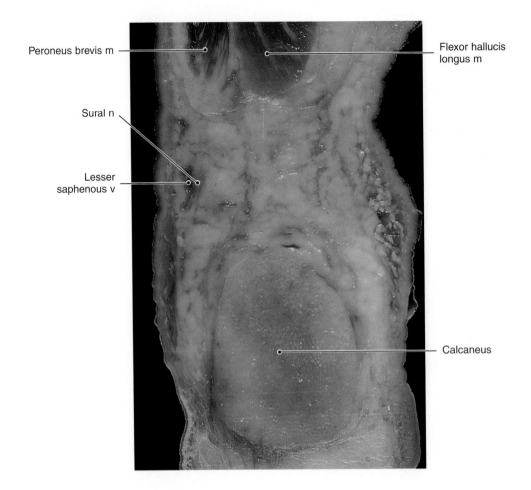

Peroneus brevis m

Sural n

Lesser
saphenous v

Flexor hallucis
longus m

Calcaneus

Ankle and Foot, Coronal

Peroneus brevis
m & t

Peroneus longus t

Lesser
saphenous v

Sural n

Calcaneus

Flexor digitorum
longus t

Tibial n

Post tibial a

Flexor hallucis
longus m & t

Abductor hallucis m

Peroneus brevis m & t

Peroneus longus t

Lesser saphenous v

Sural n

Calcaneus

Post tibial a

Tibial n

Flexor hallucis longus m & t

Abductor hallucis m

Ankle and Foot, Coronal

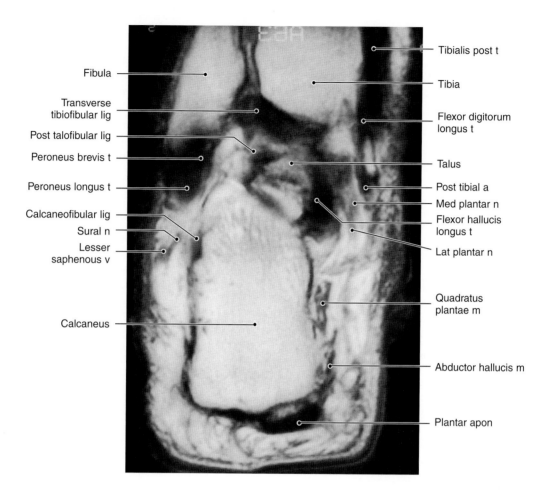

Fibula

Transverse tibiofibular lig

Post talofibular lig

Peroneus brevis t

Peroneus longus t

Calcaneofibular lig

Sural n

Lesser saphenous v

Calcaneus

Tibialis post t

Tibia

Flexor digitorum longus t

Talus

Post tibial a

Med plantar n

Flexor hallucis longus t

Lat plantar n

Quadratus plantae m

Abductor hallucis m

Plantar apon

Fibula

Transverse
tibiofibular lig

Post talofibular lig

Peroneus brevis t

Peroneus longus t

Calcaneofibular lig

Sural n

Lesser
saphenous v

Calcaneus

Tibialis post t

Tibia

Flexor digitorum
longus t

Talus

Post tibial a

Flexor hallucis
longus t

Med plantar n

Lat plantar n

Quadratus
plantae m

Abductor hallucis m

Plantar apon

Ankle and Foot, Coronal

Fibula

Talus

Post talofibular lig

Peroneus brevis t

Calcaneofibular lig

Peroneus longus t

Calcaneus

Sural n

Abductor digiti minimi m

Plantar apon, lat cord

Tibia

Post tibiotalar lig

Flexor retinaculum

Tibialis post t

Flexor digitorum longus t

Flexor hallucis longus t

Med plantar a & n

Lat plantar a & n

Quadratus plantae m

Abductor hallucis m

Plantar apon

Fibula

Talus

Post talofibular lig

Peroneus brevis t

Peroneus longus t

Calcaneofibular lig

Sural n

Calcaneus

Abductor digiti
minimi m

Plantar apon,
lat cord

Tibia

Flexor retinaculum

Tibialis post t

Flexor digitorum
longus t

Post tibial a

Flexor hallucis
longus t

Med plantar n

Lat plantar n

Quadratus plantae m

Abductor hallucis m

Plantar apon

Ankle and Foot, Coronal

Lat malleolus

Talus

Calcaneofibular lig

Peroneus brevis t

Peroneus longus t

Calcaneus

Sural n

Peroneal retinaculum

Abductor digiti minimi m

Plantar apon, lat cord

Tibia

Med malleolus

Post tibiotalar lig

Tibialis post t

Flexor retinaculum

Flexor digitorum longus t

Interosseous talocalcaneal lig

Flexor hallucis longus t

Med plantar a & n

Quadratus plantae m

Lat plantar a & n

Abductor hallucis m

Flexor digitorum brevis m

Plantar apon

Ant talofibular lig

Lat malleolus

Talus

Calcaneofibular lig

Peroneus brevis t

Peroneus longus t

Calcaneus

Peroneal retinaculum

Sural n

Abductor digiti
minimi m

Plantar apon,
lat cord

Tibia

Med malleolus

Post tibiotalar lig

Tibialis post t

Flexor retinaculum

Flexor digitorum
longus t

Interosseous
talocalcaneal lig

Flexor hallucis
longus t

Med plantar a & n

Quadratus plantae m

Lat plantar a & n

Abductor hallucis m

Flexor digitorum
brevis m

Plantar apon

Ankle and Foot, Coronal

Ant inf tibiofibular lig

Talus

Ant talofibular lig

Calcaneofibular lig

Peroneus brevis t

Calcaneus

Peroneus longus t

Peroneal retinaculum

Long plantar lig

Abductor digiti minimi m

Plantar apon, lat cord

Tibia

Med malleolus

Post tibiotalar lig

Flexor retinaculum

Tibialis post t

Tibiocalcaneal lig

Interosseous talocalcaneal lig

Flexor digitorum longus t

Sustentaculum tali

Med plantar a & n

Flexor hallucis longus t

Quadratus plantae m

Abductor hallucis m

Lat plantar a & n

Flexor digitorum brevis m

Plantar apon

Ant inf
tibiofibular lig

Talus

Ant talofibular lig

Calcaneofibular lig

Peroneus brevis t

Calcaneus

Peroneus longus t

Peroneal
retinaculum

Long plantar lig

Abductor digiti
minimi m

Plantar apon,
lat cord

Tibia

Med malleolus

Post tibiotalar lig

Flexor retinaculum

Tibialis post t

Tibiocalcaneal lig

Interosseous
talocalcaneal lig

Flexor digitorum
longus t

Sustentaculum tali

Flexor hallucis longus t

Med plantar a & n

Quadratus plantae m

Abductor hallucis m

Lat plantar a & n

Flexor digitorum
brevis m

Plantar apon

Ankle and Foot, Coronal

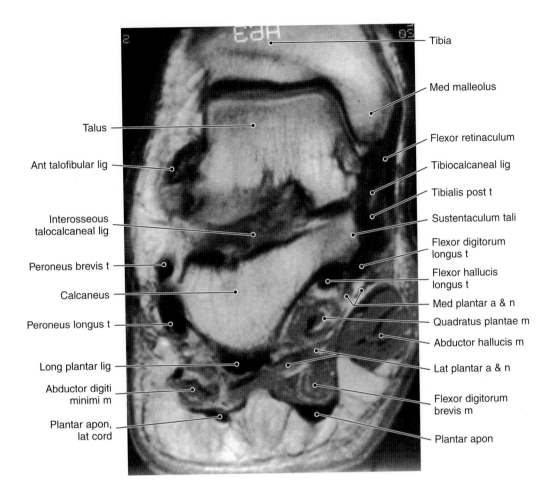

Talus

Ant talofibular lig

Interosseous talocalcaneal lig

Peroneus brevis t

Calcaneus

Peroneus longus t

Long plantar lig

Abductor digiti minimi m

Plantar apon, lat cord

Tibia

Med malleolus

Flexor retinaculum

Tibiocalcaneal lig

Tibialis post t

Sustentaculum tali

Flexor digitorum longus t

Flexor hallucis longus t

Med plantar a & n

Quadratus plantae m

Abductor hallucis m

Lat plantar a & n

Flexor digitorum brevis m

Plantar apon

Peroneus tertius m

Ant talofibular lig

Interosseous talocalcaneal lig

Peroneus brevis t

Calcaneus

Peroneus longus t

Long plantar lig

Abductor digiti minimi m

Plantar apon, lat cord

Tibia

Med malleolus

Talus

Flexor retinaculum

Tibiocalcaneal lig

Tibialis post t

Sustentaculum tali

Flexor digitorum longus t

Flexor hallucis longus t

Med plantar a & n

Quadratus plantae m

Abductor hallucis m

Lat plantar a & n

Flexor digitorum brevis m

Plantar apon

Ankle and Foot, Coronal

Tibia

Talus

Med malleolus

Flexor retinaculum

Tibiocalcaneal lig

Interosseous
talocalcaneal lig

Spring lig

Tibialis post t

Peroneus brevis t

Sustentaculum tali

Calcaneus

Flexor hallucis longus t

Flexor digitorum longus t

Peroneus longus t

Med plantar n

Quadratus plantae m

Long plantar lig

Abductor hallucis m

Abductor digiti
minimi m

Lat plantar a & n

Plantar apon,
lat cord

Flexor digitorum brevis m

Plantar apon

Extensor digitorum longus t

Peroneus tertius m & t

Talus

Interosseous talocalcaneal lig

Peroneus brevis t

Calcaneus

Peroneus longus t

Long plantar lig

Abductor digiti minimi m

Plantar apon, lat cord

Tibia

Med malleolus

Flexor retinaculum

Tibiocalcaneal lig

Spring lig

Tibialis post t

Sustentaculum tali

Flexor digitorum longus t

Flexor hallucis longus t

Med plantar n

Abductor hallucis m

Quadratus plantae m

Lat plantar a & n

Flexor digitorum brevis m

Plantar apon

Ankle and Foot, Coronal

Extensor digitorum longus t

Peroneus tertius t

Talus

Interosseous talocalcaneal lig

Calcaneus

Peroneus brevis t

Peroneus longus t

Long plantar lig

Abductor digiti minimi m

Plantar apon, lat cord

Greater saphenous v

Tibiocalcaneal lig

Spring lig

Tibialis post t

Flexor hallucis longus t

Flexor digitorum longus t

Med plantar n

Abductor hallucis m

Quadratus plantae m

Lat plantar a & n

Flexor digitorum brevis m

Plantar apon

Extensor hallucis longus m & t

Extensor digitorum longus t

Peroneus tertius t

Talus

Interosseous talocalcaneal lig

Calcaneus

Peroneus brevis t

Peroneus longus t

Long plantar lig

Abductor digiti minimi m

Plantar apon, lat cord

Tibialis ant t

Greater saphenous v

Tibiocalcaneal lig

Spring lig

Tibialis post t

Flexor hallucis longus t

Flexor digitorum longus t

Med plantar n

Abductor hallucis m

Quadratus plantae m

Lat plantar a & n

Flexor digitorum brevis m

Plantar apon

Ankle and Foot, Coronal

Extensor hallucis longus m & t

Extensor digitorum longus t

Peroneus tertius t

Interosseous talocalcaneal lig

Bifurcated lig

Calcaneus

Peroneus brevis t

Quadratus plantae m

Peroneus longus t

Long plantar lig

Abductor digiti minimi m

Plantar apon, lat cord

Tibialis ant t

Greater saphenous v

Talus

Tibionavicular lig

Spring lig

Sesamoid

Tibialis post t

Flexor hallucis longus t

Flexor digitorum longus t

Abductor hallucis m

Med plantar n

Lat plantar a & n

Flexor digitorum brevis m

Plantar apon

Extensor hallucis longus m & t

Extensor digitorum longus t

Peroneus tertius t

Interosseous talocalcaneal lig

Bifurcated lig

Calcaneus
Cuboid

Peroneus brevis t

Quadratus plantae m

Peroneus longus t
Long plantar lig
Abductor digiti minimi m

Plantar apon, lat cord

Tibialis ant t

Greater saphenous v

Talus

Tibionavicular lig
Spring lig

Sesamoid

Tibialis post t

Flexor hallucis longus t

Flexor digitorum longus t

Med plantar n

Abductor hallucis m

Lat plantar a & n

Flexor digitorum brevis m

Plantar apon

Ankle and Foot, Coronal

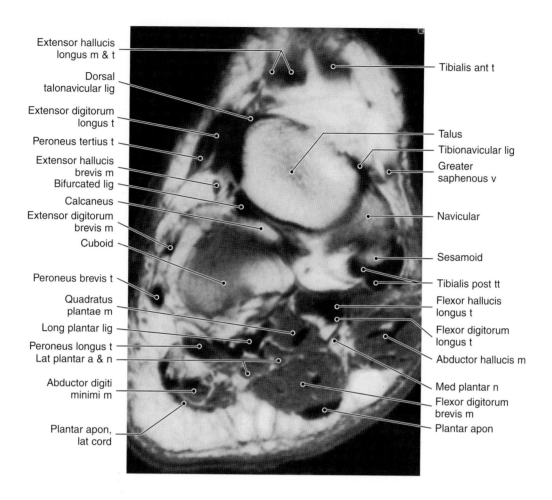

Extensor hallucis
longus m & t

Dorsal
talonavicular lig

Extensor digitorum
longus t

Peroneus tertius t

Extensor hallucis
brevis m

Bifurcated lig

Calcaneus

Extensor digitorum
brevis m

Cuboid

Peroneus brevis t

Quadratus
plantae m

Long plantar lig

Peroneus longus t

Lat plantar a & n

Abductor digiti
minimi m

Plantar apon,
lat cord

Tibialis ant t

Talus

Tibionavicular lig

Greater
saphenous v

Navicular

Sesamoid

Tibialis post tt

Flexor hallucis
longus t

Flexor digitorum
longus t

Abductor hallucis m

Med plantar n

Flexor digitorum
brevis m

Plantar apon

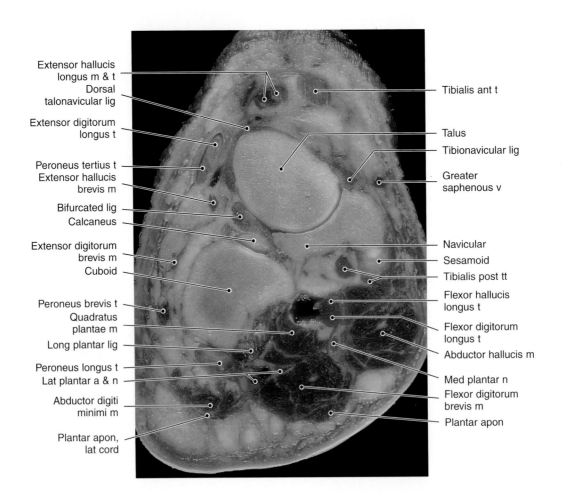

Extensor hallucis longus m & t

Dorsal talonavicular lig

Extensor digitorum longus t

Peroneus tertius t
Extensor hallucis brevis m

Bifurcated lig
Calcaneus

Extensor digitorum brevis m
Cuboid

Peroneus brevis t
Quadratus plantae m
Long plantar lig

Peroneus longus t
Lat plantar a & n

Abductor digiti minimi m

Plantar apon, lat cord

Tibialis ant t

Talus
Tibionavicular lig

Greater saphenous v

Navicular
Sesamoid
Tibialis post tt
Flexor hallucis longus t
Flexor digitorum longus t
Abductor hallucis m

Med plantar n
Flexor digitorum brevis m
Plantar apon

Ankle and Foot, Coronal

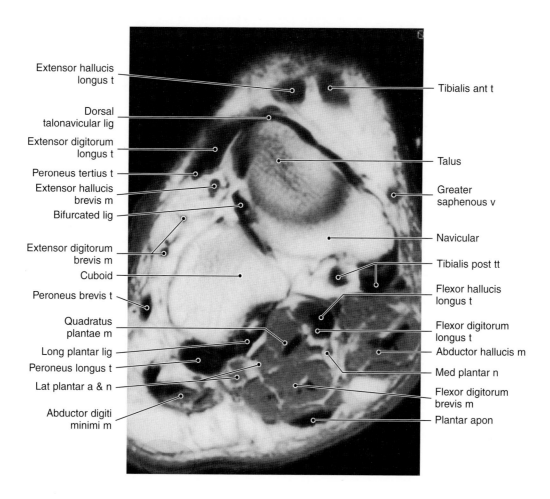

Extensor hallucis longus t

Dorsal talonavicular lig

Extensor digitorum longus t

Peroneus tertius t

Extensor hallucis brevis m

Bifurcated lig

Extensor digitorum brevis m

Cuboid

Peroneus brevis t

Quadratus plantae m

Long plantar lig

Peroneus longus t

Lat plantar a & n

Abductor digiti minimi m

Tibialis ant t

Talus

Greater saphenous v

Navicular

Tibialis post tt

Flexor hallucis longus t

Flexor digitorum longus t

Abductor hallucis m

Med plantar n

Flexor digitorum brevis m

Plantar apon

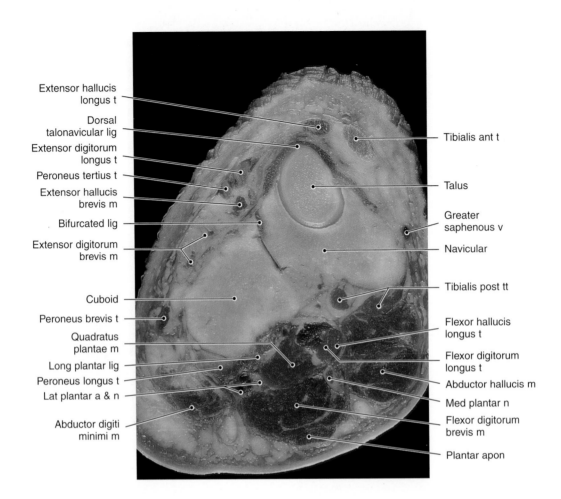

Extensor hallucis longus t

Dorsal talonavicular lig

Extensor digitorum longus t

Peroneus tertius t

Extensor hallucis brevis m

Bifurcated lig

Extensor digitorum brevis m

Cuboid

Peroneus brevis t

Quadratus plantae m

Long plantar lig

Peroneus longus t

Lat plantar a & n

Abductor digiti minimi m

Tibialis ant t

Talus

Greater saphenous v

Navicular

Tibialis post tt

Flexor hallucis longus t

Flexor digitorum longus t

Abductor hallucis m

Med plantar n

Flexor digitorum brevis m

Plantar apon

Ankle and Foot, Coronal

Dorsal talonavicular lig

Extensor digitorum longus t

Peroneus tertius t

Extensor hallucis brevis m

Dorsal cuboideonavicular lig

Extensor digitorum brevis m

Cuboid

Peroneus brevis t

Quadratus plantae m

Peroneus longus t

Lat plantar a & n

Abductor digiti minimi m

Extensor hallucis longus t

Tibialis ant t

Greater saphenous v

Navicular

Tibialis post t

Abductor hallucis m

Flexor hallucis longus t

Flexor digitorum longus t

Med plantar n

Flexor digitorum brevis m

Plantar apon

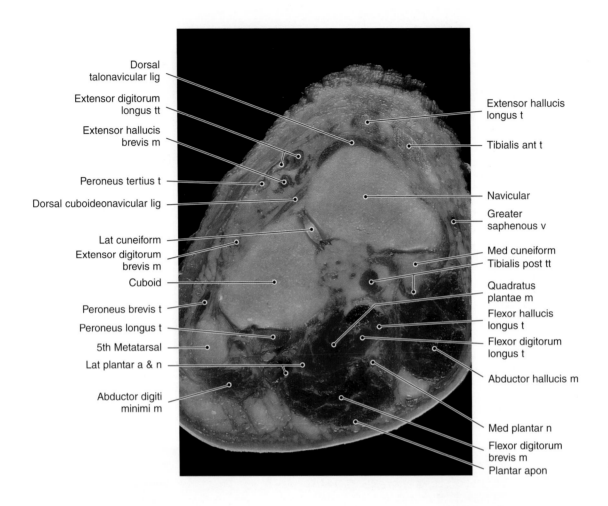

Dorsal talonavicular lig

Extensor digitorum longus tt

Extensor hallucis brevis m

Peroneus tertius t

Dorsal cuboideonavicular lig

Lat cuneiform

Extensor digitorum brevis m

Cuboid

Peroneus brevis t

Peroneus longus t

5th Metatarsal

Lat plantar a & n

Abductor digiti minimi m

Extensor hallucis longus t

Tibialis ant t

Navicular

Greater saphenous v

Med cuneiform

Tibialis post tt

Quadratus plantae m

Flexor hallucis longus t

Flexor digitorum longus t

Abductor hallucis m

Med plantar n

Flexor digitorum brevis m

Plantar apon

Ankle and Foot, Coronal

Extensor hallucis brevis m

Extensor digitorum longus tt

Peroneus tertius t

Extensor digitorum brevis m

Lat cuneiform

Cuboid

Peroneus longus t

5th Metatarsal

Lat plantar a & n

Abductor digiti minimi m

Extensor hallucis longus t

Tibialis ant t

Intermediate cuneiform

Med cuneiform

Tibialis post t

Abductor hallucis m

Flexor hallucis longus t

Flexor hallucis brevis m

Med plantar n

Flexor digitorum longus t

Flexor digitorum brevis m

Quadratus plantae m

Plantar apon

Extensor digitorum longus tt

Dorsal talonavicular lig

Extensor hallucis brevis m

Peroneus tertius t

Extensor digitorum brevis m

Lat cuneiform

Cuboid

Peroneus longus t

5th Metatarsal

Lat plantar a & n

Abductor digiti minimi m

Extensor hallucis longus t

Tibialis ant t

Navicular

Intermediate cuneiform

Med cuneiform

Tibialis post t

Flexor hallucis longus t

Abductor hallucis m

Flexor digitorum longus t

Flexor hallucis brevis m

Med plantar n

Quadratus plantae m

Flexor digitorum brevis m

Extensor hallucis brevis m

Extensor digitorum longus tt

Lat cuneiform

Peroneus tertius t

Cuboid

Peroneus longus t

5th Metatarsal

Quadratus plantae m

Lat plantar a & n

Abductor digiti minimi m

Extensor hallucis longus t

Intermediate cuneiform

Tibialis ant t

Med cuneiform

Flexor digitorum longus t

Abductor hallucis m

Flexor hallucis longus t

Flexor hallucis brevis m

Med plantar n

Flexor digitorum brevis m

Plantar apon

Extensor hallucis brevis m

Extensor digitorum longus tt

Peroneus tertius t

Lat cuneiform

Cuboid

4th Metatarsal

5th Metatarsal

Peroneus longus t

Abductor digiti minimi m

Lat plantar a & n

Extensor hallucis longus t

Intermediate cuneiform

Tibialis ant t

Med cuneiform

Tibialis post t

Flexor digitorum longus t

Abductor hallucis m

Flexor hallucis longus t

Flexor hallucis brevis m

Med plantar n

Quadratus plantae m

Flexor digitorum brevis m

Ankle and Foot, Coronal

Extensor hallucis brevis m

Extensor digitorum longus tt

Lat cuneiform

Peroneus tertius t

4th Metatarsal

Peroneus longus t

5th Metatarsal

Adductor hallucis m, oblique head

Abductor digiti minimi m

Flexor digiti minimi brevis m

Lat plantar a & n

Extensor hallucis longus t

Intermediate cuneiform

Tibialis ant t

Med cuneiform

Abductor hallucis m

Flexor hallucis longus t

Flexor hallucis brevis m

Flexor digitorum longus t

Med plantar n

Plantar apon

Quadratus plantae m

Flexor digitorum brevis m

Extensor hallucis brevis m

Extensor digitorum longus tt

Lat cuneiform

Peroneus tertius t

4th Metatarsal

5th Metatarsal

Adductor hallucis m, oblique head

Abductor digiti minimi m

Flexor digiti minimi brevis m

Lat plantar a & n

Extensor hallucis longus t

Intermediate cuneiform

Tibialis ant t

Med cuneiform

Peroneus longus t

Abductor hallucis m

Flexor digitorum longus t

Flexor hallucis longus t

Flexor hallucis brevis m

Med plantar n

Quadratus plantae m   Flexor digitorum brevis m

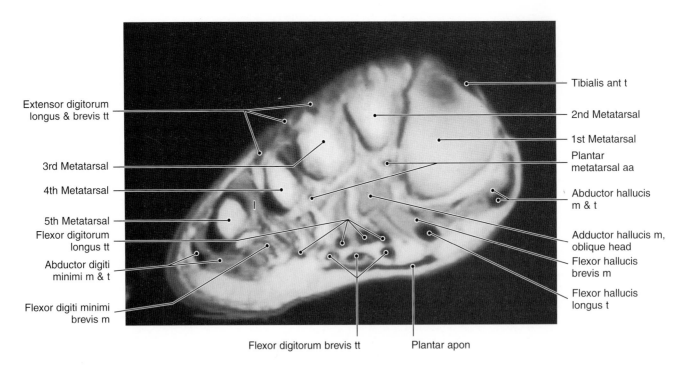

Extensor digitorum longus & brevis tt

Tibialis ant t

2nd Metatarsal

1st Metatarsal

Plantar metatarsal aa

3rd Metatarsal

4th Metatarsal

Abductor hallucis m & t

5th Metatarsal

Flexor digitorum longus tt

Adductor hallucis m, oblique head

Abductor digiti minimi m & t

Flexor hallucis brevis m

Flexor digiti minimi brevis m

Flexor hallucis longus t

Flexor digitorum brevis tt

Plantar apon

I: Interosseous m

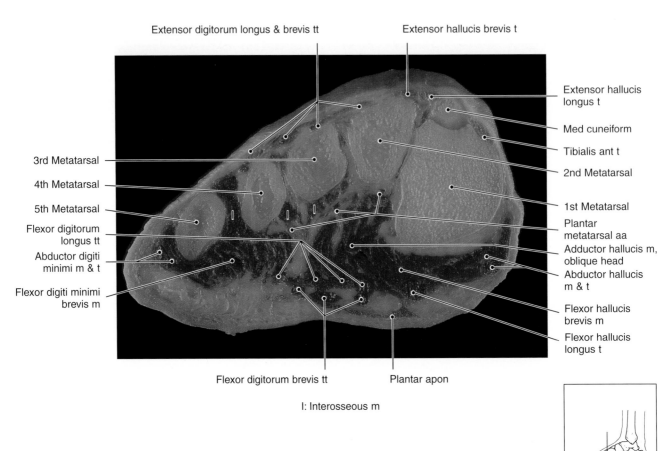

Extensor digitorum longus & brevis tt

Extensor hallucis brevis t

Extensor hallucis longus t

Med cuneiform

3rd Metatarsal

Tibialis ant t

4th Metatarsal

2nd Metatarsal

5th Metatarsal

1st Metatarsal

Flexor digitorum longus tt

Plantar metatarsal aa

Abductor digiti minimi m & t

Adductor hallucis m, oblique head

Abductor hallucis m & t

Flexor digiti minimi brevis m

Flexor hallucis brevis m

Flexor hallucis longus t

Flexor digitorum brevis tt

Plantar apon

I: Interosseous m

Ankle and Foot, Coronal

Extensor digitorum longus & brevis tt

Extensor hallucis longus t

2nd Metatarsal

1st Metatarsal

3rd Metatarsal

4th Metatarsal

Adductor hallucis m, oblique head

5th Metatarsal

Abductor hallucis m & t

Abductor digiti minimi t

Flexor hallucis brevis m

Flexor digiti minimi brevis t

Flexor digitorum longus tt

Plantar apon

Flexor hallucis longus t

Flexor digitorum brevis tt

I: Interosseous m

Arrowhead: Lumbrical m

Extensor digitorum longus & brevis tt

Extensor hallucis brevis t

Extensor hallucis longus t

2nd Metatarsal

1st Metatarsal

3rd Metatarsal

4th Metatarsal

Flexor digitorum longus tt

5th Metatarsal

Adductor hallucis m, oblique head

Abductor digiti minimi t

Abductor hallucis m & t

Plantar lig

Flexor digiti minimi brevis t

Flexor hallucis brevis m

Plantar apon

Flexor hallucis longus t

Flexor digitorum brevis tt

I: Interosseous m

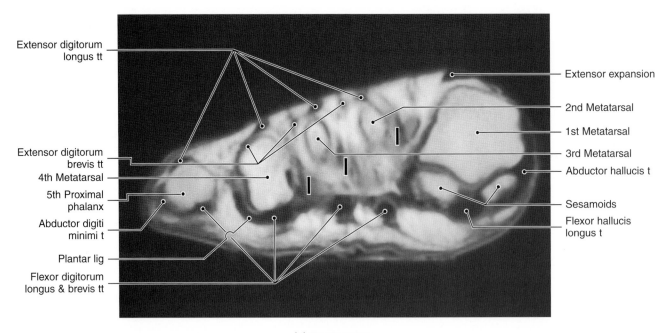

Extensor digitorum longus tt

Extensor digitorum brevis tt

4th Metatarsal

5th Proximal phalanx

Abductor digiti minimi t

Plantar lig

Flexor digitorum longus & brevis tt

Extensor expansion

2nd Metatarsal

1st Metatarsal

3rd Metatarsal

Abductor hallucis t

Sesamoids

Flexor hallucis longus t

I: Interosseous m

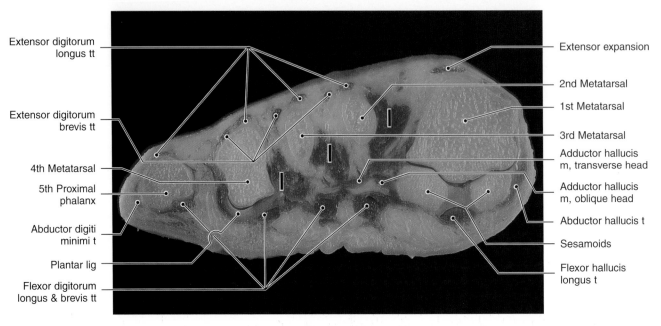

Extensor digitorum longus tt

Extensor digitorum brevis tt

4th Metatarsal

5th Proximal phalanx

Abductor digiti minimi t

Plantar lig

Flexor digitorum longus & brevis tt

Extensor expansion

2nd Metatarsal

1st Metatarsal

3rd Metatarsal

Adductor hallucis m, transverse head

Adductor hallucis m, oblique head

Abductor hallucis t

Sesamoids

Flexor hallucis longus t

I: Interosseous m

Ankle and Foot, Coronal

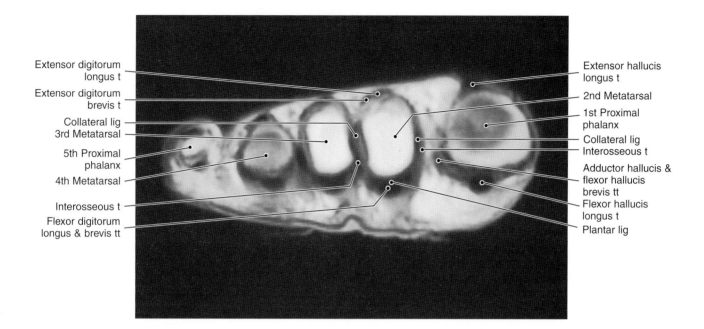

Extensor digitorum longus t
Extensor digitorum brevis t
Collateral lig
3rd Metatarsal
5th Proximal phalanx
4th Metatarsal
Interosseous t
Flexor digitorum longus & brevis tt

Extensor hallucis longus t
2nd Metatarsal
1st Proximal phalanx
Collateral lig
Interosseous t
Adductor hallucis & flexor hallucis brevis tt
Flexor hallucis longus t
Plantar lig

Extensor digitorum brevis t
Collateral lig
Extensor expansion
3rd Metatarsal
5th Proximal phalanx
4th Metatarsal
Interosseous t
Flexor digitorum longus & brevis tt

Extensor hallucis longus t
Extensor digitorum longus t
1st Proximal phalanx
Collateral lig
Interosseous t
2nd Metatarsal
Adductor hallucis & flexor hallucis brevis tt
Flexor hallucis longus t
Plantar lig

Extensor expansions

3rd Proximal phalanx

4th Proximal phalanx

5th Middle phalanx

Flexor digitorum
longus & brevis tt

2nd Proximal
phalanx

1st Proximal
phalanx

Flexor hallucis
longus t

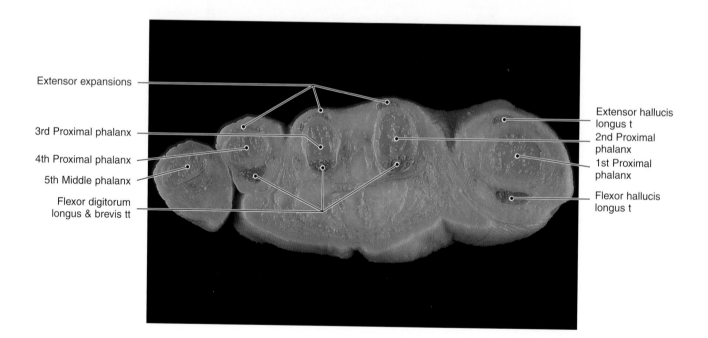

Extensor expansions

3rd Proximal phalanx

4th Proximal phalanx

5th Middle phalanx

Flexor digitorum
longus & brevis tt

Extensor hallucis
longus t

2nd Proximal
phalanx

1st Proximal
phalanx

Flexor hallucis
longus t

Ankle and Foot, Transverse

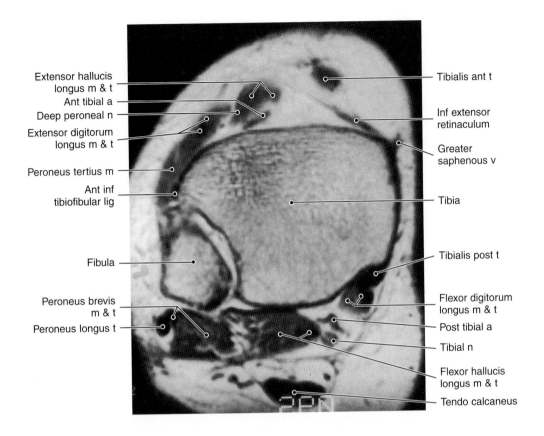

Extensor hallucis longus m & t

Ant tibial a

Deep peroneal n

Extensor digitorum longus m & t

Peroneus tertius m

Ant inf tibiofibular lig

Fibula

Peroneus brevis m & t

Peroneus longus t

Tibialis ant t

Inf extensor retinaculum

Greater saphenous v

Tibia

Tibialis post t

Flexor digitorum longus m & t

Post tibial a

Tibial n

Flexor hallucis longus m & t

Tendo calcaneus

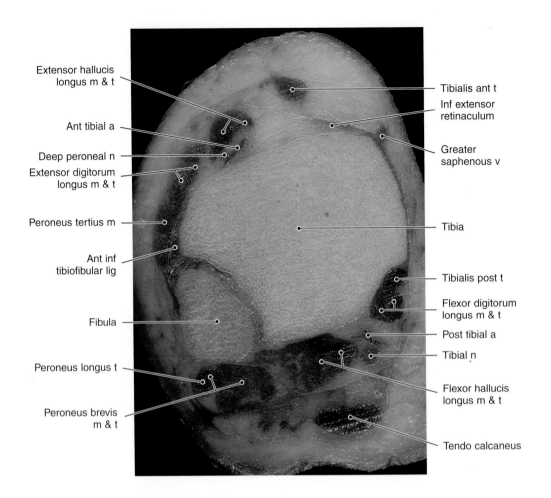

Extensor hallucis longus m & t

Ant tibial a

Deep peroneal n

Extensor digitorum longus m & t

Peroneus tertius m

Ant inf tibiofibular lig

Fibula

Peroneus longus t

Peroneus brevis m & t

Tibialis ant t

Inf extensor retinaculum

Greater saphenous v

Tibia

Tibialis post t

Flexor digitorum longus m & t

Post tibial a

Tibial n

Flexor hallucis longus m & t

Tendo calcaneus

Ankle and Foot, Transverse

Extensor hallucis longus m & t

Deep peroneal n

Extensor digitorum longus m & t

Ant tibial a

Peroneus tertius m

Ant inf tibiofibular lig

Fibula

Peroneus brevis m & t

Peroneus longus t

Tibialis ant t

Inf extensor retinaculum

Greater saphenous v

Tibia

Tibialis post t

Flexor digitorum longus t

Post tibial a

Tibial n

Flexor hallucis longus m & t

Tendo calcaneus

Extensor hallucis
longus m & t

Deep peroneal n

Extensor digitorum
longus m & t

Ant tibial a

Peroneus tertius m

Ant inf
tibiofibular lig

Fibula

Peroneus brevis
m & t

Peroneus longus t

Tibialis ant t

Inf extensor
retinaculum

Greater
saphenous v

Tibia

Tibialis post t

Flexor digitorum
longus t

Post tibial a

Tibial n

Flexor hallucis
longus m & t

Tendo calcaneus

Ankle and Foot, Transverse

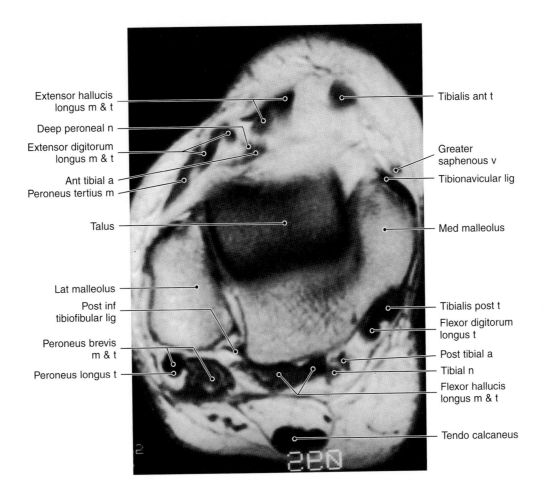

Extensor hallucis longus m & t

Deep peroneal n

Extensor digitorum longus m & t

Ant tibial a

Peroneus tertius m

Talus

Lat malleolus

Post inf tibiofibular lig

Peroneus brevis m & t

Peroneus longus t

Tibialis ant t

Greater saphenous v

Tibionavicular lig

Med malleolus

Tibialis post t

Flexor digitorum longus t

Post tibial a

Tibial n

Flexor hallucis longus m & t

Tendo calcaneus

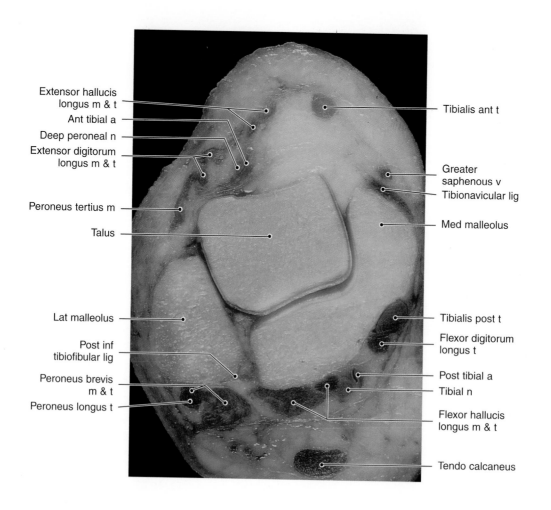

Extensor hallucis longus m & t

Ant tibial a

Deep peroneal n

Extensor digitorum longus m & t

Peroneus tertius m

Talus

Lat malleolus

Post inf tibiofibular lig

Peroneus brevis m & t

Peroneus longus t

Tibialis ant t

Greater saphenous v

Tibionavicular lig

Med malleolus

Tibialis post t

Flexor digitorum longus t

Post tibial a

Tibial n

Flexor hallucis longus m & t

Tendo calcaneus

Ankle and Foot, Transverse

Extensor hallucis longus t

Extensor digitorum longus & peroneus tertius tt

Talus

Lat malleolus

Post inf tibiofibular lig

Peroneus brevis m & t

Peroneus longus t

Peroneal retinaculum

Tibialis ant t

Greater saphenous v

Tibionavicular lig

Med malleolus

Tibialis post t

Flexor digitorum longus t

Post tibial a

Tibial n

Flexor hallucis longus m & t

Tendo calcaneus

Extensor hallucis longus t

Extensor digitorum longus & peroneus tertius tt

Talus

Transverse tibiofibular lig

Lat malleolus

Post inf tibiofibular lig

Peroneus brevis m & t

Peroneus longus t

Peroneal retinaculum

Tibialis ant t

Greater saphenous v

Tibionavicular lig

Med malleolus

Tibialis post t

Flexor digitorum longus t

Post tibial a

Tibial n

Flexor hallucis longus m & t

Tendo calcaneus

Ankle and Foot, Transverse

Dorsal talonavicular lig

Extensor digitorum longus & peroneus tertius tt

Interosseous talocalcaneal lig

Talus

Ant talofibular lig

Lat malleolus

Peroneus brevis m & t

Peroneus longus t

Peroneal retinaculum

Extensor hallucis longus t

Tibialis ant t

Greater saphenous v

Tibionavicular lig

Ant tibiotalar lig

Tibiocalcaneal lig

Tibialis post t

Flexor retinaculum

Flexor digitorum longus t

Post tibial a

Tibial n

Flexor hallucis longus m & t

Tendo calcaneus

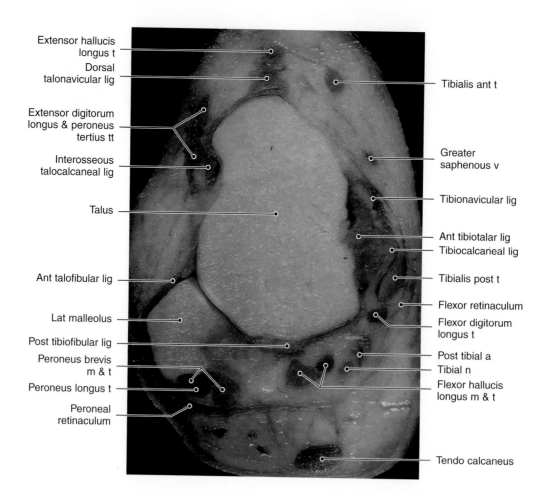

Extensor hallucis longus t

Dorsal talonavicular lig

Extensor digitorum longus & peroneus tertius tt

Interosseous talocalcaneal lig

Talus

Ant talofibular lig

Lat malleolus

Post tibiofibular lig

Peroneus brevis m & t

Peroneus longus t

Peroneal retinaculum

Tibialis ant t

Greater saphenous v

Tibionavicular lig

Ant tibiotalar lig

Tibiocalcaneal lig

Tibialis post t

Flexor retinaculum

Flexor digitorum longus t

Post tibial a

Tibial n

Flexor hallucis longus m & t

Tendo calcaneus

Ankle and Foot, Transverse

Extensor hallucis longus t

Navicular

Tibialis ant t

Extensor digitorum longus & peroneus tertius tt

Interosseous talocalcaneal lig

Talus

Ant talofibular lig

Tibionavicular lig

Tibiocalcaneal lig

Tibialis post t

Flexor digitorum longus t

Lat malleolus
Post talofibular lig

Flexor retinaculum

Peroneus brevis t

Post tibial a

Peroneus longus t

Tibial n

Peroneal retinaculum

Flexor hallucis longus t

Tendo calcaneus

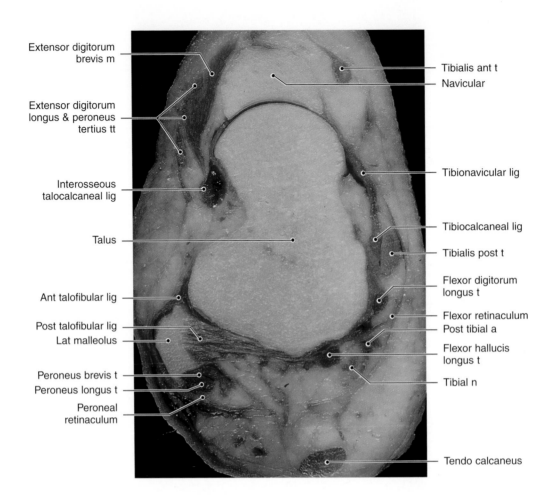

Extensor digitorum brevis m

Extensor digitorum longus & peroneus tertius tt

Interosseous talocalcaneal lig

Talus

Ant talofibular lig

Post talofibular lig

Lat malleolus

Peroneus brevis t

Peroneus longus t

Peroneal retinaculum

Tibialis ant t

Navicular

Tibionavicular lig

Tibiocalcaneal lig

Tibialis post t

Flexor digitorum longus t

Flexor retinaculum

Post tibial a

Flexor hallucis longus t

Tibial n

Tendo calcaneus

Ankle and Foot, Transverse

Dorsal cuneonavicular lig

Extensor digitorum longus tt

Extensor digitorum brevis m

Peroneus tertius t

Interosseous talocalcaneal lig

Talus

Calcaneus

Calcaneofibular lig

Peroneus brevis t

Peroneus longus t

Peroneal retinaculum

Intermediate cuneiform

Tibialis ant t

Navicular

Talus

Spring lig

Tibialis post t

Tibiocalcaneal lig

Flexor retinaculum

Flexor digitorum longus t

Post tibial a

Tibial n

Flexor hallucis longus t

Tendo calcaneus

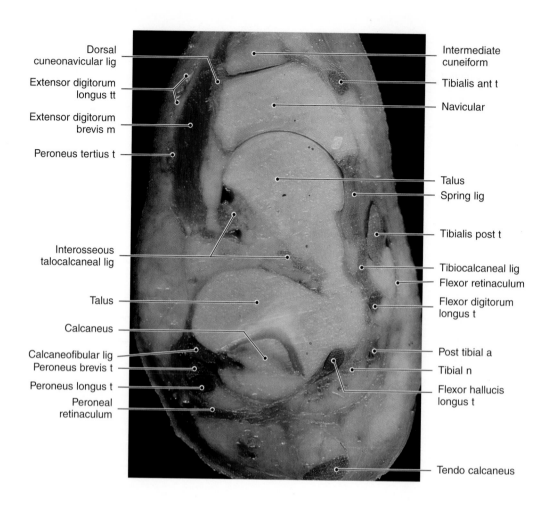

Dorsal cuneonavicular lig

Extensor digitorum longus tt

Extensor digitorum brevis m

Peroneus tertius t

Interosseous talocalcaneal lig

Talus

Calcaneus

Calcaneofibular lig
Peroneus brevis t
Peroneus longus t
Peroneal retinaculum

Intermediate cuneiform

Tibialis ant t

Navicular

Talus
Spring lig

Tibialis post t

Tibiocalcaneal lig
Flexor retinaculum

Flexor digitorum longus t

Post tibial a

Tibial n

Flexor hallucis longus t

Tendo calcaneus

Ankle and Foot, Transverse

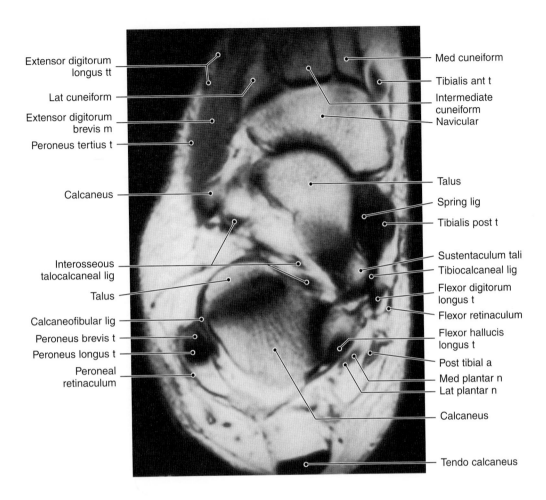

Extensor digitorum longus tt

Lat cuneiform

Extensor digitorum brevis m

Peroneus tertius t

Calcaneus

Interosseous talocalcaneal lig

Talus

Calcaneofibular lig

Peroneus brevis t

Peroneus longus t

Peroneal retinaculum

Med cuneiform

Tibialis ant t

Intermediate cuneiform

Navicular

Talus

Spring lig

Tibialis post t

Sustentaculum tali

Tibiocalcaneal lig

Flexor digitorum longus t

Flexor retinaculum

Flexor hallucis longus t

Post tibial a

Med plantar n

Lat plantar n

Calcaneus

Tendo calcaneus

Extensor digitorum longus t

Lat cuneiform

Extensor digitorum brevis m

Peroneus tertius t

Calcaneus

Interosseous talocalcaneal lig

Talus

Calcaneus

Calcaneofibular lig

Peroneus brevis t

Peroneus longus t

Peroneal retinaculum

Med cuneiform

Tibialis ant t

Intermediate cuneiform

Navicular

Talus

Spring lig

Tibialis post t

Tibiocalcaneal lig

Sustentaculum tali

Flexor digitorum longus t

Flexor retinaculum

Flexor hallucis longus t

Post tibial a

Med plantar n

Lat plantar n

Tendo calcaneus

Ankle and Foot, Transverse

Extensor digitorum longus tt

Extensor digitorum brevis m

Cuboid

Interosseous talocalcaneal lig

Peroneus brevis t

Peroneus longus t

Calcaneofibular lig

Interosseous intercuneiform lig

Med cuneiform

Tibialis ant t

Intermediate cuneiform

Lat cuneiform

Navicular

Tibialis post tt

Plantar calcaneonavicular lig

Sustentaculum tali

Flexor digitorum longus t

Calcaneus

Flexor hallucis longus t

Med plantar n

Post tibial a

Lat plantar n

Tendo calcaneus

Extensor digitorum longus tt

Lat cuneiform

Peroneus tertius t

Extensor digitorum brevis m

Cuboid

Interosseous talocalcaneal lig

Peroneus brevis t

Peroneus longus t

Calcaneofibular lig

2nd Metatarsal

Interosseous intercuneiform lig

Med cuneiform

Tibialis ant t

Intermediate cuneiform

Navicular

Tibialis post t

Plantar calcaneonavicular lig

Sustentaculum tali

Flexor digitorum longus t

Calcaneus

Flexor hallucis longus t

Med plantar n

Post tibial a

Lat plantar n

Tendo calcaneus

Ankle and Foot, Transverse

Lat cuneiform

Peroneus tertius t

Extensor digitorum brevis m

Cuboid

Peroneus brevis t

Peroneus longus t

Calcaneus

Calcaneofibular lig

Tibialis ant t

Intermediate cuneiform

Med cuneiform

Tibialis post tt

Plantar cuneonavicular lig

Plantar calcaneocuboid lig

Sustentaculum tali

Flexor digitorum longus t

Flexor hallucis longus t

Abductor hallucis m

Med palntar n

Lat plantar n

Post tibial a

Tendo calcaneus

Extensor digitorum longus tt

Lat cuneiform

Extensor digitorum brevis m

Peroneus tertius t

Cuboid

Peroneus brevis t

Peroneus longus t

Calcaneus

Calcaneofibular lig

3rd Metatarsal

2nd Metatarsal

Tibialis ant t

Intermediate cuneiform

Med cuneiform

Tibialis post tt

Plantar cuneonavicular lig

Plantar calcaneocuboid lig

Sustentaculum tali

Flexor digitorum longus t

Flexor hallucis longus t

Abductor hallucis m

Med plantar n

Lat plantar n

Post tibial a

Tendo calcaneus

Ankle and Foot, Transverse

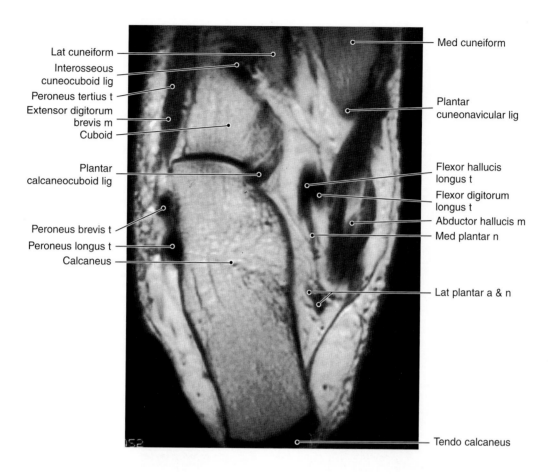

Lat cuneiform

Interosseous cuneocuboid lig

Peroneus tertius t

Extensor digitorum brevis m

Cuboid

Plantar calcaneocuboid lig

Peroneus brevis t

Peroneus longus t

Calcaneus

Med cuneiform

Plantar cuneonavicular lig

Flexor hallucis longus t

Flexor digitorum longus t

Abductor hallucis m

Med plantar n

Lat plantar a & n

Tendo calcaneus

Extensor digitorum
longus tt

1st Metatarsal

2nd Metatarsal

3rd Metatarsal

Tibialis ant t

Med cuneiform

Extensor digitorum
brevis m

Lat cuneiform

Interosseous
cuneocuboid lig

Peroneus tertius t

Plantar
cuneonavicular lig

Cuboid

Plantar
calcaneocuboid lig

Flexor hallucis
longus t

Peroneus brevis t

Flexor digitorum
longus t

Abductor hallucis m

Med plantar a & n

Peroneus longus t

Calcaneus

Lat plantar a & n

Tendo calcaneus

Ankle and Foot, Transverse

4th Metatarsal

Peroneus tertius t

Cuboid

Long plantar lig

Peroneus brevis t

Peroneus longus t

Calcaneus

1st Metatarsal

Flexor hallucis longus t

Flexor digitorum longus t

Med plantar a & n

Abductor hallucis m

Quadratus plantae m

Lat plantar a & n

Tendo calcaneus

Extensor digitorum longus t

3rd Metatarsal

Extensor digitorum brevis m

4th Metatarsal

Peroneus tertius t

Cuboid

Long plantar lig
Peroneus brevis t

Peroneus longus t

Calcaneus

2nd Metatarsal

1st Metatarsal

Med cuneiform

Flexor hallucis longus t

Flexor digitorum longus t

Quadratus plantae m

Med plantar a & n

Abductor hallucis m

Lat plantar a & n

Tendo calcaneus

Ankle and Foot, Transverse

4th Metatarsal

5th Metatarsal

Peroneus tertius t

Cuboid

Peroneus brevis t

Peroneus longus t

Long plantar lig

Calcaneus

Flexor hallucis brevis m, med head

Flexor hallucis longus t

Flexor digitorum longus t

Quadratus plantae m

Med plantar a & n

Abductor hallucis m

Lat plantar a & n

Tendo calcaneus

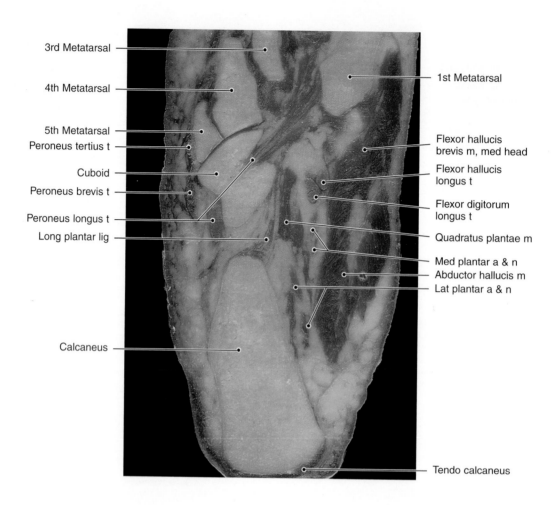

3rd Metatarsal

4th Metatarsal

5th Metatarsal

Peroneus tertius t

Cuboid

Peroneus brevis t

Peroneus longus t

Long plantar lig

Calcaneus

1st Metatarsal

Flexor hallucis
brevis m, med head

Flexor hallucis
longus t

Flexor digitorum
longus t

Quadratus plantae m

Med plantar a & n

Abductor hallucis m

Lat plantar a & n

Tendo calcaneus

Ankle and Foot, Transverse

4th Metatarsal

5th Metatarsal

Peroneus tertius t

Cuboid

Peroneus brevis t

Peroneus longus t

Long plantar lig

Calcaneus

Flexor hallucis brevis m, med head

Flexor hallucis longus t

Flexor digitorum longus t

Quadratus plantae m

Abductor hallucis m

Med plantar a & n

Lat plantar a & n

Flexor digitorum brevis m

Abductor hallucis m

4th Metatarsal

Interosseous mm

5th Metatarsal

Peroneus tertius t

Quadratus plantae m

Peroneus brevis t

Lat plantar a & n

Long plantar lig

Calcaneus

1st Metatarsal

Adductor hallucis m, oblique head

Flexor hallucis brevis m, med head

Flexor hallucis longus t

Flexor digitorum longus t

Abductor hallucis m

Med plantar a & n

Flexor digitorum brevis m

Abductor hallucis m

Ankle and Foot, Transverse

5th Metatarsal

Flexor digitorum brevis m

Abductor digiti minimi m

Plantar apon

Abductor hallucis m

Calcaneus

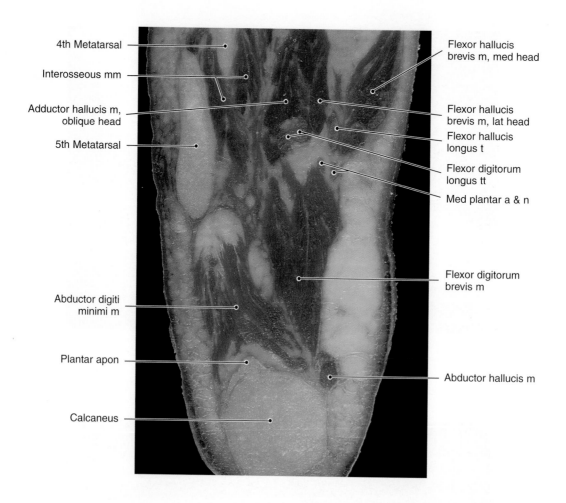

4th Metatarsal

Interosseous mm

Adductor hallucis m, oblique head

5th Metatarsal

Abductor digiti minimi m

Plantar apon

Calcaneus

Flexor hallucis brevis m, med head

Flexor hallucis brevis m, lat head

Flexor hallucis longus t

Flexor digitorum longus tt

Med plantar a & n

Flexor digitorum brevis m

Abductor hallucis m

Ankle and Foot, Sagittal

Med malleolus

Tibialis post t

Tibialis ant t

Med cuneiform

1st Metatarsal

Flexor hallucis
brevis m

Abductor hallucis m

Med malleolus

Tibialis post t

Tibialis ant t

Med cuneiform

1st Metatarsal

Flexor hallucis
brevis m

Sesamoid

Flexor hallucis
longus t

Abductor hallucis m

Navicular

Tibialis ant t

Med malleolus

Flexor digitorum longus t

Deltoid lig

Post tibial a & tibial n

Tibialis post t

Med cuneiform

1st Metatarsal

Flexor hallucis brevis m

Flexor hallucis longus t

Plantar apon

Abductor hallucis m

Navicular

Tibialis ant t

Tibialis post t

Med malleolus

Flexor digitorum longus t

Deltoid lig

Tibial n

Post tibial a

Tibialis post t

Med cuneiform

Extensor hallucis longus t

1st Metatarsal

Flexor hallucis longus t

Flexor hallucis brevis m

Plantar apon

Abductor hallucis m

Ankle and Foot, Sagittal

Navicular
Tibialis ant t
Soleus m
Tibia
Post tibial a & tibial n
Post tibiotalar lig
Talus
Spring lig
Sustentaculum tali
Flexor digitorum longus t
Tibialis post tt
Abductor hallucis m
Extensor hallucis longus t
Med cuneiform
1st Metatarsal
Flexor hallucis longus t
Flexor hallucis brevis m
Plantar apon

Navicular
Tibialis ant t
Soleus m
Tibia
Post tibial a & tibial n
Talus
Post tibiotalar lig
Spring lig
Sustentaculum tali
Flexor digitorum longus t
Tibialis post tt
Abductor hallucis m
Extensor hallucis longus t
Med cuneiform
1st Metatarsal
Flexor hallucis longus t
Flexor hallucis brevis m
Plantar apon

Extensor hallucis longus t

Navicular

Med cuneiform

Tibialis post t

Interosseous intercuneiform lig

1st Metatarsal

Flexor digitorum longus t

Peroneus longus t

Flexor hallucis brevis m

Med plantar n

Plantar apon

Flexor digitorum brevis m

Tibia

Soleus m

Tendo calcaneus

Talus

Interosseous talocalcaneal lig

Spring lig

Flexor hallucis longus t

Sustentaculum tali

Lat plantar a & n

Abductor hallucis m

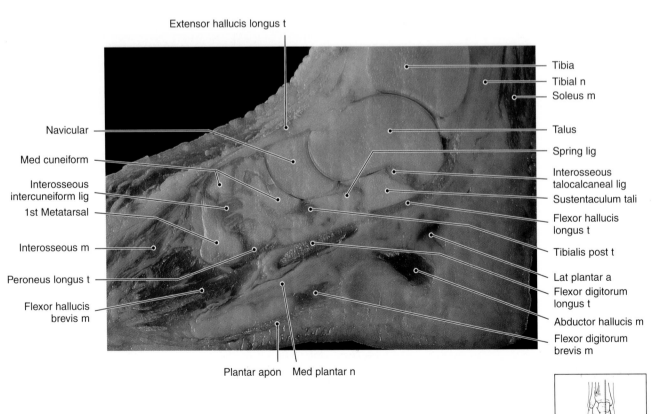

Extensor hallucis longus t

Navicular

Med cuneiform

Interosseous intercuneiform lig

1st Metatarsal

Interosseous m

Peroneus longus t

Flexor hallucis brevis m

Plantar apon

Med plantar n

Tibia

Tibial n

Soleus m

Talus

Spring lig

Interosseous talocalcaneal lig

Sustentaculum tali

Flexor hallucis longus t

Tibialis post t

Lat plantar a

Flexor digitorum longus t

Abductor hallucis m

Flexor digitorum brevis m

Ankle and Foot, Sagittal

Extensor hallucis longus m

Tibia

Ant tibial a

Flexor hallucis longus m

Soleus m

Dorsal talonavicular lig

Navicular

Intermediate cuneiform

2nd Metatarsal

Tibialis post t

Peroneus longus t

Flexor hallucis brevis m

Flexor digitorum longus t

Talus

Tendo calcaneus

Interosseous talocalcaneal lig

Calcaneus

Quadratus plantae m

Lat plantar a

Lat plantar n

Flexor digitorum brevis m

Plantar apon

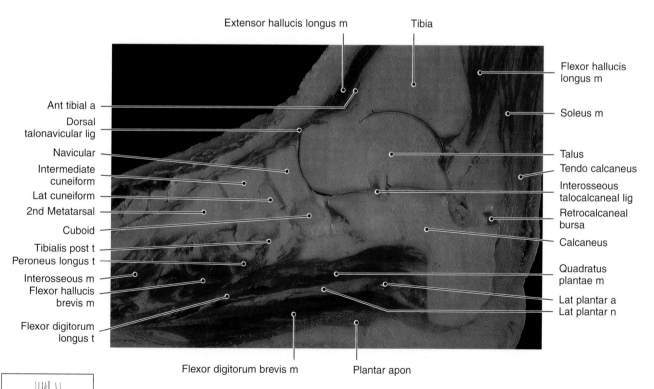

Extensor hallucis longus m

Tibia

Ant tibial a

Dorsal talonavicular lig

Navicular

Intermediate cuneiform

Lat cuneiform

2nd Metatarsal

Cuboid

Tibialis post t

Peroneus longus t

Interosseous m

Flexor hallucis brevis m

Flexor digitorum longus t

Flexor hallucis longus m

Soleus m

Talus

Tendo calcaneus

Interosseous talocalcaneal lig

Retrocalcaneal bursa

Calcaneus

Quadratus plantae m

Lat plantar a

Lat plantar n

Flexor digitorum brevis m

Plantar apon

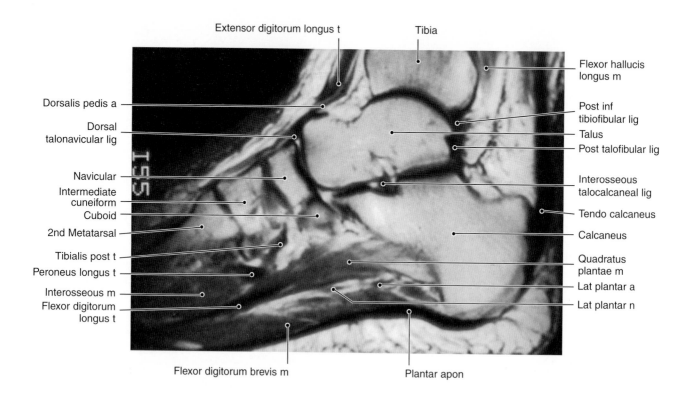

Extensor digitorum longus t

Tibia

Dorsalis pedis a

Dorsal talonavicular lig

Navicular

Intermediate cuneiform

Cuboid

2nd Metatarsal

Tibialis post t

Peroneus longus t

Interosseous m

Flexor digitorum longus t

Flexor digitorum brevis m

Plantar apon

Flexor hallucis longus m

Post inf tibiofibular lig

Talus

Post talofibular lig

Interosseous talocalcaneal lig

Tendo calcaneus

Calcaneus

Quadratus plantae m

Lat plantar a

Lat plantar n

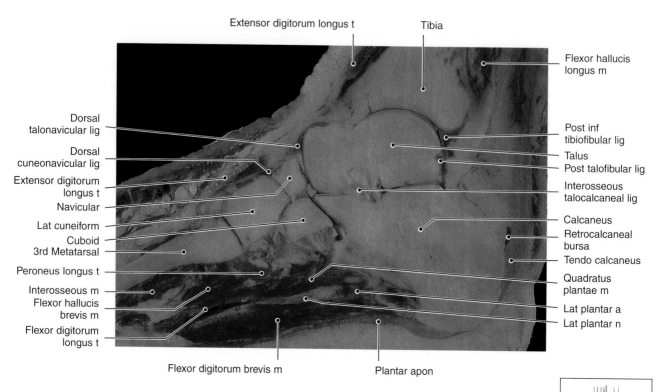

Extensor digitorum longus t

Tibia

Dorsal talonavicular lig

Dorsal cuneonavicular lig

Extensor digitorum longus t

Navicular

Lat cuneiform

Cuboid

3rd Metatarsal

Peroneus longus t

Interosseous m

Flexor hallucis brevis m

Flexor digitorum longus t

Flexor digitorum brevis m

Plantar apon

Flexor hallucis longus m

Post inf tibiofibular lig

Talus

Post talofibular lig

Interosseous talocalcaneal lig

Calcaneus

Retrocalcaneal bursa

Tendo calcaneus

Quadratus plantae m

Lat plantar a

Lat plantar n

Ankle and Foot, Sagittal

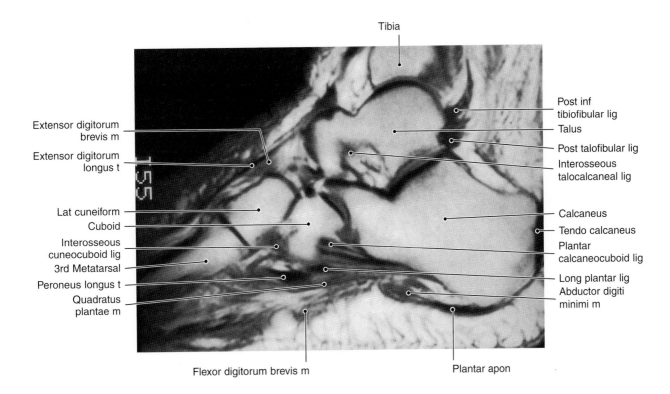

Tibia

Post inf tibiofibular lig
Talus
Post talofibular lig
Interosseous talocalcaneal lig

Extensor digitorum brevis m
Extensor digitorum longus t

Calcaneus
Tendo calcaneus
Plantar calcaneocuboid lig

Lat cuneiform
Cuboid
Interosseous cuneocuboid lig
3rd Metatarsal
Peroneus longus t
Quadratus plantae m

Long plantar lig
Abductor digiti minimi m

Flexor digitorum brevis m

Plantar apon

Extensor digitorum longus t   Tibia

Lat malleolus
Peroneus brevis m
Talus

Dorsal talonavicular lig
Extensor digitorum longus t
Extensor digitorum brevis m

Post inf tibiofibular lig
Post talofibular lig

Lat cuneiform
Cuboid
Interosseous cuneocuboid lig
3rd Metatarsal
4th Metatarsal

Interosseous talocalcaneal lig

Calcaneus

Tendo calcaneus

Peroneus longus t

Plantar calcaneocuboid lig

Interosseous m
Flexor digitorum longus t
Flexor digitorum brevis t

Long plantar lig
Quadratus plantae m

Abductor digiti minimi m

Flexor digitorum brevis m

Plantar apon

Peroneus tertius m   Tibia

Peroneus brevis m
Lat malleolus

Extensor digitorum
brevis m
Extensor digitorum
longus tt

Post inf
tibiofibular lig
Talus
Post talofibular lig

Interosseous
talocalcaneal lig

Lat cuneiform
Interosseous
cuneocuboid lig
3rd Metatarsal

Calcaneus

Cuboid
4th Metatarsal
Peroneus longus t
Interosseous m

Long plantar lig

Abductor digiti minimi m   Plantar apon, lat cord

Peroneus tertius m   Tibia

Extensor digitorum
brevis m

Peroneus brevis m

Extensor digitorum
longus t

Lat malleolus
Talus

Post inf
tibiofibular lig

Lat cuneiform

Post talofibular lig

Interosseous
cuneocuboid lig

Interosseous
talocalcaneal lig

3rd Metatarsal
Cuboid
4th Metatarsal
Interosseous mm

Calcaneus

Long plantar lig

Peroneus longus t

Plantar apon,
lat cord

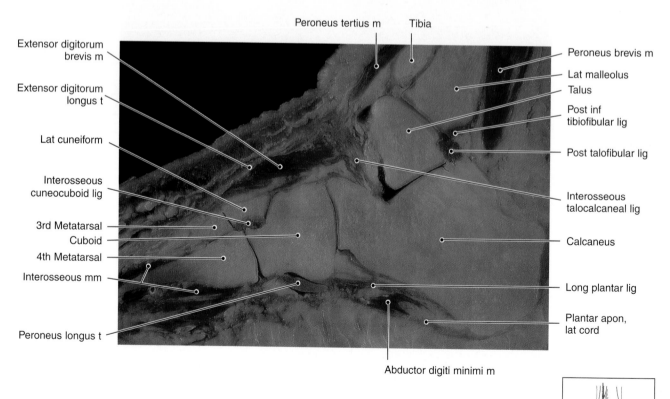

Abductor digiti minimi m

Ankle and Foot, Sagittal

Ant inf tibiofibular lig

Lat malleolus

Peroneus longus t

Post talofibular lig

Talus

Interosseous talocalcaneal lig

Calcaneus

Long plantar lig

Plantar apon, lat cord

Abductor digiti minimi m

Extensor digitorum longus t

Extensor digitorum brevis m

Cuboid

4th Metatarsal

Peroneus longus t

Interosseous m

Flexor digiti minimi brevis m

Lat malleolus

Ant inf tibiofibular lig

Peroneus longus t

Post talofibular lig

Peroneus brevis t

Talus

Interosseous talocalcaneal lig

Calcaneofibular lig

Calcaneus

Long plantar lig

Abductor digiti minimi m

Plantar apon, lat cord

Extensor digitorum longus t

Extensor digitorum brevis m

Cuboid

4th Metatarsal

Peroneus longus t

Interosseous m

Flexor digiti minimi brevis m

Extensor digitorum brevis m

Cuboid

4th Metatarsal

5th Metatarsal

Interosseous m

Flexor digiti minimi brevis m

Lat malleolus

Peroneus brevis t

Calcaneus

Peroneus longus t

Abductor digiti minimi m

Plantar apon, lat cord

Extensor digitorum brevis m

Cuboid

4th Metatarsal

5th Metatarsal

Interosseous m

Flexor digiti minimi brevis m

Lat malleolus

Peroneus brevis t

Calcaneus

Peroneus longus t

Abductor digiti minimi m

Calcaneus

Plantar apon, lat cord

Ankle and Foot, Sagittal

Lat malleolus

Extensor digitorum
brevis m

Calcaneus

Cuboid

Dorsal
interosseous m

5th Metatarsal

Flexor digiti minimi
brevis m

Peroneus brevis t

Peroneus longus t

Abductor digiti
minimi m

Lat malleolus

Extensor digitorum
brevis m

Cuboid

Dorsal
interosseous m

5th Metatarsal

Flexor digiti minimi
brevis m

Peroneus brevis t

Peroneus longus t

Abductor digiti
minimi m

Index

ISBN-0-7216-9695-3